WORKBOOK/LAB MANUAL TO ACCOMPANY

The Pharmacy
Technician Foundations
and Practices

MIKE JOHNSTON, CPhT
Chairman & CEO, National Pharmacy Technician Association
Houston, TX

CLIFFORD FRANK, CPhT
Instructor
RxTech Training, Inc.
Chugiak, AK

MICHELLE GOEKING, BM, CPhT
Instructor
Black Hawk College
Moline, IL

MICHAEL M. HAYTER, PharmD, MBA
Adjunct Instructor Pharmacy Technology and Health Information
Virginia Highlands Community College
Abingdon, VA

ROBIN LUKE, CPhT
Editorial Manager
Today's Technician Magazine
Vancouver, WA

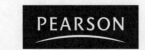
PEARSON

Upper Saddle River, New Jersey 07458

Publisher and Editor-in-Chief: Julie Levin Alexander
Assistant to Publisher: Regina Bruno
Executive Editor: Joan Gill
Development Editor: Jill Rembetski, Triple SSS Press Media Development, Inc.
Associate Editor: Bronwen Glowacki
Editorial Assistant: Mary Ellen Ruitenberg
Director of Marketing: Karen Allman
Senior Marketing Manager: Harper Coles
Marketing Specialist: Michael Sirinides
Marketing Assistant: Judy Noh
Managing Editor, Production: Patrick Walsh
Production Liaison: Julie Li
Production Editor: Kevin Bradley, GGS Book Services PMG
Media Project Manager: Stephen Hartner
Manufacturing Manager: Ilene Sanford
Manufacturing Buyer: Pat Brown
Composition: GGS Book Services PMG
Printer/Binder: Edwards Brothers Malloy
Senior Design Coordinator: Maria Guglielmo-Walsh
Creative Design Director: Christy Mahon
Cover Designer: Mary Siener
Cover Photos: (top left) iStock; (top right, bottom left and right) photos.com
Cover Printer: Edwards Brothers Malloy

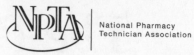

National Pharmacy Technician Association

The NPTA logo is a trademark of the National Pharmacy Technician Association

straden-schaden, inc.®

RxPRESS
PUBLICATIONS®

The Straden-Schaden and RxPress logos are both trademarks of Straden-Schaden, Inc.

Pearson Education Ltd., London
Pearson Education Singapore, Pte. Ltd
Pearson Education Canada, Inc.
Pearson Education–Japan
Pearson Education Australia PTY, Limited
Pearson Education North Asia, Ltd., Hong Kong
Pearson Educación de Mexico, S.A. de C.V.
Pearson Education Malaysia, Pte. Ltd.
Pearson Education, Upper Saddle River, New Jersey

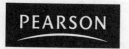

1 0 9 8
ISBN-13: 978-0-13-228291-8
ISBN-10: 0-13-228291-7

Contents

Chapter 8 Technology in the Pharmacy 110

Chapter 9 Inventory Management and Health Insurance Billing 122

Chapter 10 Introduction to Compounding 137

Chapter 11 Introduction to Sterile Products 150

Chapter 12 Basic Math Skills 184

Preface

The Pharmacy Technician: Foundations and Practices addresses today's comprehensive educational needs for one of the fastest-growing jobs in the United States: that of the pharmacy technician. The pharmacy technician career is ranked 60th among the 100 fastest-growing jobs in the United States and 19th among the 500 best jobs for people with a conventional personality type. According to the U.S. Bureau of Labor Statistics, the pharmacy technician career is growing at approximately 30 percent annually, a much higher rate than other jobs in the health professions. This equates to more than 39,000 pharmacy technician job openings available every year.

In addition to the tremendous workforce demand for pharmacy technicians, professional regulations and requirements are being established for pharmacy technicians across the United States. With many State Boards of Pharmacy either considering, or having already enacted, mandatory registration, certification, and/or formal education, the need for a comprehensive and up-to-date pharmacy technician textbook like *The Pharmacy Technician: Foundations and Practices* has never been greater.

This *Workbook/Lab Manual to Accompany The Pharmacy Technician: Foundations and Practices* is designed to give you additional practice in mastering the varied skills that will be required of you as a pharmacy technician. It is organized to correspond with the 34 chapters in the textbook. Each workbook/lab manual chapter includes:

- Learning objectives from the textbook, with references to related activities within the workbook/lab manual.

- An introduction that summarizes the main themes from the textbook chapter.

- Review Questions that evaluate your comprehension of the textbook chapter content. Question types include multiple choice, fill-in-the-blank, matching, and true/false.

- Pharmacy Calculation Problems that will give you additional practice and help increase your comfort level in using the math skills you will need on a daily basis as a practicing pharmacy technician.

- PTCB Exam Practice Questions related to the chapter's specific content that will help you prepare for the Pharmacy Technician Certification Exam.

- Activities in each chapter challenge you to explore facets of the chapter material more thoroughly and offer a variety of exercises, including anatomy worksheets, case studies with critical thinking questions, Web research problems, and role-playing scenarios.

- Hands-on Lab activities in certain chapters give you the chance to practice procedures, work with equipment, or perform additional research.

Be sure to visit the Companion website for this text. It includes an online study guide that contains helpful links, self-test questions, and an online glossary. You will be able to submit your results for a score that you can send to your professor or to yourself for further evaluation. This resource, combined with the Student CD packaged with the textbook, will give you the opportunity to put into practice those skills you are being taught in the classroom.

About NPTA

The National Pharmacy Technician Association (NPTA) is the world's largest professional organization specifically for pharmacy technicians. The association is dedicated to advancing the value of pharmacy technicians and the vital roles they play in pharmaceutical care. In a society of countless associations, we believe it takes much more than just a mission statement to meet the professional needs of and provide the necessary leadership for the pharmacy technician profession—it takes action and results.

The organization is composed of pharmacy technicians practicing in a variety of practice settings, such as retail, independent, hospital, mail-order, home care, long-term care, nuclear, military, correctional facilities, formal education, training, management, sales, and many more. NPTA is a reflection of this diverse profession and provides unparallel support and resources to members.

NPTA is the foundation of the pharmacy technician profession; we have an unprecedented past, a strong presence, and a promising future. We are dedicated to improving our profession while remaining focused on our members.

Pharmacy technician students are welcome to join more than 30,000 practicing pharmacy technicians as members of NPTA.

For more information:
call 888-247-8706
visit www.pharmacytechnician.org

CHAPTER 1
History of Pharmacy Practice

After completing Chapter 1 from the textbook, you should be able to:	Related Activity in the Workbook/Lab Manual
1. Describe the origins of the practice of pharmacy from the Age of Antiquity.	Review Questions, PTCB Exam Practice Questions Lab 1-2
2. Discuss changes in the practice of pharmacy during the Middle Ages.	Review Questions, PTCB Exam Practice Questions Lab 1-2
3. Describe changes in the practice of pharmacy during the Renaissance.	Review Questions, PTCB Exam Practice Questions Lab 1-2
4. List significant milestones for the practice of pharmacy from the 18th, 19th, and 20th centuries.	Review Questions, PTCB Exam Practice Questions Activity 1-1 Lab 1-1, 1-2
5. Discuss the role biotechnology and genetic engineering could have on the future of pharmacy practice.	Review Questions Activity 1-2

INTRODUCTION

The practice of pharmacy has ancient roots. The word *pharmacy* comes from the Greek word *pharmakon*, meaning "drug," and the origin of pharmacy practice goes back to ancient times, more than 7,000 years ago. The role of a pharmacy technician can be traced back to 2900 BCE, in ancient Egypt, where echelons were gatherers and preparers of drugs, similar to the modern-day pharmacy technician; chiefs of fabrication were the head pharmacists.

The history of pharmacy practice may seem to be unnecessary to you as you prepare to become a pharmacy technician. However, if you are to understand many of the concepts, theories, and practices covered in this workbook/laboratory manual and the textbook, you need to understand the evolution of the pharmacy profession. Many of the principles used in pharmacy thousands of years ago are still practiced today. Understanding the historic roots will also help you appreciate the areas in which the profession has evolved and how professional guidelines and regulations have developed. As you will discover, the responsibilities of and opportunities for pharmacy technicians continue to evolve, along with the profession of pharmacy itself.

REVIEW QUESTIONS

Match the following.

1. _____ pharmacogenomics
2. _____ pharmacy
3. _____ prescription
4. _____ apothecary
5. _____ biotechnology
6. _____ pharmacopoeia
7. __b__ compounding

a. Latin term for pharmacist
b. Producing, mixing, or preparing a drug by combining ingredients
c. Use of living things to make or modify a product
d. An order to prepare/dispense
e. Study of genetic differences in responses to drug therapy
f. Art/science of preparing and dispensing medication
g. Book of products, formulae, and directions for preparation

Choose the best answer.

8. The word *pharmacy* comes from which ancient Greek word for drug?
   a. pharmakos
   b. pharmakopeia
   c. pharmakon
   d. pharmakot

9. Which of the following is supposedly an abbreviation for the Latin word for *recipe*?
   a. Rx
   b. sx
   c. tx
   d. dx

10. The Age of Antiquity refers to which time period?
    a. 8000 BCE up through CE 699
    b. 5000 BCE up through CE 499
    c. 3000 BCE up through CE 899
    d. 4000 BCE up through CE 599

11. The "father of botany" is considered to be:
    a. Shen Nung.
    b. Echelon.
    c. Theophrastus.
    d. Charaka Samhita.

Match the following scientists with their accomplishments.

12. _____ Galen
13. _____ Mithridates
14. _____ Hippocrates
15. _____ Pedanios Dioscorides

a. developed the theory of humors
b. poisons and poison preventatives
c. rules for drug collection, storage, and use
d. established principles of compounding

Choose the best answer.

16. The first apothecaries, or privately owned drugstores, were established in the late eighth century by the:
    a. Arabs.
    b. Greeks.
    c. Romans.
    d. Italians.

17. The first pharmacy technicians in ancient Egypt were known as:
    a. slaves.
    b. ebers.
    c. echelons.
    d. chiefs of fabrication.

18. America's first female pharmacist was the granddaughter of:
   a. an indentured servant named Dremmell Marshall and was named Isabell.
   b. a pharmacist named Christopher Marshall and was named Elizabeth.
   c. the inventor Benjamin Franklin and was named Mary.
   d. a prominent Bostonian, Andrew Craigie, and was named Alice.

19. The first school of pharmacy was:
   a. the Philadelphia College of Pharmacy.
   b. the University of Pennsylvania Pharmacy College.
   c. Boston University.
   d. the Massachusetts School of Pharmacology.

20. The American Pharmaceutical Association was opened to "all pharmacists and druggists of good character" in:
   a. 1821.   c. 1872.
   b. 1852.   d. 1962.

21. The *United States Pharmacopoeia* (USP) was first published in:
   a. 1820.   c. 1822.
   b. 1877.   d. 1869.

22. Gregor Mendel is known as the Father of Modern Genetics. He was an Austrian:
   a. pharmacist and scientist.   c. scientist and priest.
   b. priest and pharmacist.   d. priest and author.

23. The practice of pharmacy began to be regulated by the federal government:
   a. in the early 1900s.
   b. in the late 1800s.
   c. in the late 1900s.
   d. pharmacy has always been heavily regulated by the federal government.

24. Pharmacogenomics is the use of:
   a. genomic or genetic information to predict a drug's efficacy.
   b. personal DNA information to track patients.
   c. gene splicing to produce effective medications.
   d. a study of future drugs and their possible uses.

Match the following.

25. _____ Clinical Era   a. formulating and dispensing drugs
26. _____ Pharmaceutical Care Era   b. developing and testing drugs
27. _____ Traditional Era   c. dispensing information, warnings, and advice
28. _____ Scientific Era   d. positive outcomes of therapies

PHARMACY CALCULATION PROBLEMS

Calculate the following.

1. $62.1 + 4.5 + 2.92 + 0.6 =$

2. $120 \text{ mL} + 60 \text{ mL} + 80 \text{ mL} + 40 \text{ mL} =$

3. $750 \text{ mg} - 80 \text{ mg} - 35.5 \text{ mg} =$

4. $10.5 \text{ oz.} + 11.5 \text{ oz.} - 3.25 \text{ oz.} =$

5. $9.8 \text{ mL} - 5.4 \text{ mL} + 12.9 \text{ mL} =$

PTCB EXAM PRACTICE QUESTIONS

1. Which ancient civilization provides the earliest record of apothecary practice?
   a. Babylonian
   b. Chinese
   c. Indian
   d. Aztec

2. What is the name of the first woman pharmacist in America?
   a. Wilson
   b. Marshall
   c. Washington
   d. Tyler

3. In what city was the first American school of pharmacy founded?
   a. Boston
   b. Baltimore
   c. Providence
   d. Philadelphia

4. What was the first professional pharmacy association?
   a. APHA
   b. NABP
   c. ASHP
   d. ACPE

5. Hippocrates, often referred to as the "Father of Medicine," was part of which ancient culture?
   a. Egyptian
   b. Greek
   c. Roman
   d. Chinese

ACTIVITY 1-1: History of Medicine Timeline

Instructions: List each major event in the history of medicine in its appropriate place on the timeline.

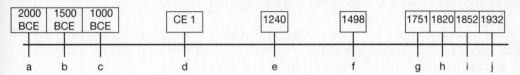

a. _____

b. _____

c. _____

d. _____

e. _____

f. _____

g. _____

h. _____

i. _____

j. _____

ACTIVITY 1-2: The Continuing Evolution of Pharmacy Practice

Chapter 1 touches on the role biotechnology and genetic engineering will play in the future of pharmacy practice, and you will learn more about these areas in Chapter 34 of the text.

What are some ways biotechnology and genetic engineering are already changing pharmacy practice? Go online and search the Internet for a current news story. Topics to search on might include recombinant DNA technology, genetic engineering, or stem cell research.

Questions

1. What is the topic of the news story you found online?

   _____

   _____

2. Was the story's coverage positive or negative in regard to biotechnology and/or genetic engineering?

   _____

   _____

3. What issues did the story raise?

   _____

   _____

   _____

   _____

4. After reading the news story, what is your opinion of this topic?

   _____

   _____

   _____

   _____

5. Now research two to three other current stories on this same topic. Did the other stories raise new issues? If so, what are they?

   _____

   _____

   _____

   _____

6. After reading all the news stories on this topic, has your opinion changed from what you described in Question #4? If so, how? If not, discuss why.

   _____

   _____

   _____

   _____

LAB 1-1: Exploring the History of Pharmacy

Objective:

Visit an online pharmacy museum and explore the history of pharmacy as preserved in the museum exhibits.

Pre-Lab Information:

Visit the History of Pharmacy Museum at the University of Arizona College of Pharmacy's website: http://www.pharmacy.arizona.edu/museum/

Explanation:

The practice of pharmacy has a rich and very interesting history. It is important for you, a future pharmacy technician, to understand how pharmacy practice has evolved. This exercise will help you gain a historical perspective on the practice of pharmacy.

Activity:

Using the Internet, go to the History of Pharmacy Museum at the University of Arizona College of Pharmacy's Web site: http://www.pharmacy.arizona.edu/museum/. Take the virtual tour, then answer the following questions.

1. What timeframe does the museum represent with the artifacts it has on display?
    _____
    _____

2. What is the significance of a red show globe?
    _____
    _____

3. What instrument was used to disinfect other instruments?
    _____
    _____

4. What was used to store the wet and dry ingredients used in pharmacy compounding?
    _____
    _____

5. What is the large box of natural products that were used in making prescriptions? (*Note:* It was produced by Parke-Davis and is one of the few remaining complete sets in the world.)
    _____
    _____

6. What is the box of homeopathic medicines called? (*Note:* A small amount was used to treat a particular malady and could be ordered by a number printed on the display box.)
    _____
    _____

7. What was the Lloyd continuous extraction apparatus used for from the 1940s through the 1970s?

_____

_____

8. What did you find most interesting?

_____

_____

_____

_____

9. What did you learn that you did not already know about pharmacy?

_____

_____

_____

_____

Student Name: _____

Lab Partner: _____

Grade/Comments: _____

_____

_____

Student Comments: _____

_____

_____

LAB 1-2: Pharmacy Pioneers

Objective:

To learn more about the origins of pharmacy practice by researching the achievements of a key pharmacy pioneer.

Pre-Lab Information:

- Review Chapter 1, History of Pharmacy Practice, in your textbook.
- Select a key pharmacy pioneer discussed in Chapter 1 of the text and presented in the following list, then perform additional online research to learn more about this person.

  Emperor Shen Nung

  Theophrastus

  Hippocrates

  Mithridates VI

  Pedanios Dioscorides

  Galen

  Savonarola

  John Winthrop

  Elizabeth Marshall

  Jonathan Roberts

  John Morgan

  Andrew Craigie

  Daniel B. Smith

  William Procter, Jr.

Explanation:

By focusing on the accomplishments of one key person in the history of pharmacy, you will gain a deeper understanding of that time period and an appreciation of how the practice of pharmacy has changed over time.

Activity:

Select a person from the preceding list, or choose another pharmacy pioneer who interests you. Go online or to the library to learn more about this person. Then answer the following questions.

1. What is the name of the pharmacy pioneer you researched?

   _____

   _____

2. In what time period did he or she live and work?

   _____

   _____

3. What was pharmacy practice like during this time period?

_____

_____

_____

_____

4. How is pharmacy practice today different from pharmacy practice in the time period in which the person you researched worked?

_____

_____

_____

_____

5. Why is the person you researched considered a pharmacy pioneer? What did he or she accomplish?

_____

_____

_____

_____

6. Are this person's accomplishments still important today? Why or why not?

_____

_____

_____

_____

7. What did you find most interesting about this person?

_____

_____

_____

_____

Student Name: _____

Lab Partner: _____

Grade/Comments: _____

_____

_____

Student Comments: _____

_____

_____

CHAPTER 2
The Professional Pharmacy Technician

After completing Chapter 2 from the textbook, you should be able to:	Related Activity in the Workbook/Lab Manual
1. Summarize the educational requirements and competencies of both pharmacists and pharmacy technicians.	Review Questions, PTCB Exam Practice Questions
2. Describe the two primary pharmacy practice settings and define the basic roles of pharmacists and pharmacy technicians working in each setting.	Review Questions Activity 2-1
3. Explain six specific characteristics of a good pharmacy technician.	Review Questions Activity 2-1, 2-2
4. Demonstrate the behavior of a professional pharmacy technician.	Review Questions Activity 2-2
5. Explain the registration/licensure and certification process for becoming a pharmacy technician.	Review Questions, PTCB Exam Practice Questions Lab 2-1

INTRODUCTION

Pharmacy is an industry consisting of professionals: pharmacists and pharmacy technicians. Many claim—with good reason—that pharmacy is the most trusted profession in America. As with any profession, employment in this field requires you to be educated, trained, diligent, and ethical. You must maintain specific competencies, undergo specialized education and training, and exhibit key personal characteristics. The process of preparing for your future includes formal education and training, registration/licensure, national certification, and involvement with a professional organization. The benefits of your hard work and dedication are the tremendous career opportunities awaiting you as a future pharmacy technician.

REVIEW QUESTIONS

Match the following.

1. _____ certification
2. _____ licensing
3. _____ registration
4. _____ attitude
5. _____ compassion
6. _____ empathy
7. _____ ambulatory pharmacy
8. _____ community pharmacy
9. _____ health system pharmacy
10. _____ institutional pharmacy

a. process of listing/being named to a list
b. government permission to do something
c. located on site where patients reside
d. common name for health system pharmacy
e. feelings of concern and understanding
f. deep awareness and sympathy
g. retail pharmacy
h. nongovernmental verification of competency
i. chain, drug/grocery store, mail-order, home health care pharmacies
j. way of acting, thinking, or believing

True or False?

11. Historically, there were only three recognized professions: law, medicine, and ministry.
    T   F

12. Pharmacy technicians must be licensed in all states.
    T   F

13. A pharmacist may advise other healthcare professionals.
    T   F

14. Most institutional pharmacies are open 24 hours.
    T   F

15. Your body language can hide your true feelings and attitudes.
    T   F

Choose the best answer.

16. Which of the following tasks is most likely to be performed by a pharmacist?
    a. insurance billing
    b. patient private information maintenance
    c. patient counseling
    d. inventory ordering

17. The set of qualities and characteristics that represent perceptions of your competence and character, as judged by your constituents, is called your:
    a. attitude.
    b. professional image.
    c. professionalism.
    d. demeanor.

18. Which of the following attire would be unacceptable for a pharmacy technician?
    a. tie
    b. lab coat
    c. shorts
    d. scrubs

19. Which is an example of adapting to change?
    a. changing priorities, strategies, or methods
    b. maintaining effectiveness
    c. handling stress properly
    d. all of the above

20. Which of the following is not a common eligibility requirement for technicians?
    a. no felony conviction(s)
    b. high school graduate or GED equivalent
    c. a two-year college degree
    d. certification

21. Pharmacy technicians are in the business of:
    a. selling drugs.
    b. patient care.
    c. patient consultations.
    d. making money.

Name four sources of CE for pharmacy technicians.

22. _____

23. _____

24. _____

25. _____

PHARMACY CALCULATION PROBLEMS

Calculate the following.

1. Bobby has completed 12 hours of CE. How many more hours does he need to complete to meet the PTCB requirements?

2. If Judy worked 38.5 hours one week and 39 hours the next week, how much would her gross pay be for those two weeks if she were paid $12.75 per hour?

3. A customer has three prescriptions and owes a co-payment of $15.00 on each one. How much will the customer be charged for all three prescriptions?

4. A technician works the third shift at a hospital for seven days in a row, followed by seven days off. She is scheduled to work Sunday through Saturday from 10:00 p.m. till 8:00 a.m., every other week. If the pay period starts on Sunday, how many hours will she work in two consecutive weeks?

5. A medication order calls for a special mouthwash that the pharmacy must make. It contains 50% diphenhydramine syrup and 50% viscous lidocaine. The physician ordered 16 ounces. How much of each ingredient will you need to make this?

PTCB EXAM PRACTICE QUESTIONS

1. When a pharmacy student graduates from an accredited college of pharmacy in the United States, what degree does she or he receive?
   a. Bachelor of Science (BS)
   b. Bachelor of Arts (BA)
   c. Doctor of Pharmacy (PharmD)
   d. Master of Science (MS)

2. In the United States, pharmacy technicians are often required to be registered or licensed before they may perform the duties of a pharmacy technician. This requirement is mandated by which government agency?
   a. Food and Drug Administration (FDA)
   b. State Board of Pharmacy (SBOP)
   c. Drug Enforcement Agency (DEA)
   d. *United States Pharmacopoeia* (USP)

3. When a pharmacy technician successfully completes a certification examination to become a CPhT, this signifies to others that he or she is:
   a. smart.
   b. polite.
   c. empathetic.
   d. competent.

4. Which of the following statements is true about the PTCB Certification Exam (PTCE)?
   a. The exam consists of 100 questions, is computer-based, and is offered 4 times each year.
   b. The exam consists of 125 questions, is computer-based, and is offered 3 times each year.
   c. The exam consists of 100 questions, is paper-based, and is offered 4 times each year.
   d. The exam consists of 125 questions, is paper-based, and is offered 3 times each year.

ACTIVITY 2-1: Case Study—Who Is Responsible?

Instructions: Read the following scenario and then answer the critical thinking questions that follow.

While processing a prescription for Bactrim DS®, the pharmacy computer system notifies you that the patient has a recorded allergy to sulfur-based drugs. Bactrim DS® is a sulfur-based antibiotic and could therefore pose a serious risk to the patient. You immediately alert the pharmacist to the situation; she determines that the prescriber has likely made a mistake and will need to select an alternative treatment.

The pharmacist explains that the pharmacy staff needs to:

- verify the allergy with the patient.
- upon confirmation of a sulfur allergy, explain to the patient that the pharmacy will have to call the prescriber to request a different prescription.
- call the doctor's office to explain the patient's allergy and to request a new, verbal prescription for the patient.

1. Who is responsible for verifying the drug allergy with the patient? Why?

   _____

   _____

   _____

   _____

2. Who is responsible for explaining to the patient that the pharmacy must call the doctor's office to request a different prescription? Why?

   _____

   _____

   _____

   _____

3. Who is responsible for calling the patient's doctor and requesting a new prescription? Why?

   _____

   _____

   _____

   _____

4. In what ways are the job functions of a pharmacist and pharmacy technician in an ambulatory setting different from those of a pharmacist and pharmacy technician in a health system pharmacy?

   _____

   _____

   _____

   _____

ACTIVITY 2-2: Case Study—Appropriate Behavior

Instructions: Read the following scenario and then answer the critical thinking questions that follow.

Ryan is a certified pharmacy technician and has worked at a local community pharmacy for seven years. He has the most seniority of the five technicians who work in the pharmacy and he takes advantage of this.

When the pharmacy is busy, Ryan takes charge and processes prescriptions with both speed and accuracy. He is typically able to have a prescription prepared for the pharmacist's review within 7 to 10 minutes, meaning that patients can generally expect only a 15-minute wait time. Ryan is always dressed professionally and he is excellent at interacting with patients.

However, Ryan refuses to help with receiving the weekly inventory order, stocking pharmacy supplies, or cleaning duties. He explains to the other technicians that those tasks are their jobs. In fact, Ryan often takes personal calls on his cell phone during slow periods, rather than assisting with these tasks.

1. List Ryan's appropriate behaviors and positive characteristics.

_____

_____

_____

_____

2. List Ryan's inappropriate behaviors and unprofessional characteristics.

_____

_____

_____

_____

3. What role, or responsibility, does the pharmacy manager have in Ryan's behavior?

_____

_____

_____

_____

4. What impact does Ryan's behavior have on the pharmacy staff?

_____

_____

_____

_____

5. List six specific characteristics of a good pharmacy technician.

_____

_____

_____

_____

_____

_____

LAB 2-1: Becoming a Certified Pharmacy Technician

Objective:

Research the process involved in becoming a certified pharmacy technician, including the continuing education requirements required to maintain certification.

Pre-Lab Information:

Visit the Pharmacy Technician Certification Board website and other suggested online resources:

- https://www.ptcb.org
- http://www.pharmacytechnician.org/
- http://www.nationaltechexam.org/

Explanation:

Certification is an important career step demonstrating that the pharmacy technician has met a set of standards. It is important for you to understand the exam process as well as the requirements for maintaining your certification.

Activity:

Using the Internet, visit the Pharmacy Technician Certification Board Web site at https://www.ptcb.org. Answer the following questions concerning technician certification.

1. What is the ATT letter and what does it mean?

   _____

   _____

2. What organization do you contact to schedule your certification exam?

   _____

   _____

3. What two requirements must you meet before registering for the PTCB certification exam?

   a. _____

   b. _____

4. How long is your initial certification valid (that is, how long before your initial certification must be renewed)?

   _____

   _____

5. How many hours of continuing education are required for each renewal period?

   _____

   _____

6. Continuing education programs must be approved by what organization?

   _____

   _____

7. When you successfully complete the PTCB National Examination, what designation can you use after your name?

   a. _____

   Can you use this same designation if you take the National Technician Exam?

   b. _____

8. Visit the National Technician Exam Web site (http://www.nationaltechexam.org/State-by-state_tech. html). Find your state and list its requirements for registration.

   _____
   _____
   _____
   _____

9. What is the cost to take the exam?

   _____
   _____

10. What testing site is located nearest to you?

   _____
   _____

Optional Activity:

Visit http://www.powerpak.com/index.asp?show=list&prof=5 and complete one of the continuing education programs.

Student Name: _____

Lab Partner: _____

Grade/Comments: _____

_____
_____

Student Comments: _____

_____
_____

Communication and Customer Care

After completing Chapter 3 from the textbook, you should be able to:	Related Activity in the Workbook/Lab Manual
1. Describe and illustrate the communication process.	Review Questions, PTCB Exam Practice Questions Activity 3-1
2. List and explain the three types of communication.	Review Questions, PTCB Exam Practice Questions Activity 3-1, Lab 3-1
3. Summarize the various barriers to effective communication.	Review Questions, PTCB Exam Practice Questions Activity 3-1, Lab 3-2
4. List and describe the primary defense mechanisms.	Review Questions Activity 3-1, Lab 3-1, Lab 3-2
5. Describe specific strategies for eliminating barriers to communication.	Review Questions, PTCB Exam Practice Questions Activity 3-1, Lab 3-2
6. Summarize the elements of and considerations in caring for patients.	Review Questions, PTCB Exam Practice Questions Activity 3-2, Lab 3-2
7. List the Five Rights of medication administration.	Review Questions Activity 3-2, Lab 3-2

INTRODUCTION

Communication is simply the process of transferring information, although it is not a simple process. You communicate to get your message across to others clearly and unambiguously. Communicating takes effort from everyone involved, including the sender (the person who initiates the communication) and the receiver (the person or group the sender is addressing). The communication process often breaks down, and errors may result in misunderstandings and confusion.

As a pharmacy technician, you will need to communicate effectively with a variety of people, including your immediate co-workers, customers or patients, healthcare personnel, suppliers, drug representatives, health insurance representatives, and many others. Pharmacy technicians work as frontline employees in the pharmacy, which means that both your management and your patients will rely on you to be an effective communicator and to identify and eliminate communication barriers as they arise. Remember that becoming an effective communicator is a lifelong process that gets easier with experience and time.

REVIEW QUESTIONS

Match the following.

1. _____ channel
2. _____ projection
3. _____ defense mechanisms
4. _____ denial
5. _____ feedback

a. unconscious mental process used to protect the ego

b. defense mechanism of refusing to acknowledge painful realities

c. gesture, action, sound, written or spoken word used in transmitting information

d. defense mechanism in which one's own attitudes are attributed to others

e. the return of information back to the sender

Choose the best answer.

6. Directly related to the effectiveness of communication are:
   a. customer service and pharmaceutical care.
   b. speed of medication delivery and customer care.
   c. patient satisfaction and sales.
   d. pharmacy profitability and customer service.

7. The situation or environment in which a message is delivered is called:
   a. channel.
   b. feedback.
   c. context.
   d. verbal.

8. In communicating with patients, it is best to use a:
   a. monotone, impersonal tone.
   b. condescending patient tone.
   c. sympathetic caring tone.
   d. tone that mimics the patient's.

9. Effective communication will involve all of the following except:
   a. pleasantness.
   b. active listening.
   c. professional tones.
   d. aggressiveness

10. When leaving a voicemail for a patient, it is important not to:
   a. provide personal patient information.
   b. provide your name.
   c. provide your pharmacy's phone number.
   d. repeat information you have already given.

11. Facial expressions, eye contact, posture, and silence, are forms of:
   a. communication barriers.
   b. nonverbal communication.
   c. intimidation.
   d. not as effective as the spoken word.

12. Which of the following is not a barrier to communication?
   a. inaccurate information
   b. language
   c. overly lengthy message
   d. translators

13. If a patient does not speak good English, a technician should:
    a. see if a translator is available.
    b. speak the patient's native language if possible.
    c. provide instructions in the patient's native language.
    d. all of the above.

14. Defense mechanisms share two common properties:
    a. repression and sublimation.
    b. denial and displacement.
    c. unconscious trigger and distortion of reality.
    d. projection and rationalization.

15. When an individual transfers his or her own negative emotions to someone who is unrelated to those feelings, it is called:
    a. rationalization.
    b. displacement.
    c. denial.
    d. projection.

16. A patient who is prejudiced against minorities, and complains that an Asian-American technician showed him disrespect, may be using:
    a. regression.
    b. sublimation.
    c. projection.
    d. displacement.

17. The best strategy a technician can use for pharmacy conflict resolution is to:
    a. hold one's ground.
    b. demand respect.
    c. identify who has a problem.
    d. involve the supervisor.

18. The Five Rights include all of the following except:
    a. right strength.
    b. right time.
    c. right patient.
    d. right price.

19. The Patient's Bill of Rights includes being treated with courtesy and respect. It was passed by Congress in:
    a. 1905.
    b. 2005.
    c. 1995.
    d. 1955.

20. In various states, technicians may, with the approval of a pharmacist, do all the following except:
    a. read the instructions for a prescription to a patient.
    b. assist the patient with OTC selection.
    c. provide verbal advice and/or clinical information.
    d. assist the patient with medical devices.

PHARMACY CALCULATION PROBLEMS

Calculate the following.

1. At retail price, two prescriptions would cost $48.00 and $125.00, respectively. The customer has insurance and only pays $15 per prescription. How much money did the customer save with her insurance?

2. It costs the pharmacy $28.48 for 32 ounces of guaifenesin syrup. How much does it cost per ounce?

3. If a customer pays 30% of the retail price for a medication, how much would the customer pay for a prescription with a retail price of $100?

4. A technician gets paid $12 per hour for the first 40 hours worked in a week. He gets traditional overtime pay that is 1.5 times more than his regular pay for the hours he works over 40 hours. How much will he get paid if he works 48 hours in one week?

5. Jane works the second shift at a hospital. Her base pay is $13.25 per hour. The hospital gives a shift differential of $1.00 per hour for every hour worked on the second shift. How much will her weekly paycheck be if she works 32 hours?

PTCB EXAM PRACTICE QUESTIONS

1. Which of the following best describes the protection of a patient's privacy (identity and health information)?
   a. Compatibility
   b. Conformity
   c. Compliance
   d. Confidentiality

2. Some patients may feel uncomfortable if the pharmacist or technician stands too close or touches them. Other patients may initiate a handshake or pat on the back. These kinds of differences might be considered:
   a. genetic differences.
   b. cultural differences.
   c. physical differences.
   d. physiological differences.

3. You have a patient who is less than 12 years old. This patient would be categorized as what kind of patient?
   a. geriatric
   b. neonate
   c. pediatric
   d. ambulatory

4. An important communication concept, which refers to the situation, environment, or circumstance in which a message is communicated, is:
   a. projection.
   b. context.
   c. intellectualization.
   d. rationalization.

5. What percentage of Americans 16 years and older have the lowest level of literacy (difficulty using certain reading, writing, and computational skills considered necessary for functioning in everyday life)?
   a. 1–3%
   b. 10–13%
   c. 20–23%
   d. 30–33%

ACTIVITY 3-1: Case Study—Overcoming Communication Barriers

Instructions: Read the following scenario and then answer the critical thinking questions.

Mrs. Lopez arrives at your pharmacy with three prescriptions that she needs to have filled. You ask her, "Have you had any prescriptions filled here before?" She gets a puzzled look on her face, but says only, "No entiendo."

None of the staff currently working speaks Spanish, including yourself, and it is clear that Mrs. Lopez does not speak English. After you look for her in the computer's database, you find that Mrs. Lopez appears to be a new patient. You provide her with a New Patient Profile form, written in Spanish, and a pen, but she once again gets a puzzled look on her face and begins shaking her head and shrugging her shoulders.

Mrs. Lopez reaches into her purse and presents you with an identity card, which has her address information, and her insurance card. It appears that Mrs. Lopez can only speak Spanish; she is unable to read or write.

You process her prescription using the information she has been able to provide with her ID card and insurance card. The label for her prescriptions is translated into Spanish, according to the pharmacist's instructions, even though she will not personally be able to read the label.

1. List the communication barriers present with Mrs. Lopez.

   _____

   _____

   _____

   _____

2. Describe the best method for explaining Mrs. Lopez's medications and how to take them properly, given the limitations on communication.

   _____

   _____

   _____

   _____

3. What additional steps can the pharmacy take to ensure that Mrs. Lopez fully understands her medications and administration instructions?

   _____

   _____

   _____

   _____

4. In addition to language barriers, what are four other examples of barriers to communication? List and discuss how you might resolve each one.

   _____

   _____

   _____

   _____

ACTIVITY 3-2: Case Study—Patient Care

Instructions: Read the following scenario and then answer the critical thinking questions.

Mr. Thomas, one of your regular customers who is in his mid-fifties, comes to the pharmacy visibly shaken and disturbed. He has just returned from his doctor's office, where he was diagnosed with diabetes.

Mr. Thomas is nervous at the mere thought of having to use a blood glucose monitor and testing his blood every day. He also shares the fact that his mother died of severe complications related to diabetes.

He has several new prescriptions to be filled. His doctor also instructed him to purchase a blood glucose meter, although there was not enough time to properly instruct him on how to use one.

1. What defense mechanisms might you potentially expect from Mr. Thomas? How would you overcome them?

_____

_____

_____

_____

2. What measures could you take to provide optimal patient care for Mr. Thomas? Explain.

_____

_____

_____

_____

3. What measures could the pharmacist take to provide optimal patient care for Mr. Thomas? Explain.

_____

_____

_____

_____

4. What rights does Mr. Thomas have as a patient?

_____

_____

_____

_____

5. What are the Five Patient Rights?

_____

_____

_____

_____

_____

6. Why do you think the Five Rights you listed in question #5 are important? In your opinion, is any one more important than the others? Why or why not?

_____

_____

_____

_____

LAB 3-1: Leaving and Receiving Voicemail Messages

Objective:

To develop proper business telephone etiquette and communication skills.

Pre-Lab Information:

Review Chapter 3, "Communication and Customer Care," in your textbook.

Explanation:

As a pharmacy technician, you will spend a lot of time communicating with patients, vendors, health insurance representatives, and others on the telephone. Conducting business on the phone is different from making personal calls. Each time you make or answer a call, you are representing your pharmacy and yourself as an employee of that facility. Remember the following tips:

- Use a pleasant and professional tone of voice.
- State your name and place of business.
- If answering a phone call, ask how you can help the caller.
- If making a phone call, explain your need or objective.
- If taking a message, document important information from the caller (see lab activity for more details).
- When leaving a voicemail message, speak slowly and clearly, to allow the receiver time to write down the information.

Example of Correct Voicemail Message

"Hello, this is Lydia Smitts from Young's Pharmacy calling for Mr. Tom Lewis regarding your refill request. Please give me a call at your earliest convenience at 333-4455. Again, this is Lydia Smitts from Young's Pharmacy, and I may be reached at 222-333-4455. Thank you."

Example of Incorrect Voicemail Message

"This is Lydia Smitts calling about your refill for Prozac. Please give me a call back at 333-4455. Thank you."

Part One

Review the steps for leaving a voicemail.

1. Provide your full name and the name of the pharmacy.
2. Provide the pharmacy telephone number and hours of operation.
3. Indicate the purpose of your phone call.
4. Make any specific requests needed.
5. Provide your name and the pharmacy telephone number a second time.

Practice these steps with a partner.

Part Two

Working with a partner, create a scenario in which you receive a patient's voicemail message, either a refill request or a question for the pharmacist. Write down the details you will provide and then compare your partner's accuracy in writing down the message after listening to the voicemail. Be creative.

Example

Patient's Name: Janice Meyers

Prescription Number or Drug Name: Rx 7786791-0245

Special Request: I need to have this refilled today before noon because I am going out of town tonight.

Part Three

Working with a partner, state your message from Part Two. Be sure to include a date and time. As one partner leaves a "message," the other should record it on the following voicemail slip. Reverse roles so that each of you has the opportunity to leave a message and retrieve a message. Once you have both taken your turns, compare your voicemail slip against the written notes your partner made in Part One for accuracy.

MESSAGES

Date: _____ Time: _____

From: _____

To: _____

Message: _____

_____

_____

_____

Taken by: _____ Date: _____

---

1. How accurate were you in retrieving the voicemail message? Describe.

_____
_____
_____
_____

2. How accurate was your partner in retrieving your voicemail message? Describe.

_____
_____
_____
_____

3. What insight(s) has this lab provided in regard to leaving and retrieving messages?

_____
_____
_____
_____

Student Name: _____

Lab Partner: _____

Grade/Comments: _____

_____
_____

Student Comments: _____

_____
_____

LAB 3-2: Practicing Effective Communication and Customer Care

Objective:

To develop effective verbal and nonverbal communication skills.

Pre-Lab Information:

Review Chapter 3, "Communication and Customer Care," in your textbook.

Explanation:

As a pharmacy technician, you will be involved in face-to-face communication nearly all day long, excluding a few specialty practice settings. This face-to-face communication will be with your pharmacists, co-workers, patients, and customers. Communicating in person with another person involves both verbal and nonverbal communication. It is also a two-way process that involves both talking and listening. Effectively doing each is critical to successful communication. Here are some tips for effective face-to-face communication.

1. Smile. Be a pleasant individual to communicate with.
2. Speak clearly and at an appropriate volume.
3. Use professional and appropriate tones of voice, inflections, and diction. Never use slang.
4. Actively listen when someone is speaking to you, and acknowledge the speaker by nodding your head.
5. Do not interrupt someone while he or she is speaking. Wait until the speaker is finished.
6. Ask questions to ensure that you both completely understand the conversation.
7. Use appropriate eye contact.

Part One

Review the tips for effective face-to-face communication.

Practice these techniques with a partner for five minutes by discussing why you each decided to become a pharmacy technician. At the end of the five-minute period, take turns relaying back the information you have learned about each other. How much of it were you able to retain? Were you surprised at all by the results?

Part Two

Using the information provided, act out the following scenarios, and then reflect on the exercise through use of the discussion questions.

Scenario 1

Cast:

- Patient
- Pharmacy Technician
- Pharmacist (optional)

Scene:

The patient arrives at the pharmacy at 4:30 in the afternoon and requests a refill of the antidepressant Zoloft. Upon looking up the patient's prescription, the pharmacy technician realizes that there are no refills remaining and that the doctor's office will have to be called for refill authorization. The technician knows that it is too late to obtain a refill authorization, but the patient is demanding and explains that the supply of the medication is completely gone.

Discussion Questions:

1. Was the pharmacy technician effective in communicating with the patient? Why?

   _____

   _____

   _____

   _____

2. What defense mechanisms, if any, were evident in the patient and the pharmacy technician?

   _____

   _____

   _____

   _____

3. Was the situation resolved in the best manner possible? What other resolutions could have been attempted?

   _____

   _____

   _____

   _____

Scenario 2

Cast:

- Pharmacy Technician 1
- Pharmacy Technician 2
- Pharmacist

Scene:

The pharmacist requests that Pharmacy Technician 1 restock the prescription vials and take out the trash. Overloaded with inventory duties, Pharmacy Technician 1 asks Pharmacy Technician 2 to take care of these duties. Two hours later, the pharmacist is outraged to discover that the vials have not been restocked and that the trash is overflowing. The pharmacist reprimands Pharmacy Technician 1, who in turn blames Pharmacy Technician 2. A heated argument ensues.

Discussion Questions:

1. What is the root cause of this argument?

   _____

   _____

   _____

   _____

2. What defense mechanisms were evident in each individual?

   _____

   _____

   _____

   _____

3. How would you have handled the situation differently? Why?

   _____

   _____

   _____

   _____

Student Name: _____

Lab Partner: _____

Grade/Comments: _____

_____

_____

Student Comments: _____

_____

_____

CHAPTER 4
Pharmacy Law and Ethics

After completing Chapter 4 from the textbook, you should be able to:	Related Activity in the Workbook/Lab Manual
1. Classify the various categories of United States law.	Review Questions Lab 4-1
2. List the regulatory agencies that oversee the practice of pharmacy and describe their function(s).	Review Questions, PTCB Exam Practice Questions Lab 4-1
3. Summarize the significant laws and amendments that affect the practice of pharmacy.	Review Questions, PTCB Exam Practice Questions Activity 4-1, Lab 4-1
4. Recognize and use a drug monograph.	Review Questions Lab 4-2
5. Define ethics and moral philosophy.	Review Questions Activity 4-1, Activity 4-2
6. List and explain the nine ethical theories.	Review Questions Activity 4-3
7. Summarize the Pharmacy Technician Code of Ethics.	Review Questions Activity 4-3

INTRODUCTION

Federal and state laws, as well as professional ethics, regulate the practice of pharmacy. The regulations on pharmacy practice in the United States have evolved over the past hundred or so years, and their number has increased as legislators responded to demands from citizens to serve and protect the public interest. The government began to take the initiative in regulating pharmacy practice toward the end of the 18th century. Over time, the profession of pharmacy has become increasingly more regulated. In the United States, a professional degree is a requirement for any individual who wishes to practice pharmacy. This requirement was established to protect the public and set minimum standards, so that citizens could rely on pharmacists having at least a standard level of education and competence.

Many of the regulations pertaining to practice as a pharmacy technician are established and enforced by your specific state's board of pharmacy. In general, federal laws govern the manufacturing of pharmaceutical products, and state laws govern the actual dispensing of those products. It is imperative that you familiarize yourself with both the federal laws and your state's laws pertaining to pharmacy practice. In addition, you should fully understand the basic ethical theories and *Code of Ethics for Pharmacy Technicians,* in preparation for ethical dilemmas and questions that will arise in the pharmacy setting.

REVIEW QUESTIONS

Choose the best answer.

1. The quality of being kind or charitable is called:
   a. beneficence.
   b. ethics.
   c. fidelity.
   d. veracity.

2. A drug that has been misleadingly or fraudulently labeled is referred to as:
   a. adulterated.
   b. a felony.
   c. a monograph.
   d. misbranded.

3. A system of principles often associated with a profession is:
   a. civil law.
   b. consequentialism.
   c. ethics.
   d. criminal law.

4. Most laws pertaining to pharmacy were enacted to:
   a. limit the scope and practice of pharmacy.
   b. protect the public interest.
   c. lower the number of drug addicts.
   d. protect drug manufacturers.

5. Which is not a type of law in the United States?
   a. legislative intent
   b. constitutional
   c. government policy
   d. statutes

6. Which set of laws would take priority?
   a. federal
   b. state
   c. municipality
   d. local codes

7. Statutes are laws that are passed by:
   a. the federal government.
   b. state governments.
   c. local governments.
   d. all of the above.

8. Legislative intent is often referred to as:
   a. common law.
   b. case law.
   c. civil law.
   d. all of the above.

9. Regulations:
   a. have the force of law.
   b. are guidelines.
   c. refine laws.
   d. are not connected to laws.

10. Crimes are classified as either _____ or _____.
    a. infractions, misdemeanors
    b. infractions, violations
    c. infractions, felonies
    d. felonies, misdemeanors

11. Professional liability insurance is:
    a. currently available only to pharmacists.
    b. available to both pharmacists and pharmacy technicians.
    c. required by most states.
    d. required by the federal government.

12. Which agency/administration is not involved in the practice of pharmacy?
    a. CMS
    b. HIPAA
    c. HCFA
    d. FEMA

13. Which agency/administration is responsible for protecting the privacy of patients?
    a. CLIA
    b. SCHIP
    c. HIPAA
    d. DEA

Match the following.

14. _____ DEA   a. regulates and registers pharmacy technicians, pharmacists, and pharmacies

15. _____ FDA   b. establishes and enforces standards for healthcare organizations

16. _____ FBI   c. assures the safety, efficacy, and security of drugs

17. _____ SBOP   d. regulates the legal trade in controlled drugs

18. _____ JCAHO   e. the administrator of the DEA reports to this chief

19. _____ OSHA   f. assures the safety and health of American workers

Choose the best answer.

20. The Food and Drug Administration was created by the:
    a. Food, Drug and Cosmetic Act of 1938.
    b. Pure Food and Drug Act of 1905.
    c. Controlled Substances Act of 1970.
    d. FBI's need to expand to combat prevalent drug abuse.

21. "A display of written, printed, or graphic matter upon the immediate container of an article" refers to the:
    a. label.
    b. labeling.
    c. package insert.
    d. patient information sheet.

22. Which of the following information is not a labeling requirement for a dispensed prescription?
    a. NDC
    b. serial number (Rx number)
    c. date of fill
    d. prescriber's name

23. Which of the following information is not required to be on the manufacturer's label of a prescription-only drug?
    a. route of administration
    b. name and quantity of active ingredients
    c. date of fill
    d. federal legend

24. Which of the following information is not required to be on the package insert?
    a. dosage
    b. indications and usage
    c. adverse reactions
    d. unique lot or control number

Fill in the blank.

25. The amendment signed in 1951 that required the "federal legend" to be printed on all prescription drugs was _____.

26. The Kefauver-Harris Amendment, signed in 1962, is also referred to as the _____.

Match the following.

27. _____ Kefauver-Harris Amendment

28. _____ Pure Food and Drug Act of 1906

29. _____ Food, Drug, and Cosmetic Act

30. _____ Durham-Humphrey Amendment

31. _____ Schedule I

32. _____ Schedule II

33. _____ Schedule III

34. _____ Schedule IV

35. _____ Schedule V

36. _____ DEA Form 224

37. _____ DEA Form 225

38. _____ DEA Form 363

39. _____ DEA Form 222

40. _____ DEA Form 41

a. limits interstate commerce in drugs to those that are safe and effective

b. established "federal legend"

c. focuses on drug manufacturers' accountability for the efficacy, or effectiveness, of drugs

d. neglected to ban unsafe drugs

e. low abuse, limited dependence

f. lowest abuse potential, lowest dependency

g. no accepted medical use, high abuse potential and high dependency risk

h. high potential for abuse and dependency

i. mostly combination drugs, moderate dependency

j. needed to compound narcotics or conduct narcotic treatment

k. used to report lost or stolen C-II drugs

l. needed to order C-II drugs from distributor

m. needed to dispense

n. needed to manufacture or distribute

True or False?

41. The patient's street address or P.O. box number is required on all C-II prescriptions.

    T   F

42. C-II prescriptions must be kept separate from all other prescriptions.

    T   F

43. All prescription drugs must be distributed in childproof containers.

    T   F

Choose the best answer.

44. The first five digits of an NDC number identify which of the following?
    a. drug
    b. manufacturer
    c. package size
    d. distributor

45. Anabolic steroids (except estrogens, progestins, and corticosteroids) are classified in which schedule?
    a. C-I
    b. C-II
    c. C-III
    d. C-IV

46. Ethics is which of the following?
  a. law
  b. religion

  c. morals
  d. none of the above

Match the following.

47. _____ indication

48. _____ warnings

49. _____ contraindications

50. _____ precautions

a. lists types of patient who should not use the drug

b. lists remaining possible side effects

c. specific conditions that the FDA has approved the drug to treat

d. serious side effects and what to do

Match the following.

51. _____ fidelity

52. _____ beneficence

53. _____ veracity

54. _____ justice

55. _____ autonomy

56. _____ ethics of care

57. _____ rights-based ethics

58. _____ principle-based ethics

59. _____ virtues-based ethics

a. acting with fairness or equity

b. acting with self-reliance

c. bringing about good

d. telling the truth

e. keeping a promise

f. the idealization of morals

g. more personal approach

h. democratic view of individuals

i. focus on kindness, tact, etc.

PHARMACY CALCULATION PROBLEMS

Calculate the following.

1. A prescription states that the patient is to take one tablet by mouth twice daily for 10 days. How many tablets will you need to dispense for a 10-day supply?

2. An antibiotic suspension is dispensed in a 150 mL bottle. If the patient takes 5 mL by mouth three times a day, how many days will the antibiotic last?

3. A customer gives herself one enoxaparin injection every day. If enoxaparin comes in a 10-count box (a box of 10 single-dose syringes), how many boxes will the customer need for 30 days?

LAB 4-1: Creating a Pharmacy Law Timeline

Objective:

Review and remember the major laws that pertain to the practice of pharmacy in the United States.

Pre-Lab Information:

Review Chapter 4, "Pharmacy Law and Ethics," in your text.

Explanation:

It is important for pharmacy technicians to have an understanding of pharmacy law. Many of our current laws were enacted because of an injury to persons using medications. The progression of laws related to the practice of pharmacy through American history can give you a better perspective on current laws and regulations.

Activity:

Using the following chart, complete the timeline by filling in the correct year in which each law was passed.

Law	Timeline
The Pure Food and Drug Act	
The Prescription Drug Marketing Act	
The Occupational Safety and Health Act	
The Orphan Drug Act	
The Medical Device Amendment	
The Poison Prevention Packaging Act	
The Omnibus Budget Reconciliation Act	
The Kefauver-Harris Amendment	
The Health Insurance Portability and Accountability Act	
The Controlled Substances Act	
The Combat Methamphetamine Epidemic Act	
The Durham-Humphrey Amendment	
The Drug Listing Act	
The Anabolic Steroids Act	
The Food, Drug, and Cosmetic Act	
The Dietary Supplement Health and Education Act	
The Drug Price Competition and Patent Term Restoration Act	

1. Name four broad categories of law in the United States and provide a brief definition of each.

_____

_____

_____

_____

2. What is the difference between criminal and civil law?

_____

_____

_____

_____

3. Name six of the regulatory agencies that oversee the practice of pharmacy in the United States and describe their function(s).

_____

_____

_____

_____

_____

_____

_____

Student Name: _____

Lab Partner: _____

Grade/Comments: _____

_____

_____

Student Comments: _____

_____

_____

LAB 4-2: Interpreting a Drug Monograph

Objective:

Recognize and use a drug monograph.

Pre-Lab Information:

- Review Chapter 4, "Pharmacy Law and Ethics," in your text.
- Gather the following materials:
  - Drug monograph, either from home or supplied by your instructor

Explanation:

Drug monographs, also called *package inserts*, are a necessary component of a drug's labeling. They provide all the clinical information about a drug as required by the FDA. As a pharmacy technician, you need to be familiar with the format, components, and content of drug monographs.

Activity:

Review the drug monograph that you brought from home or received from your instructor. Then locate all of the components listed here and answer the questions.

Drug name: _____

Description

What is the dosage form of this drug?

_____

_____

Clinical Pharmacology

Does this drug include any notes relevant to specific patient populations? If so, what are they?

_____

_____

_____

Indications and Usage

What specific conditions or symptoms has this drug been approved by the FDA to prevent or treat?

_____

_____

_____

_____

Contraindications

What types of patients should not use this medication?

_____

_____

_____

_____

Warnings

Does this drug include cautions about serious side effects that can be caused by the medication and instructions on what the patient should do if these effects are experienced? If so, describe them.

_____

_____

_____

_____

Precautions

Does the monograph list additional, possible, or potential side effects that the patient should be aware of? If so, what are they?

_____

_____

_____

_____

Drug Abuse and Dependence

Does this drug have a potential for abuse or dependence?

_____

_____

_____

_____

Adverse Reactions

Does the monograph include a description of reactions that are unexpected and potentially life-threatening? If so, what are they?

_____

_____

_____

_____

Dosage

What is the recommended dosage of this medication for an adult?

_____

_____

_____

_____

How Supplied

How is this medication supplied, including strengths, dosage formats, and storage requirements?

_____
_____
_____
_____

Student Name: _____
Lab Partner: _____
Grade/Comments: _____
_____
_____
Student Comments: _____
_____
_____

CHAPTER 5
Terminology and Abbreviations

After completing Chapter 5 from the textbook, you should be able to:	Related Activity in the Workbook/Lab Manual
1. Identify selected root words used in pharmacy practice.	Review Questions Activity 5-3, Lab 5-1
2. Identify and correctly use selected prefixes and suffixes in conjunction with root words.	Review Questions Activity 5-3, Lab 5-1
3. Recognize and interpret common abbreviations used in pharmacy and medicine.	Review Questions, Pharmacy Calculation Problems, PTCB Exam Practice Questions Activity 5-1, Activity 5-2, Lab 5-1
4. List abbreviations that are considered dangerous and explain why.	Review Questions, PTCB Exam Practice Questions
5. Recognize and list common drug names and their generic equivalents.	Review Questions, PTCB Exam Practice Questions Lab 5-1
6. Recall and define common pharmacy and medical terminology.	Review Questions Activity 5-3, Lab 5-1

INTRODUCTION

To understand the pharmacy industry and profession, you must learn its language, which consists of medical terminology, abbreviations, and drug names. Most medical terms derive from Greek and Latin and consist of a root word, prefix, and/or suffix. It is unlikely that you will remember all the information contained in Chapter 5 of the textbook, but by learning selected roots, prefixes, and suffixes, you will be able to understand words you may have never seen or heard before. Over time, with experience and practice, you will develop a strong working knowledge of medical terminology.

REVIEW QUESTIONS

Match the following.

1. _____ pneum
2. _____ arthr
3. _____ cyst
4. _____ my
5. _____ oste
6. _____ ectomy
7. _____ rhin
8. _____ brady
9. _____ dys
10. _____ hyper
11. _____ tachy
12. _____ itis
13. _____ cyte
14. _____ dipsia
15. _____ intra

a. fast
b. abnormal
c. nose
d. bone
e. bladder
f. lung
g. muscle
h. too much
i. cell
j. inflammation
k. thirst
l. too slow
m. surgical removal
n. joint
o. within

Choose the best answer.

16. The part of a word that helps identify its major meaning is the:
   a. prefix.
   b. suffix.
   c. root.
   d. origin.

17. A part of a word that is attached at the beginning of the term is a:
   a. prefix.
   b. suffix.
   c. root.
   d. origin.

18. Which of the following are on JCAHO's "do not use" list?
   a. qhs
   b. SC
   c. QOD
   d. all of the above

Fill in the blank.

19. ADR is the accepted abbreviation for _____.

Match the following.

20. _____ blood sugar   **a.** IM
21. _____ after meals   **b.** u.d.
22. _____ as needed   **c.** apap
23. _____ before meals   **d.** Fe
24. _____ as directed   **e.** gtt
25. _____ left ear   **f.** BS
26. _____ twice daily   **g.** NKA
27. _____ intramuscular   **h.** pc
28. _____ no known allergies   **i.** prn
29. _____ drop   **j.** bid
30. _____ milliliter   **k.** ac
31. _____ aspirin   **l.** AS
32. _____ potassium   **m.** Na
33. _____ penicillin   **n.** ASA
34. _____ iron   **o.** K
35. _____ acetaminophen   **p.** PCN
36. _____ sodium   **q.** mL

Match the following brand drugs with their generics.

37. _____ Accutane®   **a.** zolpidem tartrate
38. _____ Zoloft®   **b.** insulin lispro
39. _____ Flexeril®   **c.** piroxicam
40. _____ Toprol XL®   **d.** meperidine
41. _____ Allegra®   **e.** warfarin
42. _____ Zithromax®   **f.** etodolac
43. _____ Inderal®   **g.** propranolol HCl
44. _____ Feldene®   **h.** fexofenadine HCl
45. _____ Aldactone®   **i.** azithromycin
46. _____ Humalog®   **j.** clonidine HCl
47. _____ Coumadin®   **k.** donepezil HCl
48. _____ Lodine®   **l.** spironolactone
49. _____ Demerol®   **m.** celecoxib
50. _____ Ambien®   **n.** meclizine
51. _____ Fastin®   **o.** isotretinoin
52. _____ Celebrex®   **p.** phentermine
53. _____ Antivert®   **q.** clarithromycin
54. _____ Halcion®   **r.** triazolam
55. _____ Lamisil®   **s.** valsartan
56. _____ Aricept®   **t.** sertraline

57. _____ Catapres
58. _____ Phenergan
59. _____ Diovan
60. _____ Augmentin
61. _____ Plavix
62. _____ Biaxin

u. clopidogrel
v. amoxicillin and clavulanate potassium
w. promethazine HCl
x. metroprolol tartrate
y. terbinafine
z. cyclobenzaprine

PHARMACY CALCULATION PROBLEMS

Calculate the following.

1. A prescription reads: "Cephalexin 500 mg: 1 cap qid × 10d." How many capsules should you dispense?

2. If a patient takes 5 mL of albuterol syrup BID, how many mL should you dispense for a 30-day supply?

3. How many drops of timolol ophthalmic solution is a patient using per day if the instructions read: 2 gtts ou qid?

4. A prescription reads: "Azithromycin 250 mg: Take two tablets by mouth once daily for the first day, then one tablet on days 2–5." How many tablets will you dispense?

5. A bottle of fluticasone nasal spray contains 120 metered doses. If the directions state: "Use 2 sprays in each nostril QD," how many days will the spray last?

PTCB EXAM PRACTICE QUESTIONS

1. Tobrex ophthalmic ung refers to:
   a. an ointment used for the eye.
   b. a solution used for the eye.
   c. a topical ointment for external use only.
   d. an ointment used for the ear.

2. If a medication is to be taken a.c., it should be taken:
   a. in the morning.
   b. around the clock.
   c. after meals.
   d. before meals.

3. Which of the following abbreviations is considered acceptable for use when writing medication orders?
   a. Q.D.
   b. Q.O.D.
   c. Q.I.D.
   d. U

4. What is the generic name for the drug Zantac?
   a. cimetidine
   b. ranitidine
   c. zidovudine
   d. cytarabine

5. What healthcare accreditation organization has created a list of "do not use" abbreviations?
   a. APHA
   b. APA
   c. NABP
   d. JCAHO

ACTIVITY 5-1: Case Study—Lost in Translation

Instructions: Read the following scenarios and then answer the critical thinking questions provided.

Scenario 1

A patient brings in a new prescription for Glucophage XR 500 mg. When you are processing the prescription into the pharmacy computer, you quickly select Glucophage 500 mg from the drop-down list of medications as you scroll down. The prescription is filled and dispensed, as neither you nor the pharmacist notice that the prescription was written for Glucophage XR (extended release) as opposed to Glucophage.

Scenario 2

When writing up a compounding formula sheet, you put down that .5 mg of active ingredient is to be used per dose. The following month, however, another technician is reviewing the formula to prepare the patient's refill. The refill is prepared using 5 mg of active ingredient per dose, as opposed to 0.5 mg.

1. What translation error occurred in Scenario 1?

   _____

   _____

   _____

   _____

2. What effect will the error in Scenario 1 have?

   _____

   _____

   _____

   _____

3. What translation error occurred in Scenario 2?

_____

_____

_____

_____

4. What effect will the error in Scenario 2 have?

_____

_____

_____

_____

5. Who is responsible for the mistake in Scenario 2? How could it most easily have been avoided?

_____

_____

_____

_____

6. What can you do to ensure that these types of errors are avoided?

_____

_____

_____

_____

ACTIVITY 5-2: Practice with Abbreviations

For each of the following, write the meaning next to the abbreviation.

1. p _____
2. pm _____
3. ad lib _____
4. ac _____
5. po _____
6. DAW _____
7. hr _____
8. bid _____
9. u.d. _____
10. qd _____

11. s _____
12. AU _____
13. prn _____
14. qw _____
15. WA _____
16. disp. _____
17. fl. _____
18. ped _____
19. OTC _____
20. NKA _____

Now, write the appropriate abbreviation after its meaning.

21. suppository _____
22. vitamin _____
23. syrup _____
24. water _____
25. buccal _____
26. intravenous _____
27. by mouth _____
28. nasal _____
29. otic _____
30. drops _____

ACTIVITY 5-3: Defining Medical Terms

Using a medical dictionary, your text, or an online medical resource, define the following medical terms. Then, break the term into its word parts and define each word part as well.

1. gynecologist

   Definition: _____

   Word parts: _____

2. rhinoplasty

   Definition: _____

   Word parts: _____

3. epigastric

   Definition: _____

   Word parts: _____

4. arthritis

   Definition: _____

   Word parts: _____

5. abduction

   Definition: _____

   Word parts: _____

6. erythrocytes

   Definition: _____

   Word parts: _____

7. leukocytes

   Definition: _____

   Word parts: _____

8. arteriosclerosis

   Definition: _____

   Word parts: _____

LAB 5-1: Translating a Medical Record

Objective:

Reinforce your knowledge of terminology and abbreviations by completing this exercise based on a medical record entry.

Pre-Lab Information:

Review Chapter 5, "Terminology and Abbreviations," in your text.

Explanation:

It is important for pharmacy technicians to have a basic understanding of the language used in medicine. This exercise will help you gain experience by "translating" a medical record entry.

Activity:

Read the following pharmacist SOAP (Subjective, Objective, Assessment, Plan) note from a patient's pharmacist consultation and answer questions related to the content, using your knowledge of terminology and abbreviations.

S:	67 yo BF with Hx of arthritis, obesity, hyperlipidemia, hypertension. Several questions about medications and improving health status.	
O:	Type 2 DM	Morning BS 130–155+; does not test routinely, A1c 8.5% (6 mo ago)
	HTN	155/95 on ramipril 10 mg bid
	Hyperlipidemia	TC 219, LDL 143, TRG 185 (6 mo ago) on simvastatin 20 mg once daily
	Obesity	5'9" / 230 lb, BMI 34
	RA	Knee and hip pain with exercise, APAP prn only
	SCr	1.6 (6 mo ago)
	Vitals	P 78, R 19
		Not taking ASA for CVD prevention
A:	Diabetes	Poor compliance diet/meal planning; poor understanding of BS testing; above goal of A1c <7%
	HTN	Above goal of BP 125/80 with Tx
	Hyperlipidemia	Above goal of LDL ≤ 100 with Tx
	Obesity	Above goal, 25 lb gain over last 6 mo, min exercise frequency; Initial goal 10% weight loss at 1–2 lb/wk (23 lb in 4 mo)
	RA	Still not well controlled

P:	Improve medication adherence and health outcomes.
	• HTN: Recommended changing ramipril 10 mg bid to lisinopril/HCTZ 20/12.5 bid
	• Hyperlipidemia: Recommended increasing simvastatin from 20 mg to 40 mg once daily
	• RA: Recommended diclofenac XR 100 mg once daily for RA
	• Cardiovascular health: Recommended adding lo-dose ASA daily
	• Provided and instructed pt with daily BS monitoring log
	• Provided and instructed pt with personal health tracking tool
	• Reviewed "ADA Dietary Guidelines" and shopping/meal planner guide
	• Suggested pt walk 30–60 min/day
	• Schedule for 90-day F/U appt.
	• Schedule for repeat of the following labs 2 weeks prior to 90-day FU appt: SCr, fasting lipid profile, A1c, BG

Duration of appt: 45 minutes

Pharmacist's signature: _____

Questions:

1. What does the abbreviation Hx mean?

    _____

    _____

2. What does APAP prn mean?

    _____

    _____

3. In the "Objective" section, which drug (generic and brand name) did the patient take to control cholesterol?

    _____

    _____

4. In the "Objective" section, which drug (generic and brand name) did the patient take to control blood pressure?

    _____

    _____

5. What does the abbreviation BS mean?

    _____

    _____

6. What does the abbreviation HTN mean?

_____

_____

7. In the "Plan" section, what drug (generic and brand) did the pharmacist recommend changing for the patient's HTN?

_____

_____

8. In the "Plan" section, what does the abbreviation ASA mean?

_____

_____

Student Name: _____

Lab Partner: _____

Grade/Comments: _____

_____

_____

Student Comments: _____

_____

_____

Chapter 6
Retail Pharmacy

After completing Chapter 6 from the textbook, you should be able to:	Related Activity in the Workbook/Lab Manual
1. Explain the ambulatory pharmacy practice setting.	Review Questions Activity 6-2
2. Describe the two main types of retail pharmacies.	Review Questions Activity 6-2
3. List the various staff positions in retail pharmacies.	Review Questions Activity 6-2, Activity 6-5
4. Describe the typical work environment of a retail pharmacy.	Review Questions Activity 6-2
5. Discuss the two agencies that regulate retail pharmacy practice.	Review Questions, PTCB Exam Practice Questions
6. List the legal requirements of a prescription medication order.	Review Questions, PTCB Exam Practice Questions Activity 6-4, Lab 6-1
7. Describe the different ways prescriptions arrive at a retail pharmacy.	Review Questions Activity 6-1, Lab 6-4, Lab 6-5
8. List the steps required for a prescription to be filled.	Review Questions, PTCB Exam Practice Questions Activity 6-1, Activity 6-2, Lab 6-4, Lab 6-5
9. Discuss the various job duties of technicians in retail pharmacies.	Review Questions Activity 6-1, Activity 6-2, Activity 6-4, Activity 6-5, Lab 6-1, Lab 6-2, Lab 6-3, Lab 6-4, Lab 6-5
10. Discuss the importance of confidentiality for personal health information.	Review Questions, PTCB Exam Practice Questions Activity 6-3

INTRODUCTION

The two main types of pharmacy practice are ambulatory and institutional. An institutional pharmacy is located on the site of the patients' residence; pharmacies within hospitals, nursing homes, hospices, and long-term care facilities are examples. Most other pharmacies fall into the category of ambulatory. Examples of ambulatory settings, which are usually called *community-based* or *retail pharmacies,* are privately owned, chain, and franchise pharmacies, as well as clinics. Retail pharmacy is the largest category of pharmacy in the United States. These types of pharmacies serve the community in which they are located.

The staff at a retail pharmacy includes the pharmacist in charge (PIC), pharmacy manager, staff pharmacists, pharmacy technicians, and, in many cases, pharmacy clerks. It is a fast-paced work environment where pharmacy professionals interact with patients face to face. Pharmacy technicians have numerous job responsibilities, from taking care of inventory orders, rotations, returns, and billing to counting, measuring, filling, and labeling. In the retail environment, you may also help patients find OTC medications or lead them to the pharmacist for counseling, to name only a few of your daily tasks. In ambulatory pharmacy, every day is another opportunity to serve the community.

REVIEW QUESTIONS

Match the following.

1. _____ chain pharmacy

2. _____ franchise pharmacy

3. _____ neighborhood pharmacy

4. _____ retail pharmacy

a. name for all kinds of ambulatory pharmacies

b. privately owned small pharmacy

c. corporately owned, multiple-site pharmacy

d. ambulatory, multiple-site pharmacy

Fill in the blanks.

5. The process of transmitting a prescription electronically to the proper insurance carrier for approval is called _____.

6. The code DAW, when written by the prescriber, means _____.

7. An electronic record stored in the pharmacy computer system detailing the patient's personal and billing information, prescription records, and medical conditions is known as a/an _____.

8. When the patients reside where the medication is kept, the pharmacy there is described as a/an _____ pharmacy.

9. The agency that registers and regulates retail pharmacy facilities, pharmacists, and pharmacy technicians, as well as the practice of pharmacy, is known as _____.

10. The _____ conducts inspections to ensure compliance with its guidelines and also approves reimbursement for Medicare and Medicaid.

True or False?

11. Retail pharmacy practice allows a more hands-on approach.

    T   F

12. The term "PharmD" is used to designate a Director of Pharmacy.

    T   F

13. Pregnancy tests can be obtained only with a prescription.

    T   F

14. Any OTC product may be kept behind the counter if the pharmacist chooses.

    T   F

Choose the best answer.

15. Which of the following is not an approved prescriber?
- a. DDS
- b. PA
- c. DVM
- d. RN

16. Which of the following is a valid DEA number for Dr. Rebecca Carey?
- a. AC5932764
- b. BC8162753
- c. BC3791250
- d. AC79131591

17. A C-III prescription may be refilled:
- a. 6 times.
- b. 0 times.
- c. for six months from the date it was written.
- d. for one year from the date it was first filled.

18. Which of the following is not required on a prescription?
- a. route of administration
- b. patient's age
- c. strength of drug
- d. prescriber's signature

19. The prescriber wrote Mr. Mallory's prescription for Synthroid® on 12/14/2008 with prn refills. Mr. Mallory had the prescription filled for the first time on 3/09/09. He may continue receiving monthly refills until:
- a. 12/14/2009.
- b. 12/14/2008.
- c. 03/09/2010.
- d. 03/09/2009.

20. The second group of numbers in an NDC code signifies:
- a. package size.
- b. manufacturer.
- c. drug, strength, and form.
- d. cost (AWP).

21. Once a medication has left the pharmacy counter, it may:
- a. not be returned for resale.
- b. not be returned for a refund.
- c. not be returned for resale or refund.
- d. be refunded and/or resold if the pharmacist allows.

22. Most pharmacies and insurance providers require a prescription to be _____ used before it may be refilled.
- a. 50%
- b. 90%
- c. 75%
- d. 100%

23. Most states restrict controlled medications with refills:
- a. to a maximum of one transfer.
- b. to zero transfers; controlled substances may not be refilled.
- c. so that all refills written by the prescriber may be transferred.
- d. to a maximum of three refills that are transferred.

24. It is not a technician's responsibility to:
    a. verify the information in a patient's profile.
    b. counsel a patient on the use of a medication.
    c. double-count a controlled medication for accuracy.
    d. contact an insurance provider on behalf of a patient.

25. When Mrs. Rigby asked to have her Lunesta® prescription transferred from across town, the technician should have:
    a. explained to her that controlled medications cannot be transferred.
    b. informed her that the sending pharmacy has to call.
    c. checked her profile to see if the prescription had been transferred before and had refills remaining.
    d. warned her it may take up to 24 hours to complete the transfer.

PHARMACY CALCULATION PROBLEMS

Calculate the following.

1. The directions for a prescription cough medicine state: Take 5 ml po q4h prn. If the patient takes the maximum daily amount, how long will a 120 mL bottle last?

2. If the sig states "2 tabs po q hs," how many tablets will you need to dispense to last for 28 days?

3. If a patient is taking tetracycline 250 mg caps po QID, how many capsules are needed for a 30-day supply?

4. Jill is compounding a prescription that requires $\frac{3}{4}$ oz. of hydrocortisone 1% cream, $\frac{1}{4}$ oz. nystatin cream, and $\frac{1}{4}$ oz. of clotrimazole 1% cream. How many ounces will be in the finished product?

5. A technician receives a prescription for a controlled substance. The prescription is from out of state and the technician is unfamiliar with the physician and the customer. The DEA number for the physician is AG8642123. Is this a fraudulent prescription?

PTCB EXAM PRACTICE QUESTIONS

1. Which organization oversees the practice of community pharmacies in the United States?
   a. FDA
   b. DEA
   c. SBOP
   d. APHA

2. In the following number, NDC 51285-601-05, the first set (51285) represents which of the following?
   a. drug name
   b. manufacturer
   c. dosage form
   d. capsule size

3. How many times can you refill a prescription for Viagra®?
   a. As many times as indicated by the prescriber.
   b. As many times as indicated by the prescriber within one year from the date the prescription was written.
   c. Six times within six months.
   d. None.

4. Which law provides for protection of patient confidentiality?
   a. HIPAA
   b. JCAHO
   c. OSHA
   d. CSA

5. What is online adjudication?
   a. The process of transmitting prescription information electronically to the proper insurance company or third-party payor for approval and billing.
   b. The process of transmitting orders for controlled drugs.
   c. The process of transferring a prescription to another pharmacy.
   d. The process of receiving a fax from a physician's office.

ACTIVITY 6-1: Prescription Translation Worksheet

Review each of the following five prescriptions, then translate the information contained in each one.

Rx #1

Towne Center Family Medicine
40 Towne Center Drive
Pleasantville, Texas 77248-0124
Phone 281-555-0134 Fax 281-555-0125

James L. Brook, MD BB1234563   Rebecca Smith, MD AS1234563   Walter Roberts, MD AR1234563
Sharon Ortiz, NP   Beth Matthews, NP   Terri King, NP

Name _*Melvin Brooks*_   Age _____

Address _____ Date _*Nov 21*_

℞

     Isordol 10 mg

        #60

       Tpo bid

Refill _____ times   _*(signature)*_

_____
Signature

A generically equivalent drug product may be dispensed unless the practitioner hand writes the words
'Brand Necessary' or 'Brand Medically Necessary' on the face of the prescription.   6HUR133050

---

1. Patient name: _____
2. Prescriber: _____
3. Drug name and strength: _____
4. Is generic substitution permitted? _____
5. Quantity to dispense: _____
6. Directions: _____
7. Refills authorized: _____

Rx #2

Towne Center Family Medicine
40 Towne Center Drive
Pleasantville, Texas 77248-0124
Phone 281-555-0134 Fax 281-555-0125

James L. Brook, MD BB1234563   Rebecca Smith, MD AS1234563   Walter Roberts, MD AR1234563
Sharon Ortiz, NP   Beth Matthews, NP   Terri King, NP

Name _Beth Andrews_____ Age _____

Address _____ Date _03/12_____

℞

    Allegra 60 mg

           #60

    T po Bid

Refill __2___ times

_____ Signature _____

A generically equivalent drug product may be dispensed unless the practitioner hand writes the words
'Brand Necessary' or 'Brand Medically Necessary' on the face of the prescription.

6HUR133050

---

1. Patient name: _____
2. Prescriber: _____
3. Drug name and strength: _____
4. Is generic substitution permitted? _____
5. Quantity to dispense: _____
6. Directions: _____
7. Refills authorized: _____

Towne Center Family Medicine
40 Towne Center Drive
Pleasantville, Texas 77248-0124
Phone 281-555-0134 Fax 281-555-0125

James L. Brook, MD BB1234563   Rebecca Smith, MD AS1234563   Walter Roberts, MD AR1234563
Sharon Ortiz, NP   Beth Matthews, NP   Terri King, NP

Name _*Stephanie Ruiz*_____ Age _____

Address _____ Date _*March 12*_____

℞

        Azelex 308

              #1

       U UD

Refill ___*3*___ times

_____
           Becky Smith
            Signature

A generically equivalent drug product may be dispensed unless the practitioner hand writes the words
'Brand Necessary' or 'Brand Medically Necessary' on the face of the prescription.   6HUR133050

1. Patient name: _____
2. Prescriber: _____
3. Drug name and strength: _____
4. Is generic substitution permitted? _____
5. Quantity to dispense: _____
6. Directions: _____
7. Refills authorized: _____

            CHAPTER 6 *Retail Pharmacy*   **63**

Rx #4

Towne Center Family Medicine
40 Towne Center Drive
Pleasantville, Texas 77248-0124
Phone 281-555-0134 Fax 281-555-0125

James L. Brook, MD BB1234563   Rebecca Smith, MD AS1234563   Walter Roberts, MD AR1234563
Sharon Ortiz, NP   Beth Matthews, NP   Terri King, NP

Name _Algooter Prince_____ Age _____

Address _____ Date __4/20_____

℞

Leset 80mg
#30

T + D

Refill ___5___ times

_____ ~Terri King~
Signature

A generically equivalent drug product may be dispensed unless the practitioner hand writes the words
'Brand Necessary' or 'Brand Medically Necessary' on the face of the prescription.

6HUR133050

---

1. Patient name: _____
2. Prescriber: _____
3. Drug name and strength: _____
4. Is generic substitution permitted? _____
5. Quantity to dispense: _____
6. Directions: _____
7. Refills authorized: _____

Towne Center Family Medicine
40 Towne Center Drive
Pleasantville, Texas 77248-0124
Phone 281-555-0134 Fax 281-555-0125

James L. Brook, MD BB1234563   Rebecca Smith, MD AS1234563   Walter Roberts, MD AR1234563
Sharon Ortiz, NP   Beth Matthews, NP   Terri King, NP

Name _Elesabeth Beastese_____ Age_____

Address_____ Date _3/20_____

℞

Damler 25 mg

#90

TP TI D

Refill_____times

_____
                                    Signature

A generically equivalent drug product may be dispensed unless the practitioner hand writes the words
'Brand Necessary' or 'Brand Medically Necessary' on the face of the prescription.   6HUR133050

1. Patient name: _____
2. Prescriber: _____
3. Drug name and strength: _____
4. Is generic substitution permitted? _____
5. Quantity to dispense: _____
6. Directions: _____
7. Refills authorized: _____

ACTIVITY 6-2: Role Play—Retail Pharmacy Scenarios

Using the information provided, act out the scenario described, and then reflect on the exercise through use of the discussion questions.

Scenario 1

Cast:

- Customer
- Pharmacy Technician
- Pharmacist

Scene:

A customer approaches the pharmacy technician and begins to describe experiencing symptoms of fever, body aches, and chills. The customer then asks what over-the-counter product she or he should purchase to help her or him feel better.

Discussion Questions:

1. Was the pharmacy technician effective in his or her communication with the patient?

   _____

   _____

   _____

2. Did the pharmacy technician stay within his or her scope of practice while interacting with the patient?

   _____

   _____

   _____

3. At what point did the pharmacist become involved in assisting the patient? Was this appropriate?

   _____

   _____

   _____

Scenario 2

Cast:

- Pharmacy Technician
- Patient

Scene:

The patient brings in a prescription to be filled. The pharmacy technician explains that the current wait time is 30 to 45 minutes, which outrages the patient.

Discussion Questions:

1. Was the pharmacy technician professional in his or her communication with the patient?

    _____

    _____

    _____

2. How well did the pharmacy technician handle the upset customer?

    _____

    _____

    _____

3. Would you have handled the situation differently? Why? If so, what would you have done?

    _____

    _____

    _____

Scenario 3

Cast:

- Pharmacy Technician
- Patient

Scene:

The patient brings in a prescription to be filled, and the pharmacy technician explains that the current wait time is 30 minutes. The patient explains that he or she is going to run a quick errand and will then return. Upon returning, the pharmacy technician explains to the patient that the prescription will not be available until the following day at 10:30 a.m., after the pharmacy's morning delivery, because the pharmacy is out of the medication. The patient is unhappy that he or she was not informed of this when the prescription was first dropped off to be filled.

Discussion Questions:

1. What mistakes, if any, did the pharmacy technician make?

    _____

    _____

    _____

2. How did the pharmacy technician resolve the situation with the patient?

    _____

    _____

    _____

3. Would you have handled the situation differently? Why? If so, what would you have done?

    _____

    _____

    _____

ACTIVITY 6-3: Case Study—Privacy/HIPAA

Instructions: Read the following scenario and then answer the critical thinking questions.

A remodel of the workspace at the retail pharmacy in which you work has finally begun. Many people were involved in the design planning, including various construction personnel. However, no one from the pharmacy itself was included on the planning committee. Weeks pass, and it appears that the newly remodeled pharmacy will allow a more efficient use of space.

The remodel is completed on a Friday, and everyone returns to work on Monday excited to see the new space. Almost immediately, everyone notices that the redesigned space lacks an adequate area for patient counseling. HIPAA mandates that every pharmacy have a patient counseling area.

The pharmacy does not close down while this space is added, but instead remains open for business, and pharmacy personnel are asked to "work around" the inconvenience. You are told that the counseling area will be in place after two more weeks of construction. In the meantime, it seems almost impossible to find a private space to counsel patients.

1. What are some creative ways in which the pharmacy could assure patient privacy during counseling until construction is complete?

   _____

   _____

   _____

   _____

2. What effect might this inconvenience have on the pharmacy workload, in terms of time?

   _____

   _____

   _____

   _____

3. Describe what a HIPAA-compliant counseling area, which protects patient privacy, might look like or include.

   _____

   _____

   _____

   _____

ACTIVITY 6-4: Case Study—Biases

Instructions: Read the following scenario and then answer the critical thinking questions.

A gangly, unkempt, middle-aged man with a slightly offensive odor presents a prescription at your pharmacy for hydrocodone bitartrate 5 mg/acetaminophen 500 mg #120 to be taken twice daily as needed for pain. He attempts to rush you through the process, talking excessively and stating that he should be getting more than what was prescribed. His actions make you suspicious, in that he appears nervous, is constantly looking around, and becomes increasingly agitated with each question you ask, such as his address and phone number. It appears that the amount of tablets may have been altered, but you are not quite certain, as this provider's writing is not very legible.

The man becomes more and more uncooperative as you try to gain the information you need to process the prescription, but finally you have everything you need. You have been trained to notice things that may raise questions as to the validity of prescriptions and feel that this may be one such situation. You bring this to the attention of the pharmacist in charge, who in turn calls to verify the prescription. It turns out that the prescription is legitimate and the patient has some mental health issues.

1. What were some factors in this scene that made the technician suspect that this might be a fraudulent prescription?

    _____

    _____

    _____

    _____

2. Can you identify any communication barriers present with this type of patient?

    _____

    _____

    _____

3. Do you think that the way the patient was dressed or acted contributed to the assessment that his might be a fraudulent prescription?

    _____

    _____

    _____

    _____

ACTIVITY 6-5: Case Study—Patient Requests Recommendations

Instructions: Read the following scenario and then answer the critical thinking questions.

Mrs. Hornbuckle, with her 4-year-old daughter in tow, approaches the pharmacy counter and requests some assistance in locating the Children's Tylenol Liquid. You are the only person available, and state that it is located on aisle 6 toward the back of the store; you then offer to show her to the area. Mrs. Hornbuckle accepts your offer and the three of you head to aisle 6.

You point out the Children's Tylenol Liquid section, but before you can walk away, Mrs. Hornbuckle begins asking questions about the wide array of Tylenol liquid preparations. She states that her daughter has a really bad cough and wants to know which one works best, the grape- or the cherry-flavored. Meanwhile, she is picking up boxes and reading the information on the back.

You explain that a pharmacist could answer any questions she may have about the medicines. With a frustrated sigh, she says, "Forget it," and starts to walk out in a huff, obviously upset that you were not able to answer the questions yourself.

1. Why might Mrs. Hornbuckle have felt that you could (and should) have answered her questions about medications?

_____

_____

_____

_____

2. Do you think pharmacy technicians should identify themselves as such, or would it matter to the general public, who may not know the difference between pharmacy technicians and pharmacists?

_____

_____

_____

_____

3. How would you explain to a patient/customer, in an understanding way, your limited authority as a pharmacy technician?

_____

_____

_____

_____

LAB 6-1: Checking a Prescription for Completeness

Objective:

Interpret some sample prescriptions, identify their key components, and determine if the prescriptions contain all the necessary information.

Pre-Lab Information:

Review Tables 5-4, 5-5, 5-6, and 5-7 from Chapter 5 of your textbook to refamiliarize yourself with various medical terms and abbreviations.

Explanation:

Many times a legitimate prescription lacks some of the information required for processing. This exercise will help you review the key components of a prescription, practice translating prescriptions, and identify potential missing information.

Activity:

Four prescriptions have been dropped off at the pharmacy to be filled. The first step is to put the data from the prescriptions into the computer. Translate the prescription, note all key points that must be printed on the labels, and determine if the prescriptions contain all the information needed for processing.

Dr. L. MacCoy
1234 Enterprise Dr
San Francisco, CA 00000
800-555-1234

Name _Jill Johnson_   Age _____

Address _79 Holiday Rd_   Date _06/08/08_

R_x

     Metoprolol tablets

         #60

       Sig: 1 po bid

Refill ___5___ times

           L. MacCoy
             Signature

A generically equivalent drug product may be dispensed unless the practitioner hand writes the words
'Brand Necessary' or 'Brand Medically Necessary' on the face of the prescription.   6HUR133050

---

1. Does the information seem correct on the prescription for Jill Johnson? How would you translate the instructions for the prescription label? Is anything missing from this prescription?

_____

_____

_____

Dr. Fillmore McGraw
100 Hollywood Blvd.
Los Angeles, CA 00000
(800) 123-4567

Name _Britanny Spires_____ Age _____

Address _6002 Hillside Place_____ Date _07/02/08_____

℞

Xanax 0.25 mg tablet

Sig: 1 po tid prn anxiety

Refill _____0_____ times

_Fillmore McGraw_____
Signature

A generically equivalent drug product may be dispensed unless the practitioner hand writes the words
'Brand Necessary' or 'Brand Medically Necessary' on the face of the prescription.

6HUR133050

2. Does the information seem correct on the prescription for Britanny Spires? How would you translate the instructions for the prescription label? Is anything missing from this prescription?

_____

_____

_____

Elsie Kumar, MD
4605 Lakeshore Drive
Chicago, IL 00000
(819) 555-1111

Name _Sandy Deitz_____ Age_____

Address _123 Laramy Ct_____ Date _05/14/08_____

Rx

Sig: Promethazine 25 mg

1 q4-6hr prn nausea

Refill ___0___ times

_Elsie Kumar, MD_____
Signature

A generically equivalent drug product may be dispensed unless the practitioner hand writes the words
'Brand Necessary' or 'Brand Medically Necessary' on the face of the prescription.   6HUR133050

---

3. Does the information seem correct on the prescription for Sandy Deitz? How would you translate
   the instructions for the prescription label? Is anything missing from this prescription?

   _____

   _____

   _____

Name _Jeremy Jacobsen_ _____ Age _____

Address _455 Brady Street_ _____ Date _7/25/08_ _____

R

Amoxicillin 500mg

Sig: 1 po TID X 10 days

Refill ___O___ times

_____
Signature

A generically equivalent drug product may be dispensed unless the practitioner hand writes the words
'Brand Necessary' or 'Brand Medically Necessary' on the face of the prescription.

6HUR133050

---

4. Does the information seem correct on the prescription for Jeremy Jacobsen? How would you translate the instructions for the prescription label? How many capsules will be needed to fill this prescription? Is anything missing from this prescription?

_____

_____

_____

Student Name: _____

Lab Partner: _____

Grade/Comments: _____

_____

_____

Student Comments: _____

_____

_____

LAB 6-2: Counting Oral Medication in a Community Pharmacy Setting

Objective:

To demonstrate the ability to count oral medications manually and gain experience with cleaning procedures in the pharmacy.

Pre-Lab Information:

- Review Chapter 6, "Retail Pharmacy," in the textbook.
- Gather the following supplies:
  - Pill counting tray and spatula
  - Large bag of M&Ms®, Skittles®, or other small-sized hard candy
  - Prescription vials, plastic sandwich bags, or other containers for the "tablets"
  - Isopropyl alcohol (70%)

Explanation:

This exercise will give you the opportunity to practice counting "tablets" manually. In the pharmacy, tablets are generally counted in increments of five, using a pill counting tray and spatula on a clean, clutter-free counter. It requires practice to feel confident and efficient in counting tablets by fives, so until you gain experience, remember to count tablets twice before giving them to the "pharmacist."

Activity:

Part 1

For this first exercise, you will count 15 tablets.

1. Prepare a clean, clutter-free work surface, and then place a clean pill counting tray and spatula in front of you.
2. Pour a portion of your "tablets" into the counting tray, then open the lid of the pour compartment.
3. Begin counting the "tablets" in increments of five, using the counting spatula. Slide each group of five into the pour compartment of your tray. Count by fives until you reach fifteen tablets, then close the lid of the pour compartment.
4. Return any unused "tablets" that are still in your counting tray to their container or bag.
5. Select a prescription vial and place it on the counter next to the counting tray.
6. Pour the tablets you counted into the vial.
7. Now pour the tablets you counted back into your counting tray and count them again to make sure you have 15.
8. Repeat step 6. Then place the lid on the vial.

Part 2

For this next exercise, you will use the materials from the previous activity to prepare the following "prescriptions" for "dispensing."

1. Ibuprofen [M&Ms] 800 mg

   Sig: 1 tab tid x 10 days

   Count the correct number of "tablets" required to fill this prescription.

2. M&Mcycline 320 mg tabs

   Sig: 1 tab qid x 5 days

   Count the correct number of "tablets" required to fill this prescription.

3. M&Mnisone 20 mg tabs

   Sig: 1 tab qid x 2 days; 1 tab tid x 2 days; then 1 tab daily x 2 days

   Count the correct number of "tablets" required to fill this prescription.

Feel free to continue counting until all of the tablets are "gone."

Part 3

To complete this lab activity, clean your materials and work area using a disinfectant solution of water and 70% isopropyl alcohol. Spray the solution on the counting tray and spatula, then wipe them with a paper towel and return them to the shelf or appropriate storage location. Then, spray the counter with the solution and wipe the counter down.

Student Name: _____

Lab Partner: _____

Grade/Comments: _____

_____

_____

Student Comments: _____

_____

_____

LAB 6-3: Processing a New Patient

Objective:

Demonstrate ability to follow the procedure for processing a new patient.

Pre-Lab Information:

Review Chapter 6 in your textbook.

Explanation:

As a pharmacy technician working in a retail pharmacy, you will need to create a new patient profile for each new customer. The patient profile is a electronic record stored in the pharmacy computer system that details the patient's personal and billing information, prescription records, and medical conditions.

Activity:

In this exercise, you will work with a partner to create a mock patient profile and insurance card. You will then trade information and each create a new patient profile in the computer.

Materials Needed

* Pharmacy computer station
* Patient profile information
* Insurance information

Procedure

1. Complete a new patient profile form using the blank form that follows. The information you enter should be fictitious; do not use your own personal information.

2. Create an insurance card by using the template provided. Again, use fictitious information.

3. Trade information with your lab partner and add your partner's information to the pharmacy computer system as though your partner were a new patient.

4. Review the information entered for accuracy.

PATIENT PROFILE

Patient Name

_____   _____   _____
           Last   **First**   **Middle Initial**

- -

_____

Street or PO Box

_____   _____   _____

    City   State   Zip

- -

Phone   Date of Birth   Social Security No.
( )   ☐ Male ☐ Female ___ ___ ___
         Month   Day   Year

☐ Yes, I would like medication dispensed in a child-resistant container.
☐ No, I do not want medication dispensed in a child-resistant container.
Medication Insurance   Card Holder Name _____

☐ Yes ☐ No   ☐ Card Holder   ☐ Child   ☐ Disabled Dependent
                  ☐ Spouse   ☐ Dependent Parent ☐ Full Time Student

MEDICAL HISTORY

HEALTH

☐ Angina	☐ Epilepsy
☐ Anemia	☐ Glaucoma
☐ Arthritis	☐ Heart Condition
☐ Asthma	☐ Kidney Disease
☐ Blood Clotting Disorders	☐ Liver Disease
☐ High Blood Pressure	☐ Lung Disease
☐ Breast Feeding	☐ Parkinson's Disease
☐ Cancer	☐ Pregnancy
☐ Diabetes	☐ Ulcers

Other Conditions _____
_____
_____

ALLERGIES AND DRUGS REACTIONS
   ☐ No known drug allergies or
     reactions
   ☐ Aspirin
   ☐ Cephalosporins
   ☐ Codeine
   ☐ Erythromycin
   ☐ Penicillin
   ☐ Sulfa Drugs
   ☐ Tetracyclines
   ☐ Xanthines
Other Allergies/Reactions _____

Prescription Medication Being Taken
_____
_____

OTC Medication Currently Being Taken
_____
_____

Would You Like Generic Medication Where Possible? ☐ Yes ☐ No

Comments
_____

Health information changes periodically. Please notify the pharmacy of any new medications, allergies, drug reactions, or health conditions.
_____ Signature _____ Date ☐ I do not wish to provide this information.

```
United Health Care
1-800-555-3456

Subscriber No.              Group No.
_____  - _____

Name _____

Patient Code_____

Rx 10/25/50              Effective 01/09
```

Discussion Questions:

1. Did you enter the patient's information accurately on the first attempt? If not, what mistake(s) did you make?

   _____

   _____

2. Why is the information on the patient profile form so important?

   _____

   _____

   _____

   _____

3. What are the most common patient codes, and what do they represent?

   _____

   _____

Student Name: _____

Lab Partner: _____

Grade/Comments: _____

_____

_____

Student Comments: _____

_____

_____

LAB 6-4: Processing a New Prescription

Objective:

Demonstrate ability to follow the procedure for processing a new prescription.

Pre-Lab Information:

Review the steps listed in Procedure 6-2, "Entering a Prescription," in Chapter 6 of your textbook.

Explanation:

As a pharmacy technician working in a retail pharmacy, you will need to process new prescriptions for your customers. This process has many steps, including receiving the order either in person, or by phone, fax, or e-mail, depending on the regulations of your particular state. Next you must review the order for legality and correctness, and then translate the order. This all happens before the prescription may be entered into the computer system.

Activity:

In this exercise, you will enter the mock prescription that follows into the computer system and print a label.

Materials Needed

- Pharmacy computer station
- Prescription
- Printer
- Prescription labels

Procedure

1. Enter the prescription that follows into the pharmacy computer system.
2. Review the information as entered for accuracy.
3. Print a prescription label.

James L. Brook, MD BB1234563   Rebecca Smith, MD AS1234563   Walter Roberts, MD AR1234563
Sharon Ortiz, NP   Beth Matthews, NP   Terri King, NP

Name *Taylor Payne*   Age _____

Address _____   Date *April 21*

℞

 Amoxil 500 mg
  #20

  T POBFD X 10D

Refill _____ times

                              Beckey Smith
                              Signature

A generically equivalent drug product may be dispensed unless the practitioner hand writes the words
'Brand Necessary' or 'Brand Medically Necessary' on the face of the prescription.

6HUR133050

Discussion Questions:

1. Whom did you list as the prescriber?
    _____

2. What is the proper days supply for this prescription?
    _____

3. If the patient approved generic substitution, what drug name should be printed on the label?
    _____

Optional Activity:

For additional practice, process the prescriptions provided in Activity 6-1, "Prescription Translation Worksheet."

Student Name: _____

Lab Partner: _____

Grade/Comments: _____

_____

_____

Student Comments: _____

_____

_____

LAB 6-5: Processing a Refill Request

Objective:

Demonstrate ability to follow the procedure for processing a refill request.

Pre-Lab Information:

- Review Chapter 6 in your textbook.
- Review the steps listed in Procedure 6-4, "Requesting a Refill Authorization," in Chapter 6 of your textbook.

Explanation:

As a pharmacy technician working in a retail pharmacy, you will need to process prescription refills. This involves documenting patient refill orders, verifying prescription refills, processing orders with refills available, and contacting prescribers to seek approval for prescriptions for which additional refills are needed.

Activity:

Review the two prescription refill requests that follow and list the specific steps necessary to perform each one.

Rx #1

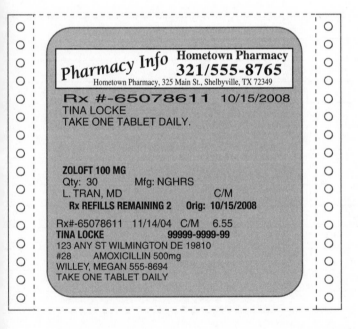

List the steps for processing this prescription refill:

_____

_____

_____

_____

_____

Rx #2

Date – April 5
For – Patient, Jim Roberts
Message – Needs a refill for his blood pressure medication

After looking up the patient's profile, you determine that he has no remaining refills for his blood pressure medication.

List the steps for processing this prescription refill:

_____

_____

_____

_____

_____

Student Name: _____

Lab Partner: _____

Grade/Comments: _____

_____

Student Comments: _____

_____

_____

CHAPTER 7
Health-System Pharmacy

After completing Chapter 7 from the textbook, you should be able to:	Related Activity in the Workbook/Lab Manual
1. Describe the health-system pharmacy practice setting.	Review Questions, PTCB Exam Practice Questions Activity 7-1, Activity 7-3, Activity 7-5
2. Describe the advantages of a unit-dose system.	Review Questions, PTCB Exam Practice Questions Activity 7-4
3. List the necessary components of a medication order.	Review Questions Activity 7-2, Lab 7-1, Lab 7-2, Lab 7-3
4. Compare the duties of a technician with those of a pharmacist in accepting a medication order in a health-system setting.	Review Questions Activity 7-2, Activity 7-3, Activity 7-5
5. Compare centralized and decentralized unit-dose systems.	Review Questions Activity 7-4
6. Compare the duties of a technician with those of a pharmacist in filling a medication order in a health-system setting.	Review Questions Activity 7-2, Activity 7-3, Activity 7-5, Lab 7-1, Lab 7-2, Lab 7-3
7. Define the tasks pharmacy technicians perform in health-system settings.	Review Questions Activity 7-1, Activity 7-2, Activity 7-3, Activity 7-5, Lab 7-1, Lab 7-2, Lab 7-3

INTRODUCTION

A health-system pharmacy, also called an *institutional pharmacy,* is designed to serve patients who live onsite. Examples of facilities that might include an institutional pharmacy are long-term care facilities, nursing homes, hospitals, correctional facilities, and hospices. Regardless of the type of facility, the onsite pharmacy is responsible for all patients' medications; pharmacy staff must ensure that drug therapies are appropriate, effective, and safe. The health-system pharmacist also identifies, resolves, and prevents medication-related problems. As a pharmacy technician working in this setting, you must understand the policies and procedures of your institution, as well as state and federal laws. In addition to filling prescriptions and medication orders, you might also work with several distribution systems, repackage bulk medications for floors and patient care areas, use unit-dose and automatic dispensing systems, and handle sterile products.

REVIEW QUESTIONS

Match the following.

1. _____ blister packs
2. _____ decentralized pharmacy system
3. _____ centralized pharmacy system
4. _____ emergency medication orders
5. _____ floor stock
6. _____ POE system
7. _____ unit dose
8. _____ STAT order
9. _____ standing order
10. _____ patient prescription stock system
11. _____ PRN order

a. a specific order required to respond to a medical emergency

b. medication order that takes priority over other orders and requests

c. orders are reviewed, prepared, verified, and delivered to the patient

d. allows prescribers to enter orders directly into the pharmacy computer system

e. scheduled order to be administered throughout the day

f. consists of central, inpatient, outpatient, and satellite pharmacies

g. unit-dose packages

h. all pharmacy-related services are performed in one location

i. order used only as necessary

j. medication order is filled for no more than a 24-hour period

k. medications stored on the same floor where patients' rooms are, for patient distribution

Choose the best answer.

12. A licensed individual who is trained to examine patients, diagnose illnesses, and prescribe/administer medication is a:
    a. doctor of medicine (MD).
    b. doctor of osteopathy (DO).
    c. licensed nursing assistant (LPA).
    d. licensed practical nurse (LPN).

13. An individual who is licensed to provide basic care, such as administering medication under the supervision of an RN, is a:
    a. doctor of medicine (MD).
    b. doctor of osteopathy (DO).
    c. licensed nursing assistant (LPA).
    d. licensed practical nurse (LPN).

14. An individual who is registered to assist physicians with specific procedures, administer medication, and provide patient care is a:
    a. licensed practical nurse (LPN).   c. registered nurse (RN).
    b. licensed nursing assistant (LNA).   d. nurse practitioner (NP).

15. An individual who is certified to assist RNs and LPNs in providing patient care, but is not permitted to administer medication, is a:
    a. licensed practical nurse (LPN).   c. registered nurse (RN).
    b. licensed nursing assistant (LNA).   d. nurse practitioner (NP).

16. An individual who is licensed to work closely with a physician in providing patient care, typically under the supervision of a physician, is a:
    a. licensed practical nurse (LPN).   c. registered nurse (RN).
    b. licensed nursing assistant (LNA).   d. nurse practitioner (NP).

17. A licensed individual, who is trained to coordinate patient care under the supervision of a medical or osteopathic doctor, is a:
    a. licensed practical nurse (LPN).   c. physician's assistant (PA).
    b. licensed nursing assistant (LNA).   d. nurse practitioner (NP).

18. A pharmacy that provides services to onsite patients 24 hours a day, 365 days each year, is called a:
    a. mail order pharmacy.   c. community pharmacy.
    b. health-system pharmacy.   d. all of the above.

19. The American Hospital Association (AHA) categorizes hospitals as community-based, federal government, psychiatric, long-term care, or institutional hospital units. Which represent 85% of the total number of registered hospitals?
    a. community-based   c. long-term care
    b. federal government   d. psychiatric

Match the following organizations/agencies/regulations to their area of influence.

20. _____ HIPAA   **a.** laboratories
21. _____ OBRA   **b.** children
22. _____ CMS   **c.** privacy
23. _____ SCHIP   **d.** counseling
24. _____ DPH   **e.** regulates hospitals
25. _____ CLIA   **f.** Medicare/Medicaid

PHARMACY CALCULATION PROBLEMS

Calculate the following.

1. A hospitalized patient needs a 24-hour supply of sucralfate 1 gm tablets. How many tablets will be dispensed if the patient takes it qid?

2. A patient on the infectious disease floor takes 10 mL of levofloxacin syrup bid. If the product is only available as a 5 mL unit-dose oral syringe, how many syringes will the patient need for a 24-hour supply?

3. A technician is checking floor stock on one of the nursing units. She notices that the floor has five acetaminophen 325 mg tablets left, but their par level is 20. How many tablets should the technician restock?

4. While checking a crash cart tray that was recently used for a code, Bill finds that there are two epinephrine syringes left in the tray. When the tray is fully stocked, it contains 12 epinephrine syringes. How many syringes should be restocked in the tray?

5. Karen is repackaging cyanocobalamin 1,000 mcg tablets into unit dosages on 2/16/08. The manufacturer's expiration date for the product is 12/09. What expiration date should Karen assign to the repackaged medication?

PTCB EXAM PRACTICE QUESTIONS

1. Which of the following healthcare practitioners is not considered a prescriber?
   a. medical doctor (MD)
   b. physician assistant (PA)
   c. nurse practitioner (NP)
   d. certified nursing assistant (CNA)

2. A unit dose is a:
   a. package that contains all noncontrolled medications for a given day.
   b. package that contains all medications for a given day
   c. controlled substance.
   d. package that contains the amount of medication for one dose.

3. Which of the following allows a patient to receive medications on an as-needed basis?
   a. STAT order
   b. standing order
   c. parenteral
   d. PRN order

4. Nurses track medication administration on a/an:
   a. PCU.
   b. PRN.
   c. STAT.
   d. MAR.

5. In the health-system setting, needles and other items that can cut or puncture the skin should be thrown away in:
   a. MSDS.
   b. designated sharps containers.
   c. red garbage bags.
   d. regular garbage cans.

ACTIVITY 7-1: Role Play—Health-System Pharmacy Scenarios

Using the information provided, act out the scenario described, and then reflect on the exercise through the use of the discussion questions.

Scenario 1

Cast:

- Pharmacy Technician
- Pharmacist
- Nurse

Scene:

The pharmacy technician is on the phone with a nurse who is complaining that the PRN floor stock medication is running low and should be refilled. While the technician is on the phone, the pharmacist brings a STAT order for the emergency room.

Discussion Questions:

1. How did the pharmacy technician prioritize his or her work? Was this correct?
   _____
   _____

2. Did the pharmacy technician remain calm and professional or become flustered?
   _____
   _____

3. What, if anything, would you have done differently?
   _____
   _____

Scenario 2

Cast:

- Pharmacy Technician
- Pharmacist

Scene:

While preparing IV bags, the pharmacy technician forgets to have the pharmacist check the measured medication before it is added to the IV bag. The technician knows that the medication is very expensive and is nervous about telling the staff pharmacist.

Discussion Questions:

1. What could have caused the pharmacy technician's error?
    _____
    _____

2. How did the pharmacist and pharmacy technician resolve the matter? Was this appropriate?
    _____
    _____

3. How else could this situation have been resolved?
    _____
    _____

Scenario 3

Cast:

- Pharmacy Technician 1
- Pharmacy Technician 2

Scene:

Pharmacy Technician 1 is training Pharmacy Technician 2 on how to establish expiration dates when repackaging medication into blister packs. They are working with ibuprofen 600 mg, which (according to the manufacturer) will expire in 18 months.

Discussion Questions:

1. Did the two pharmacy technicians establish a proper expiration date for the repackaged medication?
    _____
    _____

2. Was Pharmacy Technician 1 effective in teaching Pharmacy Technician 2?
    _____
    _____

3. Would you have handled the situation differently? Why? If so, what would you have done?
    _____
    _____

ACTIVITY 7-2: Medication Order Translation Worksheet

Review and translate each of the medication orders provided below.

Medication Order #1

PHYSICIAN'S ORDER WORKSHEET

NOTE: *Person initiating entry should write legibly, date the form using (Mo/Day/Yr.), enter time, sign, and indicate their title.*

USE BALL POINT PEN (PRESS FIRMLY)

45671001   311A
Eckels, Ruby G.
04-10-1943

Dr. C. Thomsen

Date	Time	Treatment
10/18	4:30	Dilaudid 0.5 mg IV inject q 3h prn pan
		②

 PHYSICIAN'S ORDER WORKSHEET   Distribution: (Original) Medical Record Copy (Plies 3, 2, & 1) Pharmacy   **T-5**

CHAPTER 7 *Health-System Pharmacy*

1. Patient name: _____

2. Prescriber: _____

3. Drug name and strength: _____

4. Directions: _____

Medication Order #2

PHYSICIAN'S ORDER WORKSHEET

NOTE: *Person initiating entry should write legibly, date the form using (Mo/Day/Yr.), enter time, sign, and indicate their title.*

USE BALL POINT PEN (PRESS FIRMLY)

132445855   210
Sanchez, Roberto L.
10-01-1940

Dr. L. Hubbard

Date	Time	Treatment
1/14	10:30	Vancomycin 500 mg IV infusion over 6 hr
		②

PHYSICIAN'S ORDER WORKSHEET

Distribution:
(Original) Medical Record Copy
(Plies 3, 2, & 1) Pharmacy

T-5

1. Patient name: _____

2. Prescriber: _____

3. Drug name and strength: _____

4. Directions: _____

Medication Order #3

PHYSICIAN'S ORDER WORKSHEET

NOTE: *Person initiating entry should write legibly, date the form using (Mo/Day/Yr.), enter time, sign, and indicate their title.*

USE BALL POINT PEN (PRESS FIRMLY)

```
82347665        835 A
George, Sarah M.
02-17-1961

Dr. L. Montgomery
```

Date	Time	Treatment
4/10	13:00	Ibuprofen 600 mg po q 6 hr
		②

PHYSICIAN'S ORDER WORKSHEET	Distribution: (Original) Medical Record Copy (Plies 3, 2, & 1) Pharmacy	**T-5**

1. Patient name: _____

2. Prescriber: _____

3. Drug name and strength: _____

4. Directions: _____

Medication Order #4

PHYSICIAN'S ORDER WORKSHEET

NOTE: *Person initiating entry should write legibly, date the form using (Mo/Day/Yr.), enter time, sign, and indicate their title.*

USE BALL POINT PEN (PRESS FIRMLY)

782467199   1410 B
Smith, Cody M.
11-18-1975

Dr. L. Halberdier

Date	Time	Treatment
8/14	13:15	Ranitidine 150 mg Infuse over 24 hr
		②

   PHYSICIAN'S ORDER WORKSHEET   Distribution: (Original) Medical Record Copy (Plies 3, 2, & 1) Pharmacy   **T-5**

1. Patient name: _____

2. Prescriber: _____

3. Drug name and strength: _____

4. Directions: _____

ACTIVITY 7-3: Case Study—Healthcare Professional Demands Medication

Instructions: Read the following scenario and then answer the critical thinking questions.

You are one of two pharmacy technicians working the graveyard shift at a local community hospital of 230 beds. The single pharmacist working the same evening is currently out of the pharmacy, consulting on a dosing recommendation for a powerful IV antibiotic, which must be administered to an inpatient soon. A nurse practitioner calls in to the pharmacy and frantically tells you that a loading dose of 1,500 mg IV vancomycin is needed, to be started right away on another patient. The nurse practitioner reinforces the urgent request by saying, "Have it ready when I get there in less than 2 minutes" and hangs up abruptly. Clearly, the NP is on the way to the pharmacy.

You decide to head into the IV room to start preparing the sterile solution while the other pharmacy technician attempts to contact the pharmacist, who is still out of the pharmacy.

1. What would you do if the nurse practitioner appeared at the pharmacy, demanding the IV vancomycin, while the pharmacist was still unavailable?

_____

_____

_____

2. Can you think of any situation in which a pharmacy technician would be allowed to hand over the medication before a pharmacist checks it?

_____

_____

_____

3. Is it a good idea to begin making the IV vancomycin to save time?

_____

_____

_____

4. Can you think of another way to accomplish this task other than the solution given?

_____

_____

_____

ACTIVITY 7-4: Case Study—Unit Dosing

Instructions: Read the following scenario and then answer the critical thinking questions.

Pharmacy technicians have always packaged the unit-dose medications in the nursing home where you work. In recent weeks, it seems the procedures have not been followed according to policy. In light of this information, you have been placed in charge of the unit-dosing processes for all ward stock areas. Three other pharmacy technicians also help out in this area, all working different shifts.

Numerous unit-dose medications are available for patients on the wards. You inspect the wards and notice that there are also large bottles of such items as Maalox®, Benadryl® liquid, Tylenol®, and docusate sodium. It seems that almost every patient receives these medications, and nursing staff explains that it is easier just to have these large bottles available. Besides, these are all OTC medications anyway. Your understanding of the Joint Commission on the Accreditation of Healthcare Organizations recommendations is that all medications on ward stock are to be unit-dosed, if unit doses are available from the manufacturer or when repackaging by the pharmacy into unit doses is feasible. You must decide whether to unit-dose these bulk items you find in the ward stock areas.

1. What factors would you use to determine when unit-dosing is feasible? Give examples.

   _____

   _____

   _____

2. Which of the medications mentioned in the scenario would you unit-dose? What other types of bulk medications would normally be used in a ward stock situation?

   _____

   _____

   _____

3. How would you communicate any updates to the process to the other pharmacy technicians who work with unit-dosing? How would you convey the importance of your decisions?

   _____

   _____

   _____

4. What regulations from what agencies can you find that relate to the unit-dosing of medications?

   _____

   _____

   _____

ACTIVITY 7-5: Case Study—Outside Request for Dosing Information on Patient

Instructions: Read the following scenario and then answer the critical thinking questions.

All 9 certified pharmacy technicians at the 120-bed community hospital where you work have received ongoing education through the facility monthly for the past 3 years. This CE has placed special emphasis on cyber-security and HIPAA.

An outside call comes in one evening while you are working and the person at the other end of the line begins asking a simple question. The caller goes on to explain that her father was recently a patient at the hospital and his outside doctor needs to know what dose of digoxin was prescribed while the father was a patient. The caller states that she knows it was 0.25 mg every day, but wants to verify it now. Your train of thought leads to your recent training and you inform this person that you are unable to answer that question; instead, you refer her to another source.

The person on the phone now informs you that she called the previous day and whoever answered then gave her the information that the digoxin dose was 0.25 mg per day. You ask the caller if she knows who she spoke to, and she names one of the certified pharmacy technicians who was answering phones that day.

1. Should this concern you? If so, for what reason?

   _____

   _____

   _____

2. Can you give the information requested to the outside person on the phone? Why or why not?

   _____

   _____

   _____

3. To what source did you refer this outside relative for answers to her question?

   _____

   _____

   _____

4. What regulation(s) or guideline(s), in both the cyber-security and HIPAA arenas, do you know of that would govern why you would or would not divulge this information?

   _____

   _____

   _____

LAB 7-1: Locating Basic Lab Values

Objective:

Become familiar with common lab values that the health-system pharmacist may use to monitor patients.

Pre-Lab Information:

• Review Chapter 7, "Health-System Pharmacy," in your textbook.

• Visit the following website as an introduction to normal human lab values: http://www.globalrph.com/labs.htm

Explanation:

It is important for you to have a basic understanding of the laboratory values used in the health-system and other pharmacy settings. This exercise will help you gain experience by looking up the most common "labs."

Activity:

Go to the website http://www.globalrph.com/labs.htm. Look up the information included in the following tables. Add the normal lab values for each item.

CBC		
Hemoglobin (g/dL)	Male Normal _____ g/dL	Female Normal _____ g/dL
Hematocrit (%)	Male Normal _____ %	Female Normal _____ %
Platelet Count	Normal Range _____	
White Blood Count (WBC)	Normal Range _____	

Metabolic Panel	Normal Range
Sodium	
Potassium	
Calcium (ionized)	
Chloride	
Glucose	
Blood Urea Nitrogen (BUN)	
Creatinine	
Albumin	
Alkaline phosphatase (ALP)	
Aspartate aminotransferase (AST)	
Alanine aminotransferase (ALT)	

Lipid Panel	Normal Range
Total cholesterol	
HDL cholesterol	
LDL cholesterol	
Triglycerides	

Student Name: _____

Lab Partner: _____

Grade/Comments: _____

_____

_____

Student Comments: _____

_____

_____

LAB 7-2: Filling a Medication Order

Objective:

To follow the proper procedure for filling a medication order.

Pre-Lab Information:

Review Chapter 7, "Health-System Pharmacy," in your textbook.

Explanation:

The medication order form is a multipurpose tool for communication among various members of the healthcare team working within a health system. In addition to prescribed medications, this form can be used by the physician for ordering lab values, dietary considerations, X-rays, or other medical procedures, so it is imperative that pharmacy personnel be able to properly distinguish and interpret medication orders.

Hospitals can choose to use physical, hard-copy medication order forms. Alternatives are a physician order entry system (POE) or a computerized physician order entry system (CPOE), which is a computerized system in which orders are entered electronically into the hospital's networked system.

Activity:

Review each of the following medication orders, enter them into the pharmacy computer system to generate labels, fill the medications, and label the prescriptions for the pharmacist to review.

If you do not have access to a pharmacy computer system, you can use the blank label that appears at the end of this lab.

Medication Order #1

PHYSICIAN'S ORDER WORKSHEET

NOTE: *Person initiating entry should write legibly, date the form using (Mo/Day/Yr.), enter time, sign, and indicate their title.*

USE BALL POINT PEN (PRESS FIRMLY)

63450091   105
Randall, Kristen F.
09-28-63

Dr. R. Manini

Date	Time	Treatment
3/30	10:30	Restoril 15mg po qhs prn sleep
		②

PHYSICIAN'S ORDER WORKSHEET

Distribution:
(Original) Medical Record Copy
(Plies 3, 2, & 1) Pharmacy

T-5

Medication Order #2

PHYSICIAN'S ORDER WORKSHEET

NOTE: *Person initiating entry should write legibly, date the form using (Mo/Day/Yr.), enter time, sign, and indicate their title.*

USE BALL POINT PEN (PRESS FIRMLY)

51298556   620 B
Nguyen, Kim T.
05–05–1971

Dr. K. Tran

Date	Time	Treatment
9/8	8:30	Vicodin 5/500 PO PRN PAIN
		②

 PHYSICIAN'S ORDER WORKSHEET   Distribution: (Original) Medical Record Copy (Plies 3, 2, & 1) Pharmacy   **T-5**

Medication Order #3

PHYSICIAN'S ORDER WORKSHEET

NOTE: *Person initiating entry should write legibly, date the form using (Mo/Day/Yr.), enter time, sign, and indicate their title.*

USE BALL POINT PEN (PRESS FIRMLY)

93471287   515B
Goodman, Ronald B.
06-15-1958

Dr. K. Patel

Date	Time	Treatment
4/10	11:20	Diflucan 200 mg IV over 4 hrs
		②

PHYSICIAN'S ORDER WORKSHEET

Distribution:
(Original) Medical Record Copy
(Plies 3, 2, & 1) Pharmacy

T-5

Use the following label template to perform this lab if you do not have access to a computer.

```
Hometown Pharmacy, 325 Main St., Shelbyville, TX 72349, phone 321-555-8765

Prescription #:

Patient:

Prescriber:

Prescription:

Quantity:

Directions:

Date Filled:

Refills Remaining:
```

Discussion Questions:

1. What was most the most challenging aspect of this lab for you?

   _____

   _____

   _____

2. Did you enter and fill each prescription accurately? If not, what mistakes did you make, and how can you avoid making such errors in the future?

   _____

   _____

   _____

Student Name: _____

Lab Partner: _____

Grade/Comments: _____

_____

_____

Student Comments: _____

_____

_____

LAB 7-3: Processing a New Medication Order

Objective:

To follow the proper procedure for processing a new medication order.

Pre-Lab Information:

Review Chapter 7, "Health-System Pharmacy," in your textbook.

Explanation:

As a pharmacy technician in a health-system setting, you will need to know the correct procedure for entering a new medication order into the computer.

Activity:

Materials Needed

- Pharmacy computer station
- Prescription
- Printer
- Prescription labels

Procedure

1. Enter the prescription provided below into the pharmacy computer system.
2. Review the information entered for accuracy.
3. Print a prescription label.

If you do not have access to a pharmacy computer system, you can use the blank label that appears at the end of Lab 7-2.

PHYSICIAN'S ORDER WORKSHEET

NOTE: *Person initiating entry should write legibly, date the form using (Mo/Day/Yr.), enter time, sign, and indicate their title.*

USE BALL POINT PEN (PRESS FIRMLY)

10875532   1218 A
Luke, Monica S.
01-15-1955

Dr. W. Huey

Date	Time	Treatment
12/10	6:15	Furosemide 10 mg qd
		②

PHYSICIAN'S ORDER WORKSHEET

Distribution:
(Original) Medical Record Copy
(Plies 3, 2, & 1) Pharmacy

T-5

Discussion Questions:

1. Whom did you list as the prescriber?

   _____

2. Is this prescription to be administered by mouth or intravenously?

   _____

3. What is the brand name of the medication prescribed?

   _____

Optional Activity:

For additional practice, process the prescriptions provided in Activity 7-2, "Medication Order Translation Worksheet."

Student Name: _____

Lab Partner: _____

Grade/Comments: _____

_____

_____

Student Comments: _____

_____

_____

CHAPTER 8
Technology in the Pharmacy

After completing Chapter 8 from the textbook, you should be able to:	Related Activity in the Workbook/Lab Manual
1. List the hardware and software components used in pharmacy computers and summarize their purpose.	Review Questions, PTCB Exam Practice Questions Activity 8-6
2. Describe and discuss the use of automation and robotics in community pharmacies.	Review Questions, PTCB Exam Practice Questions Activity 8-5
3. Describe and discuss the use of automation and robotics in health-system pharmacies.	Review Questions Activity 8-1, Activity 8-5
4. Summarize the uses of personal digital assistants in medicine.	Review Questions, PTCB Exam Practice Questions
5. Define and explain telepharmacy practice.	Review Questions
6. Summarize the impact of patient confidentiality regulations on the use of technology in the pharmacy.	Review Questions

INTRODUCTION

Over the past few decades, technology has revolutionized the practice of pharmacy. Today, virtually every pharmacy uses computers, automated systems, and other technology platforms for its operations and management of pharmaceutical care. Technology is used in both community and health-system pharmacies. As a pharmacy technician, it is important for you to have a basic understanding of the different technologies that are available and being used in pharmacies. These include basic tools, such as computers, printers, modems, and scanners, as well as more advanced tools, such as automatic counters, dispensing systems, bar coding, and even robots. Although you will certainly learn a lot on the job, if you enter the workplace computer literate and familiar with some basic concepts, you will be comfortable managing technological changes as they arise.

REVIEW QUESTIONS

Match the following.

1. _____ hardware
2. _____ hard drive
3. _____ database
4. _____ CPU
5. _____ applications
6. _____ input devices
7. _____ keyboard
8. _____ modem
9. _____ software
10. _____ ROM
11. _____ RAM
12. _____ operating system
13. _____ PDA
14. _____ telepharmacy

a. connects computers via phone lines or cable
b. lists of information ordered in specific ways
c. hardware that allows information to be entered
d. primary software/program of a computer system
e. uses advanced telecommunications technology
f. brain of the computer system
g. permanent memory for essential operations
h. mechanical and electrical components of a computer
i. primary input device of a computer
j. temporary memory used for inputting
k. software/programs that perform specific functions
l. main storage device
m. programs and applications that control computers
n. portable electronic device that operates like a computer

True or False?

15. Electronic counters are a threat to pharmacy technician jobs.

    T   F

16. The FDA mandates that all prescription medications contain a bar code.

    T   F

17. A faxed prescription is considered a legal document in most states.

    T   F

18. Patient profiling is a violation of federal discrimination laws.

    T   F

19. A pharmacist can now utilize a PDA as a mobile reference center.

    T   F

Fill in the blank.

20. Using telecommunications technology, pharmacists can provide care to patients in medically under-served areas at a distance. This is called _____.

PHARMACY CALCULATION PROBLEMS

Calculate the following.

1. A patient's medical order reads: "cefazolin 1 gm IVPB q8hr × 3 days." How many grams of cefazolin will the patient receive in total?

2. A patient is receiving 1,500 mg of vancomycin IVPB daily in three divided doses. How many milligrams will the patient receive in each dose?

3. A technician runs a report and finds that an automated dispensing unit in the ER only has two vials of ondansetron left. The maximum par level for that medication is 20 vials. That item also has a minimum par set of five vials. How many vials should the technician restock?

4. A patient needs 25 mg hydroxyzine IV push. The vial contains 50 mg in each mL. How many milliliters will the patient need?

5. A patient is receiving 100 mL of normal saline IV every hour. How long will a 1,000 mL IV bag last?

PTCB EXAM PRACTICE QUESTIONS

1. What part of a computer is responsible for interpreting commands and running software applications?
   a. JAZ
   b. RAM
   c. CPU
   d. ROM

2. PDAs are used by many healthcare professionals, including pharmacists. In which setting are you most likely to find pharmacists using PDAs?
   a. chain drugstore
   b. independent community pharmacy
   c. health-system pharmacy
   d. mail-order pharmacy

3. Which of the following examples of pharmacy technology has not been associated with improved patient safety?
   a. computerized patient profiles
   b. automated dispensing systems
   c. central processing unit
   d. prescription filling robot

4. What information is contained in the bar code mandated by the FDA?
   a. NDC code
   b. DEA number
   c. Social Security number
   d. AWP

5. Which of the following is considered a hardware output device?
   a. keyboard
   b. mouse
   c. printer
   d. scanner

ACTIVITY 8-1: Case Study—Bar-Coding

Instructions: Read the following scenario and then answer the critical thinking questions.

The University Teaching Hospital is buzzing about its recently purchased new technology, which will help dispense medications for patients. The new equipment that everyone is excited about will bring many conveniences to the facility, including the ability to perform electronic prescribing, which feeds into an automated medication delivery system throughout the hospital system. The system is comprised of numerous 200-draw-type units on each ward, in an area that is easily accessible to healthcare providers and requires bar-coding for medication verification.

From the point of electronic entry, once the pharmacist verifies the medication, the drug can then be withdrawn from a cabinet by healthcare personnel where the patient is located. For example, nurses are able to view and withdraw medications from a current, active medication profile.

On one particular patient's profile, a prescription for aspirin 81 mg has been entered. The patient's nurse is attempting to pull the medication from one such cabinet after it has been verified by the pharmacist. The nurse electronically logs in and looks for the aspirin. It is there, but for some reason is not available for withdrawal. A message pops up on the screen, stating "medication not found"—yet it is right there on the screen. The nurse calls in to the pharmacy and asks for help.

1. Using what you know and can research about bar-coding technology, why might this message appear?

   _____

   _____

   _____

   _____

2. What is a possible reason why the automated medication delivery system is unable to "read" the aspirin prescribed, even after verification and after it appears on the patient profile?

   _____

   _____

   _____

   _____

3. What must be done to make the medication available to the healthcare personnel from the automated medication delivery unit?

_____

_____

_____

ACTIVITY 8-2: Case Study—New Software, Not-So-New Help

Instructions: Read the following scenario and then answer the critical thinking questions.

For years your pharmacy has utilized MBC Data software for processing all its prescriptions. This system has worked flawlessly for the pharmacy as long as the data entered is correct. When the correct NDC number is entered, the prescription is just a few seconds away from being completed and a label printed, complete with auxiliary labels. Billing processes can sometimes be difficult, but overall the software gets the job done.

This is the only system most of your pharmacy staff has ever worked on, and the news that a new software application system is being installed takes them by surprise. In addition to seamless prescription processing and online billing, this new system is supposed to integrate with inventory and has the ability to create numerous valuable reports for management. Despite the apparent advantages, most, but not all, of the staff are upset with this change and actively demonstrate their resistance through actions and words. Regardless, the new system will be in place within two weeks, going live on a Monday.

The training consists of one week in a computer lab where company trainers walk your staff through various prescription scenarios. The company presents you with two user manuals. Three trainers state that they will be present when the system goes live on Monday.

Monday arrives. One trainer makes it in, but is kept busy by the data systems department, so the trainer is deemed unavailable for staff questions. As predicted, there are many problems, as the staff is too unfamiliar with this new system that must get information in certain places in order to work properly. Pandemonium breaks out and the staff becomes extremely frustrated as the day moves on due to the lack of assistance with the new system. Rejections of the new software are adding up.

1. What are some resources you could locate in a scenario such as this?

_____

_____

_____

_____

2. How would you go about calming down your fellow workers so that everyone can concentrate?

_____

_____

_____

_____

3. What person in the pharmacy should be taking the lead here?

_____

_____

_____

_____

ACTIVITY 8-3: Case Study—New Equipment Considerations

Instructions: Read the following scenario and then answer the critical thinking questions.

As a new manager in your pharmacy, you have recently acquired many hats to wear: scheduler, coordinator, trainer, counselor, and committee participant. One of the committees to which you have been assigned is the pharmacy equipment committee. This committee meets annually to evaluate the equipment/supply needs of the pharmacy.

Some of the equipment in your pharmacy is outdated; new models could be very useful. In addition, you have been assigned the task of researching any new equipment that would be beneficial to your pharmacy. Excited, you begin your search.

1. What are some ways you can learn about new or updated equipment that is available?

_____

_____

_____

_____

2. What type of equipment already in your pharmacy would most likely be outdated after one year?

_____

_____

_____

_____

3. Who can you contact to discuss pharmacy equipment?

_____

_____

_____

_____

ACTIVITY 8-4: Case Study—Online Billing

Instructions: Read the following scenario and then answer the critical thinking questions.

Third-party billing is a complicated part of pharmacy. It is not the same for every transaction. Different providers require different methods of data entry.

Both pharmacy technicians in the billing department of your facility are very efficient at what they do. It is said that if anyone can get a bill paid, it is these two pharmacy technicians. Other pharmacy technicians rotate through this billing realm periodically, but these two are the primary billers. No one person knows everything about billing except these two.

During the course of the summer, one of the pharmacy billing technicians goes on maternity leave for at least 12 weeks, leaving the one other expert biller alone. Coincidentally, within weeks the other billing person expert breaks her leg and is placed on medical leave for at least three months. Suddenly, the billing is piling up. Other pharmacy technicians are filling in, but they cannot keep pace with the workload, and there is much information that has not been disseminated.

You look around their work areas and the entire pharmacy, hoping to find something that will give you a clue as to how to perform the billing duties—but you find nothing. What do you do?

1. As you looked around the pharmacy, what did you hope to find to help?

_____

_____

_____

2. What would have been a good resource for this, and who should have provided it?

_____

_____

_____

3. What role do you think the third-party insurers have as far as providing information? What could they provide?

_____

_____

_____

_____

Activity 8-5: Exploring Technology in the Institutional Pharmacy

In a busy institutional pharmacy, it is vital that medications reach the patients as quickly and safely as possible. Modern conveniences such as phones, fax machines, and computerized physician order entry (CPOE) systems are now commonplace, and have increased the daily number of orders a pharmacy can fill. However, newer technology that has slowly been making its way into the pharmacy not only helps the staff process more orders quickly, but also decreases the drug dispensing errors that are far too common. Three different types of technology commonly used in pharmacy practice are the automated dispensing unit, bar-coding technology, and the pneumatic tube system. These three pieces of technology serve different but complementary functions. You may discover that this technology is not really all that new. You may have seen it in places outside the pharmacy in a different shape or form.

The Automated Dispensing Unit:

Automated dispensing units have become very popular in recent years. In the past, most medications for hospital patients had to come directly from the pharmacy. This entailed sending an order to the pharmacy, having the pharmacy input the order into the computer, and then filling the order. After the orders were filled, a pharmacy technician would deliver the medications to the unit on rounds. This process, multiplied hundreds of times over during a day, produced huge workloads and slow turn-around times.

An automated dispensing unit consists of a cabinet containing locked drawers and cabinets, each filled with the medications needed. This advanced computerized "vending machine" is linked to the main computer, which maintains all the patient profiles. When a nurse needs to dispense a medication, she simply enters her user name and password, accesses the patient's profile, and selects the medication that the patient needs. Then, a drawer or cabinet unlocks, and the nurse can retrieve the medication. The patient will simultaneously be billed for this medication. These automated dispensing units can be found in every major unit in the hospital, such as the OR, ER, and medical units. Each one is customized to carry a large percentage of the medications that the specific unit uses most frequently. When an item gets low or runs out, a report is generated (either automatically or manually), and a pharmacy technician is cued to restock the unit.

This system greatly decreases the amount of time it takes for a patient to receive a medication, resulting in greater customer satisfaction. With fewer phone calls and medication requests, the pharmacy can operate with much higher efficiency and pharmacy staff is able to concentrate more on other tasks. Automated dispensing units also decrease the risk of dispensing errors and reduce waste. This is accomplished by stocking the units with unit-dose medications. Unit-dose medications are individually packaged, either by the manufacturer or by the pharmacy. Each dose has all the necessary drug information on each package, such as drug, strength, lot number, expiration date, and manufacturer. Each unit dose also contains a bar code, which will indicate the same information when scanned. The nurse does not open a unit-dose medication until it is to be given to the patient, so there is little wasted medication. In addition, many institutions require the nurse to scan the bar code on the unit-dose medication along with the bar code on the patient's wristband. This practice increases safety by assuring that the right patient is receiving the right medication.

Despite the many advantages of automated dispensing systems, because of the nature of technology, sometimes things do not always work as they should. Pharmacy technicians need to be familiar with this technology, so that they will be better able to respond to unusual situations. For example: Have you ever lost a bag of chips in a vending machine because it was stuck to the coil? You only brought exact change with you, so you left it there, dangling from the coil. Then, the next person who wanted those same chips received two bags, because your bag finally fell down. Similarly, some automated units have small, removable cartridges that can hold 20 or more pills between the coils, like a smaller version of the chip vending machine. Occasionally, one pill will get hung up and will not dispense.

Overall, though, these automated dispensing units are convenient, efficient, and improve patient safety. As a pharmacy technician working at a hospital, you will most likely become familiar with this type of technology and learn how to maintain such units.

Matching Game

Even technology breaks down sometimes. Now that you have read about automated dispensing units, see if you can troubleshoot some common issues listed in Column A by matching them with the (often) simple solutions in Column B. To make this more fun, some of the solutions apply to more than one problem—and some problems have more than one solution!

CHAPTER 8 *Technology in the Pharmacy*

Problem	Solution
1. _____ Biometric (fingerprint) scanner does not work	a. Place the extra tablet back into the dispenser.
2. _____ One of the medication drawers will not open	b. Reboot the system.
3. _____ A nurse requested one tablet for a patient, but the dispenser issued two	c. Hold your finger up to your mouth and lightly breathe on it.
4. _____ While restocking, a technician found that a morphine syringe was stuck in the dispenser	d. Try inserting a long, thin object, like a ruler or a chopstick, in the crack.
5. _____ The keypad and/or the touch-screen is not responding.	e. Clean it off with an alcohol swab, then try again.
	f. Unscrew the dispenser from the unit.

Bar-Coding Technology:

Bar-coding technology has been around for decades. You can find bar codes on almost any product you buy, from food to clothing. Only recently, however, were laws passed requiring bar-code technology to be used in pharmacies. Requiring bar-code scans significantly reduces the possibility of drug errors. In all types of pharmacies, bar codes are found on all medication stock bottles and unit-dose packages. In an institutional pharmacy, every unit dose must have a bar code. If the manufacturer does not make unit-dose forms of a certain drug, the pharmacy does its own repackaging. This includes all dose forms, including oral liquids. Each unit dose, whether manufactured or repackaged by the pharmacy, has to contain a bar code indicating the drug name, strength, lot number, expiration date, and manufacturer. When a technician fills an order for a medication, a hand-held scanner can be used to scan the medication's bar code and the bar code on the patient's order. This assures that the technician has chosen the correct medication for that order. Earlier, it was mentioned that many hospitals also require the nurse to scan both the patient's ID band and the medication to be given, to guarantee that the right patient is receiving the right medication.

Bar-coding does have some minor flaws. When a medication is repackaged in the pharmacy, the technician needs to make sure to enter all the information into the repackaging/unit-dose computer correctly. If any manual overrides are performed, it greatly increases the risk of having a bar code with incorrect information. With bar-coding, the exact product must be chosen. If your usual generic brand of ibuprofen 400 mg tablets is on backorder and the procurement technician ordered a different manufacturer's brand of ibuprofen 400 mg, the bar code will not match the new brand. This is because each manufacturer uses a specific NDC (National Drug Code) number for its product. Another product from another manufacturer has its own NDC number. When this occurs, the existing medication order must be modified or changed, using the new drug or NDC number. Once this is done, the product and new label can be rescanned and will match.

Using a bar-coding system takes a little extra time, but for the most part, implementation of bar-coding is positive as well as mandatory. It significantly reduces errors in the pharmacy and on the nursing units. Because of the accuracy of bar-coding, mistakes can be caught before they ever leave the pharmacy.

Pneumatic Tube Stations:

Whether you realize it or not, you have been exposed to pneumatic tube systems for most of your life. When you use a bank drive-through, most have tube stations installed to assist in sending your transactions. It increases the number of customers they can help during busy times. Many larger hospitals have incorporated complex pneumatic tube systems that can deliver all sorts of things throughout the entire hospital. Most areas have a station from which they can receive and send medication orders, medications, X-rays, supplies, and so on. Each station has an identifying code or "address," so to speak. If you want to send something to the emergency room, you just load the item in the tube, place the tube on its launching pad, and enter in the code for the ER. These tubes or pods are heavy duty, and can withstand a heavy load, such as a one-liter bag of fluid or several piggybacks. Pneumatic tube stations are a convenient way to get something from one end of the building to the other without having to deliver it in person.

Most pharmacy items can be sent via pneumatic tube. However, most institutions have policies and procedures regarding proper use of the tube system and products that should not be tubed. Foam padding is sometimes used to help cushion fragile items during transport. Most institutions require that any sort of liquid IV bag be placed in a zip-lock plastic bag before it is placed into a tube for transport. If for any reason the IV bag breaks, the zip-lock bag will contain the spill inside. A spill that occurs within the pneumatic tube system is expensive to clean up, and the system is difficult to repair. A system that is down for repairs will also contribute to longer wait times for medication.

Policies vary from institution to institution, but most have a list of drugs/products that should not be tubed. Medications with a protein base, such as insulin vials or TPN solutions, should not be tubed. These items are sensitive to shaking, which causes the proteins within the medications to break down. Chemotherapy medications should not be tubed, because of their toxic nature. Items that could easily be broken, like glass evacuated bottles, may also be on the "do not tube" list. Other items that may be excluded from the tube system include: expensive medications, medications that are in limited supply, infected blood samples, carbonated items, and combustible items.

Pneumatic tube stations are just one of many modern conveniences that help improve patient care in hospitals. Many items can be tubed to different locations in much less time than it would take to deliver them by foot. With the implementation of automated dispensing units and bar-code technology, fewer medication errors occur, and patients receive their medications in a timely manner, thus increasing customer satisfaction. These newer technologies have greatly improved workflow in the pharmacy and contributed significantly to better patient care. Technology will continue to play a major role in the pharmacy in years to come.

Critical Thinking Questions:

1. A 200-bed private hospital is considering implementing either automated dispensing units for all of the major areas in the hospital, or a pneumatic tube system. The hospital's budget is small, so it can only afford to install either the dispensing units or the tube system. If you were on the budget committee representing the pharmacy, which system would you choose? Explain your choice.

   _____

   _____

   _____

   _____

2. Do you feel that bar-coding should be mandatory for all pharmacies? Explain your answer.

   _____

   _____

   _____

   _____

3. Can you think of any reasons why you should not tube a drug that is in limited supply? How about a syringe that is worth $12,000?

_____

_____

_____

_____

4. A nurse requested two oxycodone 5 mg tablets for John Jones, but the automated dispensing unit only dispensed one tablet. How do you think this error might affect the inventory count of this medication? How do you think it might affect Mr. Jones's billing account? Without having any experience with these units, can you think of any ways to resolve these issues?

_____

_____

_____

_____

Web Activity:

Go to the following websites to research different automated dispensing units and hospital-grade pneumatic tube systems. Navigate around each site to see the different types of units that are available for hospital use.

www.omnicell.com

www.pyxis.com

www.swisslog.com

www.pevco.com

Activity 8-6: Identifying the Parts of a Computer

You learned about the components of a computer in Chapter 8 of the textbook. Without returning to the textbook, see how much you remember by listing some examples of each of the following computer components.

1. What is hardware?

   Definition: _____

   _____

2. Name three examples of input devices.

   1. _____

   2. _____

   3. _____

3. Name three examples of processing components.

   1. _____

   2. _____

   3. _____

4. Name two examples of output devices.

   1. _____

   2. _____

5. What is software?

   Definition: _____

   _____

6. Name three examples of software you can purchase for your home computer, and briefly describe what each one does.

   1. _____

   2. _____

   3. _____

CHAPTER 9
Inventory Management and Health Insurance Billing

After completing Chapter 9 from the textbook, you should be able to:	Related Activity in the Workbook/Lab Manual
1. List and describe the various purchasing systems used in pharmacies.	Review Questions, PTCB Exam Practice Questions Lab 9-1
2. List and describe the various methods of purchasing available to pharmacies.	Review Questions Lab 9-1
3. Define and describe prescription formularies.	Review Questions Activity 9-4, Lab 9-2
4. Describe and perform the steps necessary for placing orders.	Review Questions, PTCB Exam Practice Questions Activity 9-1, Activity 9-2, Activity 9-3, Lab 9-1
5. Describe and perform the steps necessary for receiving orders.	Review Questions, PTCB Exam Practice Questions Activity 9-2
6. Classify the reasons for product returns and describe the process of making returns.	Review Questions Activity 9-1, Lab 9-3
7. Describe and differentiate Medicare and Medicaid.	Review Questions, PTCB Exam Practice Questions Lab 9-2
8. Recognize and define terms commonly used in insurance billing.	Review Questions, PTCB Exam Practice Questions Lab 9-2
9. Describe and perform the steps in collecting data for insurance purposes.	Review Questions Lab 9-2
10. Describe and perform the steps necessary to transmit a prescription for insurance.	Review Questions Lab 9-2
11. List and explain common insurance billing errors and their solutions.	Review Questions Lab 9-2

INTRODUCTION

Two of the most common duties you will perform as a pharmacy technician are inventory management and processing of third-party, or insurance, billing claims. Both tasks are vitally important to the pharmacy.

A pharmacy cannot dispense prescriptions if the proper medications are not in stock. A pharmacy obtains its inventory through a purchasing system, either as a member of a group purchasing system (GPO) or independently. The inventory is often based on an organization's formulary or the formularies approved by insurance carriers. A pharmacy's inventory must be closely and regularly monitored to ensure that adequate stock is available, to remove expired drugs, and to comply with any product recalls.

To operate effectively, the pharmacy must be reimbursed by insurance carriers in a timely fashion. Insurance billing requires a comprehensive knowledge of billing terms, codes, and policies, such as DAW codes, authorized days supply, and formularies. As a pharmacy technician, you can help prevent many insurance claim rejections by ensuring that all information is correctly entered into the pharmacy's computer system before a claim is submitted.

Although the management of inventory and health insurance billing varies by facility, as a pharmacy technician, you will be available to assist the pharmacist by handling these responsibilities and allowing the pharmacist to focus on more clinical aspects of pharmaceutical care provision.

REVIEW QUESTIONS

Fill in the blanks.

1. A request for reimbursement, from a healthcare provider to an insurance provider, for products or services rendered is known as a/an _____.

2. The portion of the cost of a service or product that a patient pays out of pocket each time the service or product is provided is called the _____.

3. _____ is the notation used by prescribers to instruct the pharmacy to use the exact drug written (usually a brand-name drug).

4. _____ is the number of days a dispensed quantity of medication will last.

5. A set amount that a client pays up front before insurance coverage applies is known as the _____.

6. Drugs that have not been dispensed as of the manufacturer's printed expiration date are classified as _____.

7. _____ are listings of drugs approved for a specific purpose.

8. A _____ is a collective purchasing system in which a pharmacy joins a GPO, which contracts with pharmaceutical manufacturers on behalf of its members.

9. A purchasing system in which the pharmacy is responsible for establishing contracts directly with each pharmaceutical manufacturer is a/an _____.

10. A federally funded, state-administered insurance program for low-income and disadvantaged persons is _____.

11. The federally funded and administered health insurance program is called _____.

12. A company hired by the insurer to process claims is a/an _____.

13. A procedure for obtaining medications, devices, and products for an organization is known as a/an _____.

14. The process through which a drug manufacturer or the FDA requires that specific drugs be returned to the manufacturer because of a specific concern is known as a/an _____.

Choose the best answer.

15. Formularies are used by:
    a. institutional pharmacies.
    b. insurance companies.
    c. ambulatory pharmacies.
    d. all of the above.

16. Inventory should be checked for "outdates":
    a. weekly.
    b. monthly.
    c. yearly.
    d. whenever there is time.

17. OTC products may be recalled by the:
    a. FDA.
    b. DEA.
    c. AFT.
    d. FTC.

18. A preferred provider organization (PPO) differs from a health maintenance organization (HMO) in that:
    a. patients have greater choice in selecting care providers in a PPO.
    b. HMOs are much larger organizations (such as Aetna) and serve more patients.
    c. both HMOs and PPOs are virtually identical in their operations.
    d. HMOs are operated by physicians and PPOs by insurance carriers.

Match the following.

19. _____ Class I Recall   a. someone has or could die from using a drug
20. _____ Class II Recall   b. a drug has been mislabeled or is noncompliant
21. _____ Class III Recall   c. a drug could cause harm, but is not deadly

PHARMACY CALCULATION PROBLEMS

Calculate the following.

1. The pharmacy's automated order system indicates that there are 240 hydrochlorothiazide 25 mg tablets left in inventory. If the system is programmed to reorder when the order point falls below 200, how many bottles of 100 tablets will the system order?

2. The pharmacy's automated order system indicates that there are 7 vials of Humulin R insulin left. How many vials will the system order if the reorder point falls below 10?

3. A small, independent pharmacy has a manual ordering system with maximum/minimum levels (in bottles) written on the shelf under the drug. If the maximum/minimum levels for nabumetone 500 mg are 4/2, and there is one bottle on the shelf, how many bottles should be reordered?

4. A customer is picking up three prescriptions and owes a co-pay of $7.50 on each one. If she hands the pharmacy clerk $30, how much change should the customer receive?

5. A pharmacy is running a special on cold medicines: buy two and get the third for 50% off. If a customer purchases three cold medicines that are all regularly $5.99 each, how much is the total cost to the customer?

PTCB EXAM PRACTICE QUESTIONS

1. A listing of the goods or items that a business will use in its normal operation is called a/an:
   a. purchasing.
   b. inventory.
   c. open formulary.
   d. closed formulary.

2. The goal of inventory management is:
   a. to ensure that drugs are available when they are needed.
   b. to maintain MSDS.
   c. to develop closed formularies.
   d. to increase use of wholesalers.

3. What do we call the minimum and maximum stock levels that are used to determine when to reorder a drug and how much to order?
   a. reorder points
   b. automatic ordering
   c. POS
   d. turnovers

4. What do we call the portion of the price of the medication that the patient is required to pay?
   a. co-insurance
   b. co-pay
   c. maximum allowable cost
   d. usual and customary price

5. Which of the following describes Medicaid?
   a. It is a federal/state program for the needy.
   b. It is a federal program for people over 65 years of age.
   c. It offers a completely open formulary.
   d. It is insurance for people with kidney failure.

ACTIVITY 9-1: Case Study—DEA Forms and Shipment Do Not Match

Instructions: Read the following scenario and then answer the critical thinking questions.

In your pharmacy, controlled medications are ordered by the vault technician. The process specifies that the vault technician fills out the DEA 222 forms and has the head pharmacist sign them. Upon arrival, two people check in the freight, matching up the shipment to the order. For many months, the two who have checked in the freight each time are the exact same pharmacist and pharmacy technician. This is acceptable because they are not the same persons who do the ordering.

One day, the pharmacy technician who checks in orders is absent and you are asked to help receive a shipment. You have the forms, and you and the pharmacist begin opening the totes. You work without incident until you get to the third tote and notice that the red locking tie is not sealed. You point it out to the pharmacist, who brushes it off, stating that it probably got caught on something. The pharmacist is also rushing you along because he has prescriptions to check. Continuing to match up the medications to the order form, you realize that you are short one #30-count bottle of Oxycontin® 10 mg. A recount brings about the same results.

You expect the pharmacist to be concerned, but he is not. He just keeps pushing you to "get on with it" and says that he will figure it out later. You are very uncomfortable with this direction; however, this is your head pharmacist giving the order.

1. What is the right thing to do here?

   _____
   _____
   _____
   _____

2. What are some possible explanations for the one missing bottle?

   _____
   _____
   _____

3. Can and should the ordering/checking-in process be altered to better prevent such situations?

   _____
   _____
   _____

4. Is there any reason why you should not do what the pharmacist directs you to do here?

   _____
   _____
   _____

ACTIVITY 9-2: Case Study—Out-of-Stock Item

Instructions: Read the following scenario and then answer the critical thinking questions.

It is late on a Saturday evening and the rural southwestern hospital where you work is the only medical facility open to the public. A middle-aged female comes into the emergency room after an assault, and the physician on duty prescribes a postexposure prophylaxis (PEP) starter pack. PEP is a course of anti-HIV drugs taken shortly after possible exposure to human immunodeficiency virus (HIV) infection; the pack includes a zidovudine (300 mg) and lamivudine (150 mg) combined tablet plus indinavir 400 mg taken over a specific time period. These medications, when taken shortly after HIV exposure, may help keep the patient from contracting HIV infection.

For some reason, either through poor supply or high demand, you discover that your pharmacy is completely out of indinavir in any dose. You are left with the task of obtaining some as soon as possible. There are only two independent pharmacies in the rural town where the hospital is located, and neither will be open on Sunday, leaving you unable to obtain a supply for at least two days. The nearest town is a two-and-a-half-hour drive away. What do you do?

1. What options do you have for obtaining the medication quickly?

_____

_____

_____

_____

2. Where do you think you can find this medication in the time allowed?

_____

_____

_____

_____

3. Detail how you would go about obtaining this medication, from time of contact to time of possession. How long does it realistically take?

_____

_____

_____

_____

ACTIVITY 9-3: Case Study—Delayed Patient Refill Date

Instructions: Read the following scenario and then answer the critical thinking questions.

Mrs. Walker is a regular customer at your retail pharmacy; today she comes in a little upset. She explains that she requested a refill of her monthly prescription for phenytoin 100 mg earlier in the day and was told that it was "too early" to get a refill. She states she was also told that her medicine could not be refilled for another 12 days, although she has no medicine left. Knowing that the customer/patient cannot go without a dose, you look up her prescription and find that indeed it appears she is not due to get a refill for 12 days.

You ask Mrs. Walker if you could call her after you have had some time to research this and find out what happened. She agrees.

Upon further research, you discover that what happened in this case was that Mrs. Walker did receive her medication on the 12th of last month, but her insurance did not accept the transaction until the 24th of that month. To the brand-new pharmacy technician who processed her prescription that day, this information made it seem that the 24th was the day she actually received it. The same pharmacy technician was the person Mrs. Walker saw earlier, who told her the refill request was too early. You diplomatically explain to Mrs. Walker, in terms she will understand, what has occurred and assure her that you have refilled her medicine.

1. How did you explain to Mrs. Walker, in lay terms, what happened?

_____

_____

_____

_____

2. Do you have a conversation with the pharmacy technician who processed the prescription? If so, what do you say?

_____

_____

_____

_____

3. Is there any way you can evaluate the process and prevent this from happening again, either with this or other future prescriptions? How?

_____

_____

_____

4. Do you think the insurance company has some accountability here?

_____

_____

_____

_____

ACTIVITY 9-4: Drug Formularies

As you learned in Chapter 9 in the textbook, a *drug formulary* is a listing of drugs. HMOs, hospitals, insurance companies, and other healthcare systems use formularies to keep track of what drugs have been approved for use. Some systems have an *open formulary* that allows the purchase of any drug a doctor prescribes. Other systems have *closed formularies* and require a physician to obtain prior approval to prescribe a drug that is not on the formulary. A quick way to get a feeling for formularies is to investigate drugs covered by Medicare Part D.

Activity:

1. Go to the Medicare website (www.medicare.gov) and follow the Formulary Finder link.
2. Choose your state.
3. Add the following drugs to your list:
   - Lipitor
   - Nexium
   - Prevacid
   - Ambien

Questions

1. How many health plans in your state have the drugs you selected on their formularies?

2. Now select one of the health plans whose formulary includes the drugs on your list. List the formulary status of each drug.

   Lipitor _____

   Nexium _____

   Prevacid _____

   Ambien _____

3. Which tier covers nonpreferred brand-name drugs?

   _____

4. Do any of the drugs on your list require prior authorization?

   _____

5. Do any of the drugs on your list have quantity limits?

   _____

6. Do you think drug formularies are a good idea? What are some benefits of using drug formularies (a) to the health plan and (b) to the patient?

   a. _____

   _____

   _____

   b. _____

   _____

   _____

LAB 9-1: Maintaining a Manual Inventory Using Par Levels

Objective:

Practice ordering medications manually using a mock par-level system.

Pre-Lab Information:

Review Chapter 9, "Inventory Management and Health Insurance Billing," in the textbook for an overview of the different types of inventory systems.

Explanation:

Some smaller institutional and retail pharmacies do not have the volume or financial means to implement an automated inventory system. When a point of sale (POS) or other automated inventory system is unavailable, inventory may be maintained through a par-level system. Generally, maximum and minimum par levels are noted on the shelf below each medication, indicating how many bottles, packages, and so forth should be kept on hand.

For example, sertraline 100 mg tablets are ordered in bottles of 100. The maximum/minimum par levels are set to 3/1, indicating that the pharmacy should have three full bottles as maximum inventory, but no less than one full bottle. When the minimum falls below one full bottle (only a partial bottle left), the pharmacy should reorder enough to bring the quantity back up to the maximum par level (three bottles). If inventory is somewhere between one and three bottles, no stock is reordered, as it is in the acceptable par-level range. Depending on the company's reorder policies, this technique could vary (perhaps the facility keeps only a minimum or an ideal par level).

Activity:

In this activity, you will be given information regarding the par levels of certain medications along with the current level of inventory. Based on these quantities, determine whether a product should be reordered and, if so, how many bottles/packages should be reordered.

> ✔ **Tip:** If an item is in the range of the maximum/minimum par level, you do not need to reorder. If an item falls below the recommended minimum par level, you should reorder enough to bring the inventory back up to the maximum level of full bottles/packages.

1. Fluticasone 0.05% nasal spray (each)

   Max/min: 5/2

   On hand: 3

   How many nasal sprays should be reordered? _____

2. Furosemide 40 mg tablets (bottle)

   Max/min: 3/1

   On hand: partial bottle

   How many bottles should be reordered? _____

3. Hydralazine 25 mg tablets (bottle)

   Max/min: 2/1

   On hand: 1 bottle

   How many bottles should be reordered? _____

4. Enoxaparin 30 mg syringes (box)

Max/min: 4/2

On hand: 1 box

How many boxes should be reordered? _____

5. Nifedipine 10 mg capsules (bottle)

Max/min: 4/1

On hand: 1 bottle

How many bottles should be reordered? _____

6. Albuterol 17 g inhalers (each)

Max/min: 12/4

On hand: 2 inhalers

How many inhalers should be reordered? _____

7. Nystatin ointment, 15 g tube (each)

Max/min: 3/1

On hand: 2 tubes

How many tubes should be reordered? _____

8. Clonidine 0.2 mg transdermal patches (box)

Max/min: 5/2

On hand: 2 boxes

How many boxes should be reordered? _____

9. Valacyclovir 500 mg tablets (bottle)

Max/min: 2/1

On hand: partial bottle

How many bottles should be reordered? _____

10. Metoprolol 100 mg tablets (bottle)

Max/min: 3/2

On hand: 1 full bottle and a partial bottle

How many bottles should be reordered? _____

Student Name: _____

Lab Partner: _____

Grade/Comments: _____

_____

_____

Student Comments: _____

_____

_____

LAB 9-2: Insurance Billing

Objective:

Practice looking at insurance information and calculating prices in different insurance situations.

Pre-Lab Information:

Read Chapter 9, "Inventory Management and Health Insurance Billing," in your textbook.

Explanation:

As a pharmacy technician, you will be involved with billing and insurance on a daily basis. It is important for you to understand where to find the information required to bill accurately. It is equally important for you to understand the impact of billing on the pharmacy business. These exercises are designed to help you experience working with this type of information.

Activity:

Review the following three scenarios and answer the associated questions.

Scenario 1

Some insurance companies have contracts with participating pharmacies that include a monthly capitation fee for each patient. This means that the pharmacy gets paid the same amount every month for each patient member of that plan, regardless of the number or cost of prescriptions filled for that patient.

For example, the pharmacy may have two patients with the same HMO for which the monthly capitation fee is $100. That means the pharmacy will receive $100 for each patient. The patients each have a $5.00 co-pay for each prescription filled.

Mr. Smith has three monthly prescriptions that cost $23, $36, and $32. Mrs. Lee has two prescriptions costing $13 and $128. In questions A–H below, calculate the patient's cost as well as the pharmacy's total profit or loss for the two patients.

  A. Mr. Smith's monthly prescription cost: $_____

  B. Mr. Smith's capitation fee + co-pays: $_____

  C. Mrs. Lee's monthly prescription cost: $_____

  D. Mrs. Lee's capitation fee + co-pays: $_____

  E. Pharmacy profit or loss from Mr. Smith's prescriptions: $_____

  F. Pharmacy profit or loss from Mrs. Lee's prescriptions: $_____

  G. Combined profit or loss from both patients: $_____

  H. Did the pharmacy have a profit or a loss? _____

Scenario 2

Mr. Thomas's insurance company reimburses the pharmacy using the formula AWP minus 10% plus a $5.00 dispensing fee. Mr. Thomas pays a $10 co-pay for each prescription. The actual acquisition cost of his medicine is $95 for 100 tablets, and the AWP is $125 for 100 tablets.

In questions A–F below, calculate how much the pharmacy will receive from the insurance company for a 30-day supply if Mr. Thomas takes one tablet bid. Calculate the pharmacy's gross profit for each prescription.

A. Acquisition cost for 60 tablets: $_____

B. AWP for 60 tablets: $_____

C. Insurance reimbursement for 60 tablets: $_____

D. (AWP – 10%): $_____

E. Plus $5.00 dispensing fee = _____ = insurance reimbursement

F. Plus patient's co-pay = $_____

G. Less acquisition cost (from above) = gross profit: $_____

Scenario 3

Consider the following insurance card. Fill in the information for the patient on the attached patient profile. Then, fill in the blanks labeled A–J in the chart.

ACME HMO	Group: 00001681
	Member#: 00004568
	Effective: 01/01/2010
Member: Mary T. Smith	
PCP: James S. Thomas, MD	
Phone#: 321-123-3231	Co-Pays
Network: Mountain Medical Group	RX: Generic $10, Brand $30

Patient Profile

Patient	Address	Phone	D.O.B.	Allergie	Insurance	Plan/Group #	ID #	Co-Pay
Smith, Mary T	11334 Park NY, NY	444-3457	02/01/43	Sulfa	A.	B.	C.	D.

Rx #	Date	Drug	Directions	Quantity	AWP	Prescriber	Charge to Patient
60456	03/15/10	furosemide 40 mg	1 tab PO q.a.m.	30	$1.75	Thomas	E.
60457	03/15/10	Plavix 20 mg	1 tab PO q.a.m.	30	$124.74	Thomas	F.
60458	03/15/10	lisinopril 10 mg	1 tab PO bid	60	$6.45	Thomas	G.
60458	03/15/10	Lantus insulin	10 Units S.CUT. QHS	10 mL	$86.76	Thomas	H.
				TOTAL COST	J.	TOTAL CHARGE	I.

Student Name: _____

Lab Partner: _____

Grade/Comments: _____

_____

_____

Student Comments: _____

_____

_____

LAB 9-3: Drug Recalls

Objective:

To become familiar with the drug recall process.

Pre-Lab Information:

Review the FDA website: http://www.recalls.gov/medicine.html

Explanation:

As a pharmacy technician, you may be involved with a drug recall and have to deal with "pulling" a drug from the shelves and discontinuing dispensing of that drug. This exercise is designed to help you become familiar with the FDA's definitions and processes used when a drug is recalled.

Activity:

Review the following website and read "FDA 101: Product Recalls–From First Alerts to Effectiveness Check": http://www.recalls.gov/medicine.html

Review the following website and answer the questions: http://www.fda.gov/oc/po/firmrecalls/recall_defin.html

1. Define a Class I recall.

   _____
   _____
   _____

2. Define a Class II recall.

   _____
   _____
   _____

3. Define a Class III recall.

   _____
   _____
   _____

4. Define a market withdrawal.

   _____
   _____
   _____

5. Define a medical device safety alert.

   _____
   _____
   _____

Student Name: _____

Lab Partner: _____

Grade/Comments: _____

_____

_____

Student Comments: _____

_____

_____

CHAPTER 10
Introduction to Compounding

After completing Chapter 10 from the textbook, you should be able to:	Related Activity in the Workbook/Lab Manual
1. Explain the purpose and reason for compounding prescriptions.	Review Questions
2. Discuss the basic procedures involved in compounding.	Review Questions, PTCB Exam Practice Questions Lab 10-1, Lab 10-2, Lab 10-3
3. List and describe the equipment, supplies, and facilities required for compounding.	Review Questions, PTCB Exam Practice Questions Activity 10-2, Lab 10-1, Lab 10-2, Lab 10-3
4. List the major dosage forms used in compounding.	Review Questions, PTCB Exam Practice Questions Activity 10-2, Lab 10-3
5. Discuss the considerations involved in flavoring a compounded prescription.	Review Questions, PTCB Exam Practice Questions Activity 10-2

INTRODUCTION

Pharmaceutical *compounding* is the practice of extemporaneously preparing medications to meet the unique need of an individual patient according to the specific order of a physician or prescriber. Compounded medications may be either sterile or nonsterile and include suspensions, capsules, suppositories, topically applied medications, intravenous admixtures, and parenteral nutrition solutions.

Extemporaneous compounding is a special service provided by a number of community-based pharmacies. To assist the pharmacist in compounding medications, you will require additional training, skills, and practice. However, this unique area of pharmacy practice offers a number of advanced professional opportunities for those who pursue these skills.

REVIEW QUESTIONS

Match the following.

1. _____ comminuting
2. _____ compounding
3. _____ emulsion
4. _____ excipient
5. _____ geometric dilution
6. _____ suspension
7. _____ titration

a. contains nonsoluble ingredients

b. another word for titration

c. contains two unmixable liquids

d. substance added to make suitable consistency

e. reducing particle size by grinding

f. starts with smallest ingredient

g. extemporaneously preparing medication to meet needs of individual patients

Choose the best answer.

8. Which of the following is not a compounding resource?
   a. *United States Pharmacopoeia*
   b. Merck book of brand and generic drugs
   c. *Veterinary Drug Handbook*
   d. *Remington's Pharmaceutical Sciences*

9. Which of the following compounding steps should be completed before the others?
   a. Collect all necessary ingredients.
   b. Write up a compounding worksheet.
   c. Weigh each ingredient.
   d. Follow the formula.

10. Which of the following is more appropriate for melting bases?
    a. magnetic stir plate
    b. heat gun
    c. hotplate
    d. electronic mortar and pestle

11. When using geometric dilution, one should start with the:
    a. ingredient needed in the smallest amount.
    b. ingredient needed in the largest amount.
    c. equal amounts of each ingredient.
    d. the liquid or binding base.

12. Assuming that only the following dosage forms were suitable, which is the desirable choice for animal patients?
    a. cream
    b. ointment
    c. transdermal gel
    d. injection

Match the following.

13. _____ capsule
14. _____ emulsion
15. _____ stick
16. _____ troche
17. _____ cream
18. _____ suspension
19. _____ paste
20. _____ ointment

a. topical application of anesthetics or antivirals

b. dissipates into the skin when applied

c. liquid preparation that contains insolubles

d. oral dosage form used for more than 100 years

e. oral form that disintegrates over time

f. liquid/semisolid form that can be taken orally or applied topically

g. stiff, viscous ointment

h. semisolid preparation that stays on top of skin

True or False?

21. Otic preparations may be used ophthalmically.

    T   F

22. The most common form of compounded transdermal gel therapy is a two-phase vehicle made from pluronic lecithin organogel.

    T   F

23. Using the proper coloring and flavoring in medications is important for patient compliance.

    T   F

24. One of the five basic flavoring techniques is physiological.

    T   F

25. Aseptic, or sterile, technique should be used in all compounding.

    T   F

PHARMACY CALCULATION PROBLEMS

Calculate the following.

1. Tom is compounding a prescription that calls for 15 g betamethasone 0.05% cream, 15 g diphenhydramine cream, then qsad 60 g with aquaphilic ointment. How much aquaphilic ointment will he need to add to this compound?

2. A prescription was brought to the pharmacy for a product that is not commercially available. It calls for clindamycin 4,500 mg qsad 120 mL with lubricating lotion. If the clindamycin is available in 300 mg capsules, how many capsules should be opened for use in this compound?

3. How many sucralfate 1 g tablets will you need for an oral suspension that calls for 20 g sucralfate as the active ingredient?

4. A pharmacy received a faxed order from a veterinarian for celecoxib 25 mg chicken dog treats, #100. If the celecoxib comes in 100 mg capsules, how many capsules should be mixed in the chicken base to make 100 treats?

5. A special compound requires equal parts zinc oxide 20% ointment, nystatin ointment, and hydrocortisone 0.5% ointment. If the prescription calls for 60 grams, how many grams of each ointment will be needed?

PTCB EXAM PRACTICE QUESTIONS

1. A two-phase system consisting of a finely divided solid dispersed in a liquid is a/an:
   a. suspension.
   b. emulsion.
   c. solution.
   d. trituration.

2. What is the on-demand preparation of a drug product according to a physician's prescription?
   a. IVPB
   b. extemporaneous compounding
   c. trituration
   d. spatulation

3. The fine grinding of a powder is called:
   a. extemporaneous compounding.
   b. suspension.
   c. emulsion.
   d. trituration.

4. Clear liquids in which the drug is completely dissolved are called:
   a. sublimations.
   b. suspensions.
   c. solutions.
   d. emulsions.

5. A system containing two immiscible liquids with one dispersed in the other is called a/an:
   a. emulsion.
   b. suspension.
   c. syrup.
   d. solution.

ACTIVITY 10-1: Case Study—Compounded Laser Gel

Instructions: Read the following scenario and then answer the critical thinking questions.

Note: Based partly on an actual event.

A 22-year-old college student decides she would like to use laser treatment to remove the hair from her legs. She hears that the benefits of laser treatment include a much longer time for hair to grow back. The negative, however, is that it can be a painful procedure. She finds a local "medical spa" that performs this procedure. The spa provides her with two tubes of anesthetic gel to apply just before her procedure; the gel was compounded in an outside compounding pharmacy. She is also told to wrap her legs in cellophane for better absorption. She is told that it is a numbing gel, but receives no counseling or patient information sheet about the product.

She applies the gel and cellophane wrap in anticipation of her appointment. As she is driving down the road, she begins to feel dizzy and pulls over. When she is found, she is unconscious and convulsing; she then goes into a coma.

The numbing product she received was called Laser Gel 10-10 and consisted of 10 percent lidocaine and 10 percent tetracaine with phenylephrine. After much media attention, several other cases are discovered in which people have gone into comas after using the anesthetic gel.

The spa's lawyer said the spa owners never knew that a prescription was needed for the gel, and they thought it was a safe and approved product. So did the 22-year-old college student.

1. In this case, from the information you have, what key elements are absent from the staff persons' knowledge about the gel?

_____

_____

_____

_____

2. Should the patient have questioned the product, or do you feel the responsibility lies with the medical spa?

_____

_____

_____

_____

3. What disciplinary measures, if any, do you think should be levied against the medical spa in this case? Against the compounding pharmacy?

_____

_____

_____

_____

ACTIVITY 10-2: Case Study—Veterinary

Instructions: Read the following scenario and then answer the critical thinking questions.

The veterinary compounding pharmacy where you work consists of three pharmacist/pharmacy technician teams. Pharmacists help with dosing for the patients while pharmacy technicians prepare the formulations and perform administrative tasks. It is an optimum arrangement in which both staff members can practice their skills. This pharmacy also encourages and provides yearly training to update skills and learn new information. It does this through seminars, videos, and the purchase of materials such as books.

Calculations must be done for proper dosing and various drug forms may have to be created for better acceptance from the animal patients. Compounding for animals is a specialty area and can sometimes require some creativity. For example, when a dog will not swallow a necessary medicine, a flavoring might be added to help make it more palatable. Your team has been assigned a few cases today, each of which requires you to call upon your creativity:

- An elephant has recently had major eye surgery and has not eaten for days afterward. Elephants are notorious for not accepting oral medications. The elephant has been prescribed a sterile ophthalmic solution that must be compounded to acquire the correct dose. After consulting with the pharmacist, you now have a "recipe" or SOP to compound. However, you are told that elephants dislike having their eyes manipulated and will do anything to prevent access.

- A horse with equine Cushing's syndrome is prescribed pergolide mesylate and you are told that the horse can accept oral medications.

- A cat with leukemia has been prescribed chlorambucil. Although the cat can take medications orally, the owner has tried numerous times and failed to administer them successfully.

1. Can you think of a way to access the elephant's eye to administer the medication without touching any of the eye area?

   _____

   _____

   _____

   _____

2. What oral drug forms could be used to compound the pergolide medication for administration to the horse?

   _____

   _____

   _____

   _____

3. Can you think of anything to do to the cat's medication to help the cat accept it?

   _____

   _____

   _____

   _____

ACTIVITY 10-3: Case Study—Childproof Containers

Instructions: Read the following scenario and then answer the critical thinking questions.

Mrs. Gaynor has been on estrogen therapy for a short time now and is beginning to feel much better. Her premenopausal hot flashes and night sweats have subsided. She receives an 8 oz. jar of a custom-compounded estrogen cream made specifically for her. She uses it daily and keeps the jar under a sink in the bathroom.

While her prepubescent grandson is visiting, he becomes curious and applies some of the cream. He thinks it must be something special because of the claims made on the jar about feeling much better. The grandson continues to do this, without anyone's knowledge, as he visits on a weekly basis. Meanwhile, Mrs. Gaynor is receiving more frequent refills through the compounding pharmacy.

Soon the grandson develops gynecomastia (the development of abnormally large mammary glands that can sometimes secrete milk). A doctor's visit confirms that the grandson has been exposed to large amounts of estrogen and enlists the family's help in finding the source.

1. What steps could the compounding pharmacy take to help prevent this situation?

   _____

   _____

   _____

   _____

© 2009 Pearson Education, Inc.

2. What steps could the grandmother take to help prevent easy access by the grandson?

_____

_____

_____

_____

3. From the information provided, what signs or "flags" were present to indicate that there might be a problem?

_____

_____

_____

_____

LAB 10-1: Measuring Liquids Accurately

Objective:

Gain experience in measuring liquids using graduated cylinders.

Pre-Lab Information:

- Review Chapter 10 in the textbook and visit http://pharmlabs.unc.edu/
- Gather the following materials:
  - 20, 50, and 100 mL graduated cylinders
  - chilled grape juice
  - chilled cranberry juice
  - chilled apple juice
  - paper cups to contain the liquid "medication"

Explanation:

This exercise gives you the opportunity to experience measuring liquids. You must be careful when pouring liquid medications, and it takes practice to accurately find the meniscus.

Activity:

Using the materials listed previously, prepare the following "prescriptions" for "dispensing":

1. apple juice 30 mL
   cranberry juice 20 mL
   grape juice 50 mL
   Sig: Mix together and enjoy UD

2. grape juice 55 mL
   apple juice 35 mL
   cranberry juice 80 mL
   Sig: Mix together and enjoy UD

Student Name: _____

Lab Partner: _____

Grade/Comments: _____

_____

_____

Student Comments: _____

_____

_____

LAB 10-2: Using the Prescription Balance

Objective:

Review use of the prescription balance, including taring the balance and using weights.

Pre-Lab Information:

- Review Chapter 10 in your textbook.
- Gather the following materials:
  - prescription torsion balance
  - prescription weights
  - weighing papers or boats
  - spatula
  - powder to weigh (could be flour, cake mix, or other kitchen ingredient)

Explanation:

Extemporaneous compounding has become increasingly important. Accurate use of the prescription balance is a vitally important aspect of compounding. The following exercise will help you develop a basic understanding of the process.

Activity:

Using the materials listed previously, weigh out 6.5 grams of the powder.

Steps

1. Place the balance on a clean, flat surface away from moving air (windows, doors, etc.).
2. Check the balance pans for any residue left from previous use.
3. Move the calibration dial to zero.
4. Place a weighing boat or paper in the center of each pan.
5. Unlock the arrest knob and check that the balance is level.
6. If the pointer is not in the center, carefully rotate the leveling screws to bring the pointer to a level position. Lock the arrest knob.
7. Move the calibration dial to the 0.5 g mark.
8. Using tweezers, add a 5 g and 1 g weight to the boat or paper on the *right side* of the balance.
9. With the arrest knob still in the locked position, add a small amount of powder to the weighing boat on the *left side* of the balance.
10. Unlock the arrest knob and observe the balance pointer to see if the amount of powder added was too much or too little.
11. If the pointer rests to the left of the index center, you have added too much powder. If the pointer is to the right of the center, you have added too little powder.
12. Lock the arrest knob before adding or removing powder. When the pointer is near equilibrium, it will move back and forth within the index. At this point, you may leave the knob unlocked and add very small amounts of powder by placing a small amount of powder on the spatula and gently tapping the spatula.
13. Lock the arrest knob and remove the weighing boat or paper with the powder on it.

Questions

1. Why do you think it is necessary to use weigh boats or paper?

   _____

   _____

   _____

2. Why do you need to adjust the balance after a weigh boat has been placed on each pan?

   _____

   _____

   _____

3. Why is it a good idea to lock the pans in place before adding or removing weight from either pan?

   _____

   _____

   _____

Student Name: _____

Lab Partner: _____

Grade/Comments: _____

_____

_____

Student Comments: _____

_____

_____

LAB 10-3: Compounding Exercise—Capsules

Objective:

To give you experience in filling capsules using the punch method.

Pre-Lab Information:

- Review Chapter 10 in your textbook.
- Gather the following materials:
  - prescription torsion balance
  - prescription weights
  - weighing papers or boats
  - spatula
  - powder to weigh (could be flour, cake mix, or other kitchen ingredient)
  - gelatin capsules, size 0
  - ointment slab
  - powder paper or wax paper
  - nonsterile gloves

Explanation:

As a pharmacy technician, you should be familiar with the punch-filling of capsules to deliver custom-compounded medications to patients. This exercise is designed to give you practical experience with filling capsules.

Activity:

Using the materials outlined previously, follow these steps:

1. Using the steps from Lab 10-2, place the powder on the ointment slab that has been covered with powder paper or wax paper.
2. Using a spatula, form a smooth block that is about half the length of the capsule body.
3. Wearing gloves to prevent hand contact, separate 5 capsules and place them in an empty weighing boat.
4. Begin "punching" the capsules by taking the body of a capsule and holding it in an upright position. Punch the open end repeatedly into the powder until the capsule is full.
5. Replace the capsule cap and weigh each capsule, using an empty capsule on the other pan of the balance. Each capsule should weigh 500 mg; each must be between 90% and 110% of 500 mg.
6. Clean the capsules with a soft tissue and place them in an appropriate container.

Student Name: _____

Lab Partner: _____

Grade/Comments: _____

_____

_____

Student Comments: _____

_____

_____

CHAPTER 11
Introduction to Sterile Products

After completing Chapter 11 from the textbook, you should be able to:	Related Activity in the Workbook/Lab Manual
1. List the equipment and supplies used in preparing sterile products.	Review Questions, PTCB Exam Practice Questions Activity 11-1, Activity 11-2, Activity 11-3, Activity 11-4, Lab 11-1, Lab 11-2, Lab 11-3, Lab 11-4, Lab 11-5, Lab 11-6
2. List the routes of administration associated with sterile products.	Review Questions, PTCB Exam Practice Questions Activity 11-1, Activity 11-2, Activity 11-3, Activity 11-4, Lab 11-4, Lab 11-5, Lab 11-6
3. Discuss special concerns regarding chemotherapy and cytotoxic drugs.	Review Questions, PTCB Exam Practice Questions Activity 11-5

INTRODUCTION

Sterile compounding is the preparation of compounded medications using aseptic technique, or the process of performing a procedure under controlled conditions in a manner that minimizes the chance of contamination of the preparation. Following proper aseptic techniques ensures that all compounded products remain free of bacteria, fungi, pyrogens, infectives, and other microorganisms. To ensure sterility, these products are prepared in laminar flow hoods, including horizontal flow hoods and biological safety cabinets, which contain a high-efficiency particulate air (HEPA) filter.

Patients generally receive sterile products parenterally through various administration sites, such as veins (IV) and muscle tissue (IM). Other sterile products include total parenteral nutrition (TPNs), as well as ophthalmic and otic preparations.

Sterile product preparation can be a complex, high-risk process in the healthcare setting. As a pharmacy technician with proper training, you can play an integral role in the procurement, storage, preparation, and distribution of sterile products.

REVIEW QUESTIONS

Match the following.

1. _____ antineoplastics
2. _____ intradermal
3. _____ infusion
4. _____ pH
5. _____ buffer capacity
6. _____ intramuscular
7. _____ isotonicity
8. _____ precipitate
9. _____ intrathecal

a. a larger volume of solution given at a steady rate
b. injection into a muscle
c. the same tonicity as red blood cells
d. injection into the spine
e. medications to treat cancer
f. injection into the skin
g. solid that forms in a solution
h. ability of a solution to resist a change in pH
i. the degree of acidity

Choose the best answer.

10. A bevel is:
    a. an angle cut to measure cc/mL.
    b. a rounded-edge needle.
    c. the sharp pointed end of a needle.
    d. the only part of a needle that can be touched.

11. Medication used to treat cancer is called:
    a. antitoxin.
    b. chemotherapy.
    c. radiation.
    d. cytoblast.

12. Class 100 environment is:
    a. a classification of airflow units.
    b. a dimensional measurement of the floor plan.
    c. an airflow of 100 psi.
    d. the best level of sterility available.

13. HEPA refers to:
    a. patient privacy rights.
    b. a large insurance group.
    c. a type of air filter.
    d. the government group that inspects air filters.

Identify and indicate the parts of a needle.

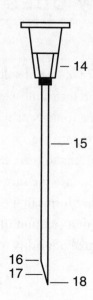

14. _____
15. _____
16. _____
17. _____
18. _____

Identify and indicate the parts of a syringe.

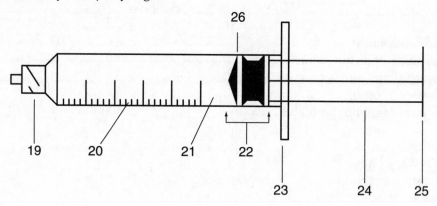

19. _____
20. _____
21. _____
22. _____
23. _____
24. _____
25. _____
26. _____

Identify and indicate the parts of an IV bag system.

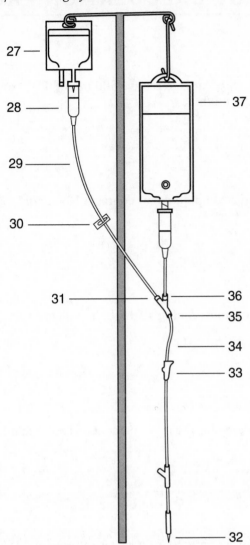

27. _____

28. _____

29. _____

30. _____

31. _____

32. _____

33. _____

34. _____

35. _____

36. _____

37. _____

CHAPTER 11 *Introduction to Sterile Products*   **153**

PHARMACY CALCULATION PROBLEMS

Calculate the following.

1. A medical order states that a patient is to receive 500 mL of 0.9% sodium chloride IV over 2 hours. How fast is the IV running in mL/hr?

2. A technician prepares a sterile compound that contains 100 mg/mL of active drug. How many mL are required for a dose of 800 mg?

3. If a bulk bottle of IV multivitamins contains 50 mL, how many 10 mL doses can be obtained from the bottle?

4. After reconstitution, ceftriaxone for IM injection contains 350 mg/mL. How many milligrams are in 2.5 milliliters?

5. A 1,000 mL bag of 5% dextrose with 20 mEq KCl is infusing at 125 mL/hr. How many hours will the bag last before it must be replaced?

PTCB EXAM PRACTICE QUESTIONS

1. When using a horizontal laminar airflow hood, how far should the technician work inside the hood?
   a. at least two inches
   b. at least four inches
   c. at least six inches
   d. at least eight inches

2. In a laminar airflow hood, the air flows in how many direction(s)?
   a. four
   b. three
   c. two
   d. one

3. In horizontal laminar airflow hoods, the air blows in which direction?
   a. down toward the work area
   b. away from the operator
   c. toward the operator
   d. up toward the HEPA filter

4. Large-volume parenterals (LVPs) usually have what kind of infusion rates?
   a. intermittent
   b. rapid
   c. slow
   d. instantaneous

5. Vertical airflow hoods have what characteristic?
   a. vertical airflow down toward the product
   b. horizontal airflow away from the operator
   c. vertical airflow up toward the HEPA filter
   d. horizontal airflow toward the operator

ACTIVITY 11-1: Case Study—USP 797 and Training Personnel

Instructions: Read the following scenario and then answer the critical thinking questions.

All the sterile compounding areas in your facility have recently finalized plans to bring them up to USP 797 standards in the pending remodel. The rooms are constructed according to the guidelines and you have been placed in charge of providing training to the certified pharmacy technicians who will be preparing sterile products in this area.

Your manager tells you that there are some training supplies left over in the pharmacy storage area and that you are welcome to look through it to find anything you could use. The manager also states that a pharmacist will be available for any questions you may have.

While searching through the storage area, you find a written manual 755 pages thick that appears to encompass numerous sterile preparation products. Continuing your search, you also find a sterile preparation workbook; however, it does not relate to the written manual you already found. You also discover a video that you viewed yourself when you were hired about nine years ago. A box of leftover products contains various syringes, IV bags, packages, needles, dispensing pins, and gloves. You also find a dusty poster illustrating the steps for proper handwashing techniques when preparing to compound a cream.

1. Which of the items found in the storage room do you think you could use for the current training?
   _____
   _____
   _____
   _____

2. Why did you choose to use or not use each item?
   _____
   _____
   _____
   _____

3. What are the basic requirements for training personnel in sterile preparation, according to USP 797? Do you think these requirements are realistic?
   _____
   _____
   _____
   _____

4. What are the barriers to USP 797 compliance in this scenario?

_____

_____

_____

_____

ACTIVITY 11-2: Case Study—IV Pump Machine and Shortcuts

Instructions: Read the following scenario and then answer the critical thinking questions.

Your 200-bed hospital incorporates automated sterile preparation pumps to help mix the large number of IV orders that arrive in your pharmacy each day. It is a very efficient system, which helps reduce errors, increases accuracy, and reduces time of preparation. Four pharmacy technicians are quite skilled at using these pumps, including for complicated orders such as the total parenteral nutrition (TPN) orders. Good aseptic technique is used in a USP 797-compliant sterile compounding area.

The process is simple: Pharmacy technicians prepare all the IVs according to the times they are due, then pharmacists check off the preparations when they are all finished. This is a round-the-clock operation broken up into eight-hour sections.

Time is of the essence for the new orders that arrive all day long. The same person must process these immediate requests along with the 24-hour IV orders. It can be quite hectic at times, and the staff is always looking for better ways to do things.

One such person is the pharmacy technician who is processing the TPNs for the day. The procedures clearly state that all the ingredients can be mixed through the machine with the exception of the potassium chloride. This must be added last, through a syringe, once the bag is detached from the automated sterile preparation pump.

To cut corners on a particularly busy day, the pharmacy technician decides to add the potassium chloride through the pump. The technician feels that this is acceptable because he is right there to watch and make sure the correct amount is added.

1. Why do you think the potassium chloride is not to be pumped along with the other ingredients?

_____

_____

_____

2. Is it acceptable for the pharmacy technician to add the potassium chloride to the pump as long as he is standing right there?

_____

_____

_____

_____

3. Since the pharmacists check off the final product, are they at all liable for the shortcuts that the pharmacy technician took to make the TPN?

_____

_____

_____

_____

ACTIVITY 11-3: Case Study—IV Education and Skills

Instructions: Read the following scenario and then answer the critical thinking questions.

The IV pharmacy technicians at University Hospital where you work are at different levels of skill and experience in this area. All are learning, and the hospital provides ongoing training. Most of you take this position seriously, but unfortunately there are some who do not.

The majority of the IV staff follows the guidelines and utilizes resources provided by the pharmacy for the sterile preparations that come their way. Everything from small-volume reconstitution, piggybacks, and large-volume IVs are prepared by this staff. Different drugs require specific diluents based on compatibility, stability, and other factors.

As most of the IV pharmacy technicians have progressed in their skill, they also have helped other IV staff learn as well. They all realize that some people take a little longer than others to grasp ideas and sometimes need extra assistance—but how long is too long? For about six months now, most of the IV pharmacy technicians have used the resources mentioned. However, three continue to ask the same questions repeatedly without attempting to apply what they have learned.

1. What pharmacy resources might be available to the IV pharmacy technicians to assist them with preparation and drug knowledge?

_____

_____

_____

_____

2. What are the benefits of these resources?

_____

_____

_____

_____

3. How often do you think education and/or training should take place for IV pharmacy technicians? What medium or media would be good to utilize?

_____

_____

_____

_____

4. How would you address the problem with the IV pharmacy technicians who seem apathetic?

_____

_____

_____

_____

ACTIVITY 11-4: Case Study—Identifying Errors in Aseptic Technique

Read the following scenario and identify at least 10 aseptic errors that the pharmacy technician made. Describe ways to improve her technique.

As a student, you are assigned to observe the aseptic technique of the IV room technician. Mindy is scheduled to work in the IV room this morning, but she stayed up too late the night before and had to rush to get to work on time. Before leaving home, she quickly put on some makeup to cover up the circles under her eyes. After punching in late, she began by washing her hands for 10 seconds, missing the dirt she had under her fingernails. After drying her hands with a paper towel, she threw the towel away and then shut off the faucet with her right hand. Next, she put on her gloves, a face mask, and a gown.

Once gowned, Mindy began cleaning the laminar airflow hood with blue window cleaner, using paper towels. She randomly wiped down the hood in circular patterns, and then began preparations for compounding some IV orders. She piled several syringes and needles in the hood, as well as several vials of various medications for the prescriptions that had to be prepared.

At this point, Mindy told you she needed a cup of coffee to perk herself up, so she excused herself to grab some coffee in the break area. A few minutes later, she returned to the clean room with the coffee. She resumed preparing the IVs, selecting several small-volume bags that she would need for the medications. She put those in the hood next to the syringes and began removing the caps to the vials. She assembled a needle and syringe, pulled out the appropriate volume from one of the vials, and immediately injected it into a small-volume bag. It was at this point that you recognized she would need more aseptic training.

Critical Thinking Questions:

1. List at least 10 aseptic errors made in this scenario, then describe the correct solutions to the errors.

   Mistake 1: _____

   Correct Procedure: _____

   _____

   _____

   _____

   Mistake 2: _____

   Correct Procedure: _____

   _____

   _____

Mistake 3: _____
Correct Procedure: _____
_____
_____
_____

Mistake 4: _____
Correct Procedure: _____
_____
_____
_____

Mistake 5: _____
Correct Procedure: _____
_____
_____
_____

Mistake 6: _____
Correct Procedure: _____
_____
_____
_____

Mistake 7: _____
Correct Procedure: _____
_____
_____
_____

Mistake 8: _____
Correct Procedure: _____
_____
_____
_____

Mistake 9: _____
Correct Procedure: _____
_____
_____
_____

Mistake 10: _____

Correct Procedure: _____

_____

_____

_____

2. How could this pharmacy technician's negligent technique result in serious harm to a patient?

_____

_____

_____

_____

_____

ACTIVITY 11-5: Hazardous Drugs

As you learned in Chapter 11 in your textbook, healthcare personnel who work with chemotherapy and cytotoxic drugs face damage to their own health unless they take precautions to protect themselves.

Part One

Find out more about hazardous drugs by discovering what some of the key terms mean. Use your text, a medical dictionary, or a reliable online resource to help you define the following terms.

antineoplastic

_____

_____

cytotoxic

_____

_____

genotoxicity

_____

_____

carcinogenicity

_____

_____

teratogenicity

_____

_____

Part Two

Visit the OSHA website (http://www.osha.gov/dts/osta/otm/otm_vi/otm_vi_2.html) and locate the OSHA Technical Manual, Section VI: Chapter 2. Then answer the following questions.

1. What are some examples of activities in the pharmacy that might cause splattering, spraying, or aerosolization of hazardous materials?

   _____

   _____

   _____

   _____

2. What does the abbreviation HD mean?

   _____

   _____

   _____

   _____

3. Why are horizontal airflow hoods not used or recommended for use when preparing HDs?

   _____

   _____

   _____

   _____

4. To prevent exposure of personnel who are working with HDs, what does OSHA require that every facility have on hand?

   _____

   _____

   _____

   _____

LAB 11-1: Proper Hand Hygiene and Aseptic Gowning

Objectives:

Demonstrate the proper techniques for handwashing and aseptic gowning.

Explain why hand hygiene is a key component of aseptic technique.

Pre-Lab Information:

- Review Chapter 11 in your textbook.
- Go to www.usp.org and search for "General Chapter 797." You will find a document that explains all of the latest national guidelines for preparing sterile products. This bulletin is related to pharmaceutical compounding and sterile preparations and has specific information under "Personal Cleansing and Garbing."
- Gather the following materials:
  - germicidal, microbial soap such as Hibiclens or chlorohexidene
  - lint-free paper towels or gauze
  - lint-free gowns, head/hair covers, shoe covers, gloves, and face masks

Explanation:

Proper hand hygiene and aseptic garbing are essential for maintaining cleanliness and sterility while preparing IV and other sterile medications in a clean room. All surfaces of our bodies have bacteria on them, called *normal bacterial flora,* which are harmless if we are healthy. However, patients who are ill or whose immune systems are not working properly (immunocompromised) can be harmed by these normal bacteria. Washing your hands with a germicidal, microbial soap before entering the clean room, and after eating, performing personal hygiene, or doing anything that could cause contamination, is critical to maintaining asepsis.

When working in a sterile preparation area, you also need to wear the proper attire to maintain asepsis. At the minimum, this means clean hospital scrubs or surgical gowns, regardless of whether you are working under the hood or checking IVs. Proper garb also includes disposable hair and shoe covers, masks, and gloves. You will not necessarily need to wear all of these items every time. Your facility will have guidelines on what should be worn and when.

Activity:

Part 1

Review the information from the USP website, then answer the following questions.

1. Chapter 797 suggests that handwashing should be done for how many seconds?

   _____

   _____

2. Describe the hand hygiene techniques discussed in the Chapter 797 bulletin.

_____

_____

_____

_____

_____

_____

3. Describe the order in which you should don your sterile garb and perform hand hygiene before working with sterile products.

_____

_____

_____

_____

4. What should you do if you accidentally touch your face after you have already cleansed yourself and dressed aseptically?

_____

_____

_____

_____

5. Describe the exiting or degarbing procedure when leaving the compounding area for the day.

_____

_____

_____

_____

6. Although Chapter 797 does not address this issue specifically, you should be able to apply its principles: After you wash your hands thoroughly, what do you feel would be the best method for turning off the faucet without risking recontamination?

_____

_____

_____

_____

Part 2

Now that you have reviewed the techniques for hand hygiene and gowning and degowning, it is time to practice each technique. Practice first with a lab partner. When you are ready, ask your instructor to observe.

Student Name: _____

Lab Partner: _____

Grade/Comments: _____

_____

_____

Student Comments: _____

_____

_____

LAB 11-2: The Horizontal Laminar Airflow Hood

Objective:

Review the technique involved in using a horizontal laminar airflow hood.

Pre-Lab Information:

• Read Chapter 11, "Introduction to Sterile Products," in your textbook.

• Visit the website http://www.globalrph.com/aseptic.htm

Explanation:

Nonhazardous sterile products are compounded inside a horizontal laminar airflow hood (LAH). The LAH contains a prefilter in the front of the hood that removes large contaminants from the air inside the room. After the air has been filtered by the prefilter, it travels to the back of the LAH, where it is filtered next by the HEPA filter. This removes particles that are 2 microns or larger (the size of most bacteria, fungi, and viruses). The filtered air is then blown back to the front of the hood. The LAH also maintains a constant airflow out of the hood which prevents the entry of contaminants. The hood must be turned on 30 minutes in advance of use in aseptic compounding.

If you perform aseptic compounding as a pharmacy technician, you must know how to clean and disinfect the LAH properly. At a minimum, the hood must be cleaned every eight hours, or sooner if it becomes dirty. To prevent cross-contamination of products, always wipe down the hood if you have finished compounding one product and need to switch to another.

Here are the steps for cleaning a LAH:

1. Turn on the LAH and allow the blower to run for 30 minutes.
2. Follow proper hand washing procedure and technique and wear appropriate apparel. Keep your head on the outside of the hood to prevent contamination.
3. Wash the entire hood—all walls and surfaces—with sterile water to remove salt, starch, sugars, and/or proteins. Soak stubborn spots for 5 to 10 minutes, then wipe clean.
4. To disinfect, wipe all surfaces of the hood with 70% isopropyl alcohol, using a lint-free fabric such as special paper towels or gauze. Never use regular paper towels, as they produce lint and create particulates.
5. Clean the IV pole first, if applicable.
6. Second, clean the sides of the LAH, starting at the top and working side-to-side with overlapping strokes. Alternatively, the sides of the hood can be cleaned from top to bottom.
7. Last, clean the work surface, starting at the back and working side-to-side with overlapping strokes. Do not block airflow to or from the HEPA filter, and be careful not to contaminate any previously cleaned surface.
8. Dispose of the towels or gauze and document the hood cleaning.

Note that the prefilter is normally changed monthly, and the HEPA filter is tested every six months for efficiency.

Activity:

Part One

Review the technique for cleaning a LAH described in the preceding list and visit the website http://www.globalrph.com/aseptic.htm. Then, answer the following questions about the proper use of a horizontal laminar airflow hood.

1. What are the three functions of a horizontal laminar airflow hood?

   _____

   _____

   _____

   _____

2. What is the most important part of the horizontal laminar airflow hood?

   _____

   _____

3. What should be used to clean a horizontal laminar airflow hood?

   _____

   _____

4. Describe the technique used to disinfect the laminar airflow hood (e.g., where to start, what kind of motion to use, etc.).

   _____

   _____

   _____

   _____

Part Two

Now it is your turn to try cleaning a LAH. Review the procedure described earlier for cleaning a laminar airflow hood. Practice the technique with a partner, then perform the procedure for your instructor.

Student Name: _____

Lab Partner: _____

Grade/Comments: _____

_____

_____

Student Comments: _____

_____

_____

LAB 11-3: The Vertical Laminar Airflow Hood

Objective:

Review the technique involved in using a vertical laminar airflow hood.

Pre-Lab Information:

- Read Chapter 11, "Introduction to Sterile Products," in your textbook.
- Visit the website at http://www.ibc.arizona.edu/BSC TRAINING/Working in a BSC.htm

Explanation:

A vertical laminar airflow hood, also known as a chemo hood or biological safety cabinet (BSC), is used for compounding hazardous agents. A BSC has four sides with an 8- to 12-inch opening in the front, and a sliding glass door that can be brought down to the proper opening level. In a BSC, the room air enters the front opening and moves into the BSC grills, which are located in the front and back of the inside of the hood's work surface area. This air is then filtered and circulated to the HEPA filter, which filters the air to 0.3 micron. The filtered air is blown from the top of the hood vertically downward to the work surface area. The air is then filtered again and either eliminated back into the room air or to an outside vent.

Work with chemotherapy drugs or other sterile products using a vertical laminar airflow hood requires knowledge of proper techniques for cleaning and disinfecting the laminar airflow hood. The procedure for cleaning a BSC is essentially the same as the one used when cleaning a laminar airflow hood, although the class or level of the BSC may require some additional steps or precautions.

Activity:

Part One

Visit the website listed in the "Pre-Lab Information" section, then answer the following questions about the proper use and disinfection of a vertical laminar airflow hood.

1. In what ways does the BSC differ from the laminar airflow hood? Why do these differences make the BSC more appropriate for use with cytotoxic or hazardous agents?

   _____

   _____

   _____

   _____

2. What condition should never exist when operating a vertical laminar flow hood or biological safety cabinet?

   _____

   _____

   _____

   _____

3. When should you disinfect the BSC?

_____

_____

_____

_____

4. What are two appropriate disinfectants?

_____

_____

_____

_____

5. Biological safety cabinets are available in three different classes. Use the Internet to research the three different classes, then describe what you discover about each class and its different uses. Which one do you think you would be most likely to use in the pharmacy setting?

_____

_____

_____

_____

Part Two

Now it is your turn to try cleaning a BSC. Review the procedure described earlier for cleaning a laminar airflow hood. Practice the technique with a partner, then perform the procedure for your instructor.

Student Name: _____

Lab Partner: _____

Grade/Comments: _____

_____

_____

Student Comments: _____

_____

_____

LAB 11-4: Withdrawing Medication from a Vial or Glass Ampule

Objective:

Demonstrate the techniques involved in withdrawing medications from vials or ampules.

Pre-Lab Information:

- Review Chapter 11 in your textbook for review of aseptic compounding, needles, and syringes.
- Gather the following materials:
  - sterile vials and ampules of 0.9% sodium chloride
  - 10 mL syringes
  - 18 gauge, 1-1/2 inch needles
  - filter needles
  - gloves
  - alcohol swabs

Explanation:

You will learn the proper aseptic techniques for withdrawing medication from vials and ampules. If your instructor is unable to provide a lab component, your local hospital pharmacy may provide a demonstration for students upon request.

Activity:

Your instructor will take you through the proper procedures for withdrawing medication from vials and glass ampules. You will then have the opportunity to practice some of these techniques in class. If a laminar airflow hood is not available, you will need to use a little imagination regarding true aseptic technique.

Key points for working with vials:

1. Always observe the six-inch rule and critical areas when working with sterile products in a laminar airflow hood.
2. Always disinfect the top of the vial with an alcohol swab. One single swipe in one direction should be adequate to disinfect the vial and its stopper. Wait a moment for the alcohol to evaporate before entering the vial with a needle.
3. Attach a needle to a syringe of appropriate size. Before entering the vial, always draw some air into the syringe, to a volume that is slightly less than you want to withdraw from the vial. This extra air will be pushed into the vial before withdrawing the contents to help equalize the air pressure and make the withdrawal easier to accomplish.
4. Use care entering the vial with the needle. Using too large a needle or the wrong entry technique could result in "coring" of the stopper, which could leave fragments of the stopper in the medication. Adding too much air to the vial could also cause some of the medication to accidentally spray out, reducing the volume available for use and contaminating the hood.
5. With the bevel facing up, press the needle into the middle of the stopper until it has completely broken the seal. Be careful not to interrupt any of the airflow between the hood and the entry point shared between the vial and the needle. This process can be challenging for the beginner. Carefully tip the vial upside down, maintaining aseptic technique, and gently push some of the air from the syringe into the vial. The syringe will usually start to withdraw some of the fluid on its own. Repeat the process until all the air is out of the syringe and you have withdrawn the correct amount of fluid.
6. The syringe is now ready either to be capped or to be added to an IV bag for further dilution.

Key points for working with ampules:

1. Always observe the six-inch rule and critical areas when working with sterile products in a laminar airflow hood.

2. Always disinfect the narrow portion of the ampule with an alcohol swab.

3. Make sure that no liquid is trapped in the neck of the ampule. Tapping the ampule gently with a finger usually releases any liquid from the neck, allowing it to settle in the bottom.

4. Break the ampule open at the weakest part around the neck, usually indicated by a dot or a stripe. Be sure to break it open toward the side of the hood and not into the back of the hood. Glass fragments can damage the HEPA filter, which is located behind the grate at the back of the hood.

5. When withdrawing medication from a glass ampule, you must use a filter needle in order to filter out any glass particles that may have gotten into the medication. You do not need to withdraw air into the syringe before withdrawing medication from an ampule, because there is no longer a vacuum once you have broken open the ampule.

6. Using a filter needle attached to an appropriate syringe, tilt the ampule slightly in order to withdraw the amount of medication desired. You may need to adjust the volume in the syringe and repeat until you have the correct amount.

7. If the contents of the syringe are to be added to an IV bag, you must first change to a new, nonfiltered needle. If you keep the same needle, all of the glass particles you trapped will be pushed into the IV bag along with the medication, negating the whole filtering process.

8. Alternatively, some technicians prefer to draw the medication from the ampule with a regular needle, and then change to a filter needle before injecting the medication into an IV bag. Either method prevents glass particles from getting into the IV.

Questions:

1. Why do you need to pull air into the syringe before withdrawing medication from a vial?

2. Why do you need to swab off the top of a vial or an ampule with alcohol?

3. Why is it important to use a filter needle when working with glass ampules?

4. Why should you break open an ampule toward the side of the hood instead of toward the back of the hood?

5. Why do you not need to pull air into the syringe before withdrawing medication from an ampule?

LAB 11-5: Reconstituting Sterile Dry Powder Medications

Objectives:

Determine the diluents and amount of diluents required to reconstitute sterile dry powder medications.

Determine the storage requirements for the reconstituted medication.

Pre-Lab Information:

- Reread Chapter 11 in your textbook for review of aseptic technique and sterile compounding.
- Gather the following materials:
  - miscellaneous package inserts from sterile powder medications that require reconstitution

Explanation:

Some drugs contained in vials are in powder form. Before they can be used in patient treatment, they have to be reconstituted, which simply means that one must add a diluent, like sterile water, to the vial to make a liquid. Every sterile drug that requires reconstitution contains directions for reconstitution either directly on the vial and/or on the package insert.

Activity:

Your instructor will provide you with miscellaneous package inserts that accompanied sterile dry powder medications. Read through the package inserts to see what kind of information is provided about the medication. Stability and reconstitution requirements are usually found toward the end of the insert.

Questions:

Find the following information from each of the inserts provided to you.

1. Drug name and strength (example: vancomycin, 1 g):

   _____

   _____

2. Preferred diluent(s) (examples: sterile water, 0.9% sodium chloride, etc.):

   _____

   _____

3. Amount of diluent needed (example: 20 mL):

   _____

   _____

4. Concentration of the medication after reconstitution (example: 50 mg/mL):

   _____

   _____

5. Stability of the reconstituted medication (example: 72 hours):

   _____

   _____

6. Storage requirements for the reconstituted medication (example: Keep refrigerated or at room temperature):

   _____

   _____

7. What do you think might happen if you were to reconstitute a medication with the wrong diluent?

   _____

   _____

   _____

   _____

8. When comparing the amount of diluent needed to the concentration obtained, did you notice any trends?

   _____

   _____

   _____

   _____

Student Name: _____

Lab Partner: _____

Grade/Comments: _____

_____

Student Comments: _____

_____

_____

LAB 11-6: Transferring Liquid into an IV Bag

Objective:

Understand the technique involved in transferring liquid medication from a syringe into an IV bag so that you are able to apply the technique in a pharmacy setting.

Pre-Lab Information:

Review Chapter 11 in your textbook for information regarding aseptic technique and IV medications.

Explanation:

Many IV medications have to be further diluted before they are administered to patients. This process, also known as *sterile compounding,* is most often done with one or more syringes and an IV bag containing an isotonic fluid. In this activity, you will learn the proper aseptic technique for transferring solutions from a syringe into the IV bag, identify which port on the IV bag is used for the transfer, and learn how to add multiple products to the same bag.

Activity:

When compounding sterile products, follow these simple guidelines:

1. Read the prescription label to determine which products you need to use.

2. Select the correct IV bag and size (example: dextrose 5%, 100 mL) and the correct medication that will be transferred to this bag (example: diltiazem 125 mg/25 mL).

3. Remove the outer packaging and wipe down the entire bag with alcohol (in a clean room, parts of these processes may be done by a co-worker).

4. Place the disinfected bag on a hanger in the laminar airflow hood.

5. Strip off the seal to the center port of the IV bag and disinfect the port with an alcohol swab. (The port is usually in the middle with a blue seal, but certain IV bags have more than one port for pharmacy use.)

6. Prepare the medication for transfer to the IV bag. If it comes in a sterile powder, first follow the directions for reconstitution; then draw the appropriate amount of medication into a syringe, using aseptic technique.

7. Taking care to observe the critical areas of the hood and the six-inch rule, insert the needle (which is still attached to the syringe of medication from step 6) straight into the center of the port. You will need to pass the needle through the outer core and through an inner membrane. Try to keep the needle straight so as not to puncture the side of the port or the bag. A puncture will void the sterility of all the products involved and you will have to start over with new supplies.

8. Once the needle has passed the inner membrane, gently push the fluid from the syringe into the bag; then carefully pull out the needle and the syringe.

9. If your pharmacist has not double-checked your work at this point, some pharmacies allow you to pull the empty syringe back with air to the volume that you placed in the bag, to indicate how much drug you used.

10. After your work has been checked by a pharmacist, place a cap or seal over the port you just used (this step may be omitted depending on the pharmacy). Remove the IV from the hook, gently shake the bag to distribute the drug, and then label the bag appropriately.

11. If multiple drugs are used in the same bag, gently shake the IV bag between medications to avoid possible precipitation. "Banana bags," which got their nickname from their yellow color, are a multivitamin/mineral infusion and are a good example of a prescription for which you would use more than one drug in a bag.

These step-by-step instructions can be used to prepare most sterile products that require further dilution in an IV bag. You or your instructor may be able to get permission from a local hospital to demonstrate these techniques or allow you to practice.

Questions:

1. What might happen if a punctured bag accidentally made it out of the pharmacy and were hung for a patient?

   _____

   _____

   _____

   _____

2. What might happen if you added several products to an IV bag without mixing in between additions?

   _____

   _____

   _____

   _____

3. Why is it so important to practice aseptic technique when preparing IV medications?

   _____

   _____

   _____

   _____

4. While you are performing a fluid transfer, you accidently lose your grip on the syringe and it falls onto the hood. You discover that the needle has touched the surface of the hood. What should you do?

   _____

   _____

   _____

   _____

Forms

The following forms are for use in logging aseptic technique practice and skill validations.

Aseptic Technique Training Log	
Student Name	
Date	
Start Time	
End Time	
Contact Hour(s)	
Location	
Trainer's Name	
Trainer's Lic. #	
State of License	
Daytime Phone (trainer)	
Skill(s) Covered	

By signing below, I validate that the information listed above is complete and fully accurate.

_____   _____   _____   _____
Student Signature   Date   Trainer Signature   Date

Process Validation Record
Aseptic Handwashing Technique

Student Name: _____   Date: _____

PROCEDURE	YES	NO
Removed all jewelry, watches, and objects up to the elbow		
Did not have on acrylic nails or nail polish		
Starts water and adjusts to the appropriate temperature		
Avoided unnecessary splashing during process		
Used sufficient disinfecting agent/cleanser		
Cleaned all four surfaces of each finger		
Cleaned all surfaces of hands, wrists, and arms up to the elbows in a circular motion		
Did not touch the sink, faucet, or other objects that could contaminate hands		
Rinsed off all soap residue		
Rinsed hands holding them upright and allowing water to drip to the elbow		
Did not turn off water until hands were completely dry		
Turned water off with a clean, dry, lint-free paper towel		
Did not touch the faucet while turning off the water		

By signing below, I certify that the student has demonstrated 100% competency at the above task.

_____
Trainer Name (printed)

_____
Trainer Signature

_____
Trainer Daytime Phone

_____   _____
Date   Trainer's License #

                                    _____
                                    State Licensed

Process Validation Record
Horizontal Laminar Flow Hood

Student Name: _____   Date: _____

PROCEDURE	YES	NO
Hood was turned on and running at least 30 minutes prior to preparation		
Followed proper handwashing procedure and technique		
Wore appropriate apparel		
Used clean, sterile gauze/sponge and plenty of disinfectant to clean the hood		
Cleaned the IV pole first (if applicable)		
Cleaned the sides of the hood second, starting at the top and working side-to-side with overlapping strokes		
Cleaned the work surface last, starting at the back and working side-to-side with overlapping strokes		
Did not contaminate previously cleaned surfaces		
Did not block airflow from HEPA filter		
Did not utilize outer 6 inches of the hood opening		
Properly stood outside the hood without allowing the head to enter the inside		
Knows that hood certification is every 6 months, if moved, or if damaged		
Knows that prefilters should be changed monthly		

By signing below, I certify that the student has demonstrated 100% competency at the above task.

_____
Trainer Name (printed)

_____
Trainer Signature

_____   _____
Trainer Daytime Phone   Trainer's License #

_____   _____
Date   State Licensed

Process Validation Record
Vertical Laminar Flow Hood

Student Name: _____   Date: _____

PROCEDURE	YES	NO
Hood was turned on and running at least 30 minutes prior to preparation		
Followed proper handwashing procedure and technique		
Wore appropriate apparel		
Used clean, sterile gauze/sponge and plenty of disinfectant to clean the hood		
Cleaned the IV pole first (if applicable)		
Cleaned the sides of the hood second, starting at the top and working side-to-side with overlapping strokes		
Cleaned the back wall and inside the glass shield, starting at the top and working up and down with overlapping strokes		
Cleaned the work surface last, starting at the back and working side-to-side with overlapping strokes		
Did not contaminate previously cleaned surfaces		
Did not lower the glass shield more than 8 inches from the work surface prior to preparation		
Did not block airflow from HEPA filter or air intake grills at any time		
Did not utilize outer 6 inches of the hood opening		

By signing below, I certify that the student has demonstrated 100% competency at the above task.

_____
Trainer Name (printed)

_____
Trainer Signature

_____   _____
Trainer Daytime Phone   Trainer's License #

_____   _____
Date   State Licensed

Process Validation Record
Vial Preparation

Student Name: _____   Date: _____

PROCEDURE	YES	NO
Followed proper handwashing procedure and technique		
Wore appropriate apparel		
Followed proper procedure and technique in cleaning the hood		
Performed all necessary calculations correctly, prior to drug preparation		
Brought the correct drugs and concentrations into the hood for preparation		
Brought the correct supplies into the hood prior to preparation		
Inspected all products for particulate matter/contamination prior to use		
Removed dust covers and cleaned rubber diaphragms correctly		
Inserted needle correctly to prevent coring		
Used proper milking technique or venting device, and did not aspirate at any time		
Did not remove needle from vial until all air bubbles were removed and amount verified		
Removed air bubbles correctly and did not spill any liquid Withdrew needle correctly from vial to prevent spilling or aspiration		
Cleaned additive port on final container prior to injecting drug		
Did not core or puncture side of additive port when adding drug to the final container		
Properly mixed contents of container and inspected for incompatibilities or particulate matter		
Properly sealed additive port of container		
Did not contaminate the needle or syringe during preparation		
Did not contaminate the hood		
Did not block airflow from HEPA filter or air intake grills at any time		
Did not utilize outer 6 inches of the hood opening		
Properly discarded all waste, including sharps		

By signing below, I certify that the student has demonstrated 100% competency at the above task.

_____
Trainer Name (printed)

_____
Trainer Signature

_____
Trainer Daytime Phone

_____   _____
Date   Trainer's License #

                                                          _____
                                                          State Licensed

Process Validation Record
Ampule Preparation

Student Name: _____   Date: _____

PROCEDURE	YES	NO
Followed proper handwashing procedure and technique		
Wore appropriate apparel		
Followed proper procedure and technique in cleaning the hood		
Performed all necessary calculations correctly, prior to drug preparation		
Brought the correct drugs and concentrations into the hood for preparation		
Brought the correct supplies into the hood prior to preparation		
Inspected all products for particulate matter/contamination prior to use		
Ampule neck was cleared of fluid before breaking		
Ampule neck was cleaned correctly before breaking		
Ampule neck was wrapped correctly before breaking		
Ampule was broken correctly		
Attached filter device to syringe correctly		
Ampule was drawn up correctly, without spilling contents		
Filter needle was removed and replaced with new needle prior to injecting final container		
Drew up the correct amount of drug and checked measurement prior to injecting into container		
Cleaned additive port on final container prior to injecting drug		
Did not core or puncture side of additive port when adding drug to the final container		
Properly mixed contents of container and inspected for incompatibilities or particulate matter		
Properly sealed additive port of container		
Did not contaminate the needle or syringe during preparation		
Did not contaminate the hood		
Did not block airflow from HEPA filter or air intake grills at any time		
Did not utilize outer 6 inches of the hood opening		
Properly discarded all waste, including sharps		

By signing below, I certify that the student has demonstrated 100% competency at the above task.

_____
Trainer Name (printed)

_____
Trainer Signature

_____   _____
Trainer Daytime Phone   Trainer's License #

_____   _____
Date   State Licensed

Process Validation Record
Vial Preparation—Hazardous Drugs

Student Name: _____   Date: _____

PROCEDURE	YES	NO
Followed proper handwashing procedure and technique		
Wore appropriate apparel		
Followed proper procedure and technique in cleaning the hood		
Knew location of spill kit		
Knew location of eyewash station		
Performed all necessary calculations correctly, prior to drug preparation		
Placed prep-mat/paper drape correctly, prior to drug preparation		
Brought the correct drugs and concentrations into the hood for preparation		
Brought the correct supplies into the hood prior to preparation		
Inspected all products for particulate matter/contamination prior to use		
Removed dust covers and cleaned rubber diaphragms correctly		
Inserted needle correctly to prevent coring		
Used proper milking technique or venting device, and did not aspirate at any time		
Did not remove needle from vial until all air bubbles were removed and amount verified		
Removed air bubbles correctly and did not spill any liquid		
Withdrew needle correctly from vial to prevent spilling or aspiration		
Cleaned additive port on final container prior to injecting drug		
Did not core or puncture side of additive port when adding drug to the final container		
Properly mixed contents of container and inspected for incompatibilities or particulate matter		
Properly sealed additive port of container		
IV container was placed in a ziplock bag before removal from the hood		
Used any and all appropriate hazardous labeling (for product and waste)		
Did not contaminate the needle or syringe during preparation		
Did not contaminate the hood		
Did not block airflow from HEPA filter or air intake grills at any time		
Did not utilize outer 6 inches of the hood opening		
Properly discarded all waste, including sharps		

By signing below, I certify that the student has demonstrated 100% competency at the above task.

_____
Trainer Name (printed)

_____
Trainer Signature

_____   _____
Trainer Daytime Phone   Trainer's License #

_____   _____
Date   State Licensed

CHAPTER 12
Basic Math Skills

After completing Chapter 12 from the textbook, you should be able to:	Related Activity in the Workbook/Lab Manual
1. Determine the value of a decimal.	Review Questions Pharmacy Calculation Problems PTCB Exam Practice Questions
2. Add, subtract, multiply, and divide decimals.	Review Questions Pharmacy Calculation Problems PTCB Exam Practice Questions Activity 12-1
3. Recognize and interpret Roman numerals.	Review Questions Pharmacy Calculation Problems PTCB Exam Practice Questions
4. Change Roman numerals to Arabic numerals.	Review Questions Pharmacy Calculation Problems PTCB Exam Practice Questions
5. Change Arabic numerals to Roman numerals.	Review Questions Pharmacy Calculation Problems PTCB Exam Practice Questions
6. Describe the different types of common fractions.	Review Questions Activity 12-4
7. Add, subtract, multiply, and divide fractions.	Review Questions Pharmacy Calculation Problems PTCB Exam Practice Questions Activity 12-2
8. Define a ratio.	Review Questions Activity 12-4
9. Define a proportion.	Review Questions Activity 12-4
10. Solve math problems by using ratios and proportions.	Review Questions Pharmacy Calculation Problems PTCB Exam Practice Questions Activity 12-3

INTRODUCTION

Knowledge of basic arithmetic is essential for today's pharmacy technician. You need basic math skills to understand and perform drug preparations. Nearly every aspect of drug dispensing requires a consideration of numbers. All advanced pharmacy calculations, which are explained throughout this text, rely on a solid understanding of basic math principles. Remember that Chapter 12 in your textbook is designed to serve as a review of these general principles and as an assessment of your basic math skills; the activities in this workbook/lab manual will provide you with additional review.

REVIEW QUESTIONS

Match the following.

1. _____ common fractions
2. _____ complex fractions
3. _____ cross-multiplication
4. _____ decimal fractions
5. _____ denominator
6. _____ fraction line
7. _____ improper fraction
8. _____ numerator
9. _____ proper fraction
10. _____ proportion
11. _____ ratio
12. _____ Roman numerals
13. _____ simple fractions

a. bottom value of a fraction; placed beneath the fraction line

b. setting up two ratios or fractions in relationship to each other as a proportion and solving for the unknown variable

c. symbol representing the division of two values; placed between the numerator and denominator of a fraction

d. fractions written with a numerator separated by a fraction line from and positioned above a denominator

e. fraction in which both the numerator and the denominator are themselves common fractions

f. fractions written as a whole number with a zero and a decimal point in front of the value

g. a fraction in which the value of the numerator is smaller than the value of the denominator

h. letters and symbols used to represent numbers

i. the top value of a fraction; placed above the fraction line

j. the expression of a relationship of two numbers, written with a colon (:) between the numbers

k. proper fraction, with both the numerator and denominator reduced to lowest terms

l. fraction in which the value of the numerator is larger than the value of the denominator

m. two or more equivalent ratios or fractions that both represent the same value

Choose the best answer.

14. Which of these decimals has the highest value?
    a. 0.21
    b. 0.35
    c. 0.31
    d. 0.42

15. Which of these decimals has the highest value?
    a. 1.37
    b. 1.43
    c. 1.89
    d. 1.25

16. Which of these decimals has the lowest value?
    a. 12.4
    b. 12.006
    c. 12.03
    d. 12.891

17. Which of these decimals has the lowest value?
    a. 0.15
    b. 0.16
    c. 0.016
    d. 0.22

Multiply the following decimals.

18. $8.6 \times 0.24 =$ _____

19. $6.58 \times 2.26 =$ _____

20. $5.5 \times 4.986 =$ _____

Divide the following decimals.

21. $0.98 \div 0.3 =$ _____

22. $5.5 \div 0.4 =$ _____

23. $6.0 \div 0.66 =$ _____

Change these Roman numerals to Arabic.

24. XXVII _____

25. MDLXVI _____

26. XC _____

27. CL _____

28. XXI _____

29. LX _____

30. CCCLXV _____

PHARMACY CALCULATION PROBLEMS

Calculate the following.

1. Add the following fractions: $\frac{2}{4} + \frac{1}{8} + \frac{3}{16} =$

2. Solve for X: $\frac{50}{2} = \frac{30}{X}$

3. Solve for X: 250 mg/1 mL $= \frac{X}{5}$ mL

4. Solve for X: $1{,}000 \text{ mcg}/1 \text{ mL} = \frac{X}{2.5} \text{ mL}$

5. A physician writes a prescription for CXX tablets. If the patient takes 11 tablets qid, how many days will the supply last?

PTCB EXAM PRACTICE QUESTIONS

1. How many capsules will be taken in three days if a prescription order reads tetracycline 250 mg/capsule, one capsule qid?
    a. 16   c. 3
    b. 12   d. 6

2. How would you express 33.3% as a decimal?
    a. 33.3   c. 3.33
    b. 0.333   d. 333

3. What is 20% of 30?
    a. 6   c. 3
    b. 60   d. 300

4. How would you express 49 as a Roman numeral?
    a. IL   c. XXXXVIIII
    b. XLVIIII   d. XLIX

5. How would you round 145.1155 to the nearest hundredth?
    a. 145.1   c. 145.12
    b. 145.11   d. 145.116

ACTIVITY 12-1: Case Study—How Much?

Instructions: Read the following scenario and then answer the critical thinking questions.

Ms. Kipsky is an older woman who is on a very tight budget. She has worked at the local fabric store part time since her children all moved out of the house. In addition to this part-time job she receives an overdue child support check every now and then that helps her make it to the next payday. Luckily, she does not have any health conditions that require her to be on medicine and she is very glad about that; she just would not be able to afford it on top of her bills and bus fare to get to work every day.

It is deep into winter in the small town Ms. Kipsky works in when she comes to the independent pharmacy where you work, bearing a prescription for a mild bacterial infection. She tried to beat this infection for about a week and finally she went to the free clinic, where they prescribed amoxicillin suspension 250 mg/5 mL, 2 teaspoonfuls every 8 hours until gone (times 10 days).

Unfortunately for Ms. Kipsky, payday is not until next Friday and today is only Saturday. She brings the prescription to the pharmacy to be filled and asks the cost. You calculate the amount for her as $30.

1. Ms. Kipsky is uninsured and is paying cash. She asks you how much of the medication she will get if she can only pay for half right now.

   _____

   _____

   _____

2. Ms. Kipsky checks her purse and finds that she has only $5.00. She wants to know how much medicine that will buy. (Use the formula based on $30 for the entire prescription amount.)

   _____

   _____

   _____

3. She next asks how many doses she could get for $10.

   _____

   _____

   _____

   _____

ACTIVITY 12-2: Case Study—A Tapering Dose

Instructions: Read the following scenario and then answer the critical thinking questions.

Mr. Mindes is a regular customer at your retail pharmacy. His medication profile seems to be a who's-who of allergy medicines. Your pharmacy typically begins to see Mr. Mindes in early spring when the rain slows down and the flowers start to bloom. He has tried a variety of medications to help relieve allergy symptoms, such as fexofenadine, chlorpheniramine, and loratadine. He also has a nasal spray that keeps his sinuses clear during allergy attacks.

In spite of Mr. Mindes's preparation for each spring's natural bounties, this year he finds that he has actually acquired an infection that makes it tough for him to breathe. He has an uncomfortable case of bronchitis. His provider is prescribing a course of prednisone to help reduce the inflammation in his lungs.

The prescription is as follows: 5 tablets daily for 5 days, then 4 tablets daily for 5 days, then 3 tablets daily for 5 days, then 2 tablets daily for 5 days, then 1 tablet daily for 6 days.

1. What is the total number of tablets needed to fill the complete prescription?

   _____

   _____

2. At exactly halfway through his course of prednisone treatment, how many tablets will Mr. Mindes have left in the bottle?

   _____

   _____

3. With three days to the end of his treatment and last dose, how many tablets are left in his prescription bottle?

_____

_____

ACTIVITY 12-3: Case Study—Cream Compound

Instructions: Read the following scenario and then answer the critical thinking questions.

Sebastian, a very nice old man, has a very not-nice skin condition. He always has some rash or major itching problem that just will not go away. Over the years he has tried it all: a multitude of moisturizers, none of which seem to keep his skin from getting all these bumps that make him itch constantly.

Sebastian put up with this after the doctors told him it was not a medical condition like psoriasis or eczema. He has tried a variety of home remedies and herbal concoctions to make it go away, but it persists. Once in a while it will move around, but basically the active area remains on his lower left and right arms near the elbows.

One day Sebastian is with his doctor and the rash is just a little bit worse. The doctor decides to try a compound of two ingredients that he thinks might help alleviate the itching and add more moisture to the skin. Sebastian brings the prescription to your pharmacy to have it filled. The prescription is for 60% of ingredient A and 40% of ingredient B. The total amount is 155 grams.

1. How many grams of each of the ingredients will be used to make the compound?

_____

_____

_____

_____

2. If Sebastian wants to pick up only 80% of his prescription today, how many grams is he going to get?

_____

_____

3. Sebastian has 3.5 refills on his prescription. He is going out of town for 3 months and would like to pick up the entire amount today. How many grams is he going to get with all the refills?

_____

_____

ACTIVITY 12-4: Math Definitions

Match the math term in the left-hand column with its definition in the right-hand column.

Term

1. _____ proportion

2. _____ common fraction

3. _____ improper fraction

4. _____ simple fraction

5. _____ proper fraction

6. _____ ratio

Definition

a. can be expressed as one number that is set on a fraction line above another number

b. the value of the numerator is smaller than the value of the denominator

c. expresses the relationship of two numbers

d. two or more equivalent ratios or fractions that both represent the same value

e. the value of the numerator is larger than the value of the denominator

f. cannot be reduced to any lower terms

CHAPTER 13
Measurement Systems

After completing Chapter 13 from the textbook, you should be able to:	Related Activity in the Workbook/Lab Manual
1. List the three fundamental systems of measurement.	Review Questions Pharmacy Calculation Problems PTCB Exam Practice Questions
2. List the three primary units of the metric system.	Review Questions Pharmacy Calculation Problems PTCB Exam Practice Questions
3. Define the various prefixes used in the metric system.	Review Questions Pharmacy Calculation Problems PTCB Exam Practice Questions
4. Recognize abbreviations used in measurements.	Review Questions Pharmacy Calculation Problems PTCB Exam Practice Questions Activity 13-1, Activity 13-2, Activity 13-3
5. Explain the use of International Units and milliequivalents.	Review Questions Pharmacy Calculation Problems PTCB Exam Practice Questions
6. Convert measurements between the household system and the metric system.	Review Questions Pharmacy Calculation Problems PTCB Exam Practice Questions Lab 13-1
7. Convert measurements between the apothecary system and the metric system.	Review Questions Pharmacy Calculation Problems PTCB Exam Practice Questions
8. Perform temperature conversions.	Review Questions Pharmacy Calculation Problems PTCB Exam Practice Questions Activity 13-3

INTRODUCTION

Three fundamental systems of measurement are used to calculate dosages: the metric, apothecary, and household systems. Most prescriptions are written using the metric system. Regardless of your practice setting as a pharmacy technician, you must understand each system and how to convert from one system to another. With practice, the conversions you need to calculate dosages will become second nature to you. Until that time, use the charts and formulas from Chapter 13 as a guide. Remember that although miscalculating a conversion may seem to be a minor issue, it could have irrevocable effects on a patient's health.

REVIEW QUESTIONS

Match the following.

1. _____ apothecary system
2. _____ avoirdupois system
3. _____ household system
4. _____ International Units
5. _____ metric system
6. _____ Celsius
7. _____ Fahrenheit
8. _____ grain
9. _____ milliequivalent
10. _____ gram
11. _____ liter
12. _____ meter

a. measurement of a drug in terms of its action
b. unit of length in the metric system
c. based on the number of grams in 1 milliliter
d. metric unit of volume
e. international temperature unit
f. metric unit of weight
g. international and scientific system of measurement
h. common system of measurement in the United States
i. Old English system of weight measurement
j. American measurement of temperature
k. American measurement for weight
l. primary unit of the apothecary system

Choose the best answer.

13. If you are denoting 2 tenths of a milligram, you would write:
    a. 2/10 mg
    b. 0.2 mg
    c. 2 mg
    d. .2 mg

14. 2 g is equivalent to:
    a. 2,000 mg
    b. 20,000 mg
    c. 200 mg
    d. 20 mg

15. 8 ounces is equivalent to how many mL?
    a. 16
    b. 24
    c. 240
    d. 160

16. There are 16 ounces in a pint. How many milliliters is that?
    a. 480
    b. 48
    c. 4.8
    d. 4,800

17. If Mary is to take 2 teaspoonfuls bid for 10 days, how many mL should be dispensed?
    a. 20,000
    b. 2,000
    c. 200
    d. 20

Match the following.

18. _____ micro
19. _____ kilo
20. _____ milli
21. _____ centi

a. one-hundredth of the base
b. one thousand of the base
c. one-millionth of the base
d. one-thousandth of the base

PHARMACY CALCULATION PROBLEMS

Calculate the following.

1. According to the prescription, a patient uses latanoprost ophthalmic drops "1 gtts os qd." If the bottle only comes in 2.5 mL, how many days will the supply last?

2. Metronidazole IV comes in a 500 mg/100 mL concentration. If the patient received 100 mL × 8 doses, how many grams of metronidazole were given in total?

3. A prescription calls for 8 fl. oz. of guaifenesin a.c. syrup. If the patient is to take 5 mL po qid, how long will the bottle last?

4. A patient is to take 1 g valacyclovir po bid × 5 days. If the medication comes in 500 mg tablets, how many tablets will the patient need?

5. A TPN contains 2.25 L and is running at 120 mL/hr. How many hours will the TPN last?

PTCB EXAM PRACTICE QUESTIONS

1. A prescription is written for hydrocortisone 5% in zinc oxide—dispense 50 g. How many hydrocortisone 50 mg tablets are needed to prepare this compound?
   a. 2,500
   b. 2.5
   c. 5
   d. 50

2. Potassium chloride 30 mEq is to be given in 1,000 mL of IV fluid. Available vials contain 40 mEq/20 mL. How many mL of the drug would you use?
   a. 1.5
   b. 15
   c. 60
   d. 6

3. You receive an order for 0.2 g of Tigan IM. You have a 5 mL vial labeled 100 mg/mL. How many mL are required?
   a. 0.5
   b. 0.002
   c. 2
   d. 5

4. You check the pharmacy refrigerator and it is 40 degrees Fahrenheit. What is the temperature in degrees Celsius?
   a. 4
   b. −4
   c. 104
   d. 72

5. How many mg of phenobarbital are in one tablet of 2 grain phenobarbital?
   a. 65
   b. 6.5
   c. 13
   d. 130

ACTIVITY 13-1: Case Study—Kilograms

Instructions: Read the following scenario and then answer the critical thinking questions.

Mrs. Sarnoto is probably one of the world's best mothers. In addition to her three biological children, she has adopted four boys. Her days are full of chores, activities, driving, and homework, but many people say Mrs. Sarnoto would not have it any other way.

Mrs. Sarnoto also takes care of all the children's healthcare needs, from vaccinations to outbreaks of poison oak exposure. For this reason, she is a frequent visitor at the retail pharmacy where you work. Over the past five years alone, she has probably purchased at least half of the products in the pharmacy.

As luck would have it, five of the seven children have come down with a terrible bronchial infection. Everyone in the household is miserable, including Mrs. Sarnoto, who is also sick. She knows she has to be the strong one, though, and heads to the pharmacy to fill the amoxicillin prescriptions she has gotten for the family. Each person weighs a different amount and the amoxicillin prescription doses are based on weight in the following formula: 40 mg/kg/day in divided doses every 8 hours. The amoxicillin you have available in the pharmacy is 250 mg/5 mL.

1. One of the children weighs 28 pounds. How much amoxicillin suspension (in mL) will this child receive for a 7-day course of treatment?

_____

_____

_____

_____

2. One of the children weighs 83 pounds. How much amoxicillin suspension (in mL) will this child receive for each dose?

_____

_____

_____

_____

3. Mrs. Sarnoto has been prescribed amoxicillin capsules 500 mg three times daily, but she has a sore throat and wants the suspension. How much suspension (in mL) does she need to complete a 10-day course of treatment?

_____

_____

_____

_____

4. Mrs. Sarnoto had to travel 3 kilometers to get to the pharmacy. How many miles is her round trip?

_____

_____

_____

_____

ACTIVITY 13-2: Case Study—Milliliters

Instructions: Read the following scenario and then answer the critical thinking questions.

Carlene is the most experienced IV pharmacy technician at the Children's Hospital on the hill. She has been making IVs of all types for more than 11 years. She is in charge of all the specialty formulations that require precise measuring of multiple ingredients. Carlene takes great pride in what she does and shares all the little tricks she knows with the other pharmacy technicians who mix IVs. She has found a way to manipulate fluids when measuring so that they come out with exactly the volume the doctor has ordered, regardless of the IV contents. Some of the tricks she has learned include ways to use milliliters and liter measurements interchangeably, taking into account displacement of added items.

1. From a 2.5 liter volume, Carlene removes 325 mL. What is the final volume in mL?

_____

_____

_____

_____

2. Carlene adds 6,700 mL to a volume of 2 liters. How many total liters are there?

_____

_____

_____

_____

3. A formulation of 3.2 liters requires Carlene to remove 1,600 mL of fluid. How many mL are left after this?

_____

_____

_____

_____

ACTIVITY 13-3: Case Study—Drug Storage

Instructions: Read the following scenario and then answer the critical thinking questions.

Note: False medication names are used in this case study.

Sam is the inventory pharmacy technician at one of the biggest compounding pharmacies in his home town. He is in charge of medication purchasing, rotation, budget, and destruction, to name just a few of his tasks. His inventory is very large, accommodating more than 10,000 types of drugs in various forms.

Many of the drugs used for compounding in Sam's pharmacy are in raw and bulk forms. This is the optimum mixing in the situations that constantly arise in this type of business. Proper storage of medication is very important to prevent the breakdown of the active components in each medication. With the volume of inventory Sam has to manage, it is difficult to remember the storage instructions for each medication or product, so he refers to storage data books in each section of the pharmacy.

It is the end-of-the-year inventory and all items must be counted. In addition to counting all the products, Sam uses this time to ensure that all medications are stored within their optimum temperature ranges. For some medications, the manufacturers periodically issue updates on storage instructions.

1. The product ectium is a fine powder that must be kept in a temperature-controlled environment of 40–48 degrees Fahrenheit. What is this temperature in degrees Celsius?

_____

_____

_____

_____

2. Another product, silicutitum, is composed of small 4 cm balls that will melt if left at a temperature above 55 degrees Fahrenheit. What is this temperature in degrees Celsius?

_____

_____

_____

_____

3. A liquid known as pasitoxel will release a vapor if stored in an area above 3.333 degrees Celsius. What is this temperature in degrees Fahrenheit?

_____

_____

_____

_____

4. The lab where the mixing takes place is kept at a steady 72 degrees Fahrenheit. When the staff need to mix basculum, they have to drop the temperature by 11.11 degrees Celsius. After the reduction for mixing basculum, what is the lab temperature in degrees Fahrenheit?

_____

_____

_____

_____

LAB 13-1: Measuring Liquids Using Different Measurement Systems and Units

Objectives:

Demonstrate the ability to measure liquids using common pharmacy measurement systems.

Describe the relationship between the metric and household systems.

Use ordinary kitchen tools to understand and visualize the relationship between the most common pharmacy measurement systems.

Pre-Lab Information:

• Review Chapter 13 in the textbook.
• Gather the following materials:
  • kitchen measuring spoons
  • kitchen measuring cup
  • 10 mL and 20 mL syringes
  • 100 mL graduated cylinder
  • container of water

Explanation:

It is important for you to understand the relationship between the different liquid measurements used in pharmacy. This exercise will help you visualize the differences and relate them to more familiar kitchen measurements. This knowledge will also help you assist your patients in understanding how to measure certain medications.

Activity:

Using the equipment you have collected, complete the following exercises.

1. Take the 10 mL syringe and draw up 5 mL of water.

2. Now use the 5 mL of water from the syringe to fill up the teaspoon.

3. How much of the water fits into the teaspoon? Describe the relationship between 5 mL and 1 teaspoon.

   _____

   _____

   _____

   _____

4. Take the 20 mL syringe and draw up 15 mL of water.

5. Now use the 15 mL of water to fill up the tablespoon.

6. How much of the water fits into the tablespoon? Describe the relationship between 15 mL and 1 tablespoon.

_____

_____

_____

_____

7. Add 2 tablespoons of liquid (water) to the 100 mL graduated cylinder.

8. Describe the relationship between 2 tablespoons and 1 fl. oz. (30 mL).

_____

_____

_____

_____

9. Using the 100 mL graduated cylinder from question 8, pour the liquid into the measuring cup.

10. Describe the relationship between 1 fl. oz. (30 mL) and 1 cup.

_____

_____

_____

_____

Student Name: _____

Lab Partner: _____

Grade/Comments: _____

_____

_____

Student Comments: _____

_____

_____

CHAPTER 14
Dosage Calculations

After completing Chapter 14 from the textbook, you should be able to:	Related Activity in the Workbook/Lab Manual
1. Calculate the correct number of doses in a prescription.	Review Questions Pharmacy Calculation Problems PTCB Exam Practice Questions Activity 14-1, Activity 14-2
2. Determine the quantity to dispense for a prescription.	Review Questions Pharmacy Calculation Problems PTCB Exam Practice Questions Activity 14-1, Activity 14-2, Activity 14-3
3. Calculate the amount of active ingredient in a prescription.	Review Questions Pharmacy Calculation Problems PTCB Exam Practice Questions
4. Determine the correct days supply for a prescription.	Review Questions Pharmacy Calculation Problems PTCB Exam Practice Questions Activity 14-1, Activity 14-2
5. Perform multiple dosage calculations for a single prescription.	Review Questions Pharmacy Calculation Problems PTCB Exam Practice Questions Activity 14-2, Activity 14-3
6. Calculate accurate dosages for pediatric patients.	Review Questions Pharmacy Calculation Problems PTCB Exam Practice Questions Activity 14-1
7. Convert a patient's weight from pounds to kilograms.	Review Questions Pharmacy Calculation Problems PTCB Exam Practice Questions Activity 14-1
8. Perform dosage calculations based upon mg/kg/day.	Review Questions Pharmacy Calculation Problems PTCB Exam Practice Questions

INTRODUCTION

Proper dosing of medications is important to ensure patient safety. Dosage calculations include calculating the number of doses and dispensing quantities and ingredient quantities. These calculations are performed in the pharmacy on a daily basis. As a pharmacy technician, you must have a full working knowledge of how to perform these calculations. To perform dosage calculations, you will draw upon the knowledge you have mastered in previous chapters in the textbook, such as setting up ratios and proportions, keeping like units consistent, and cross-multiplying to solve for an unknown.

REVIEW QUESTIONS

Match the following.

1. _____ Clark's Rule   a. pediatric dose based on age in months
2. _____ dispensing quantity   b. number of days the medication will last
3. _____ dose   c. pediatric dose based on weight
4. _____ Fried's Rule   d. total amount of medication to be given
5. _____ days supply   e. amount of medication taken at one time

Write the correct sig. codes.

6. every 6 hours _____
7. every day _____
8. 4 times daily _____
9. every other day _____
10. twice daily _____
11. every 8 hours _____
12. as needed _____
13. every 4 hours _____
14. every 12 hours _____
15. every 4–6 hours _____
16. 6 times daily _____
17. 3 times daily _____
18. 4–6 times each day _____

Choose the best answer.

19. When figuring the quantity to dispense you should always:
    a. round up, so the patient gets enough medication.
    b. round down, so the patient will not overdose.
    c. dispense the exact quantity, including a $\frac{1}{2}$ tablet if necessary.
    d. not worry too much about quantity if the patient has refills.

20. A 5 mL bottle of eyedrops will last how long if the patient is using 1 gtt OU bid?

    a. 30   c. 20

    b. 25   d. 15

Fill in the blanks.

Mr. Mestophel has a prescription for cephalexin 500 mg, #60, with the sig code "1 po bid ug."

21. The dose is _____ capsules.

22. The days supply is _____ days.

23. The daily dose is _____ mg.

24. The dispensing quantity is _____.

25. If Tyra's emergency inhaler contains 200 puffs and she uses 1 puff up to 4 times daily, how long should her inhaler normally last? _____

PHARMACY CALCULATION PROBLEMS

Calculate the following.

1. How many grams are in a 4 fl. oz. bottle of levetiracetam 100 mg/mL oral solution?

2. A patient takes 2 teaspoonfuls of citalopram hydrobromide 2 mg/mL. How many mcg are in each dose?

3. A medical order states that a patient is to receive 2 mg/kg/day of a medication. The patient weighs 185 lbs. How many milligrams will the patient receive?

4. A child needs a medication that does not have a pediatric formula available. The usual adult dosage for this medication is 800 mg. If the child weighs 60 lbs, how many mg would constitute an appropriate pediatric dose?

5. A patient weighing 215 lbs is receiving a medication dosed at 5 mcg/kg/day in three divided doses. How many mcg are in each dose?

1. A prescription reads: Amoxicillin 250 mg/10 mL, 1 tsp bid × 10d. How many mL will you need to dispense?
   a. 50
   b. 100
   c. 150
   d. 200

2. The doctor orders vancomycin 10 mg/kg q12h IV for a newborn. The infant weighs 4,000 g. How many mg should be given per dose?
   a. 18.2
   b. 80
   c. 4
   d. 40

3. Calculate a single dose, in milliliters, for a 22-pound child receiving gentamicin 2 mg/kg of body weight IVPB q8h. Gentamicin is available in 20 mg/2 mL concentration.
   a. 2
   b. 10
   c. 15
   d. 20

4. You have a prescription for Vioxx® 25 mg/5 mL, dispense 150 mL. The patient is to take 12.5 mg once daily. What is the days supply for this prescription?
   a. 60
   b. 30
   c. 6
   d. 15

5. A parent of a 5-year-old child weighing 47 lbs needs to give an oral dose of Tylenol® elixir. The literature states that the dose for a child of this age and weight should not exceed 70 mg/kg per day. This daily maximum is to be divided into six doses. Tylenol® elixir contains 125 mg/mL. How many teaspoonfuls would the parent give for a single dose?
   a. 1
   b. 1.25
   c. 1.5
   d. 2

ACTIVITY 14-1: Case Study—Pediatric Dosing

Instructions: Read the following scenario and then answer the critical thinking questions.

Jimmie is a cute 8-year-old boy who weighs 55 pounds and presents with all the symptoms of a cold. The primary symptoms he exhibits are a fever and constant tugging at his ears. The doctor diagnoses acute otitis media and prescribes a 7-day course of amoxicillin capsules and acetaminophen for fever.

As Jimmie is waiting in the lobby with his mother to have his prescription filled, you notice that in spite of his illness, he is quite actively chewing and pulling on his gum. Cute as he is, his gum-smacking is annoying other patients, so the pharmacy attempts to expedite his prescription.

When Jimmie's mother hands the prescription to you, you notice that the doctor has forgotten to write in the dose.

1. What does the pharmacist need to know to correctly dose the amoxicillin for Jimmie?

_____

_____

_____

_____

2. While turning the prescription in, the mother mentions that Jimmie's throat is very sore and he has had a hard time swallowing. You realize that capsules will be too difficult for the boy to swallow. How is Jimmie going to take his medicine?

_____

_____

_____

_____

3. The dose turns out to be 500 mg 3 times daily (one capsule). If you were to provide a suspension of 250 mg/5 mL, how much would Jimmie receive per dose, and how much would you need to dispense for the full seven days?

_____

_____

_____

_____

ACTIVITY 14-2: Case Study—Tablets

Instructions: Read the following scenario and then answer the critical thinking questions.

Ms. Kelsey, two-time award-winning journalist, has worked for the newspaper for more than 22 years. She absolutely loves her job because of the places it has taken her and the people she has met. Ms. Kelsey has interviewed so many different people that it truly has made her feel like she has lived a rewarding life.

Ms. Kelsey has taken one particular medication all through her life in tablet form. She has a form of asthma and this medication helps her breathe. In addition to this one tablet, she has a rescue inhaler. A few times in the past she has been treated with maintenance inhalers, but luckily does not have to be on them most of the time. The tablets seem to work very well. Occasionally, depending on age and situation, her doctor has increased or decreased the amount of medication in the tablets to prevent flare-ups.

1. In her 20s, Ms. Kelsey was instructed to take 3 tablets twice a day for 28 days at a time. How many tablets did she need to complete one course of treatment?

_____

_____

_____

2. When she turned 30 years of age, Ms. Kelsey was instructed to take 3.5 tablets 3 times a day for 28 days. How many tablets did she need for one course of treatment?

_____

_____

_____

3. Now that Ms. Kelsey is over 40 years of age, she is instructed to take 3.75 tablets twice a day for 34 days. How many does she need to complete this course of treatment?

_____

_____

_____

4. When Ms. Kelsey turns 50 years old, she will need to take 272 tablets over 32 days with twice-daily dosing. How many tablets will she be taking per dose?

_____

_____

_____

ACTIVITY 14-3: Case Study—Cream

Instructions: Read the following scenario and then answer the critical thinking questions.

Note: False medication names are used in this case study.

Sharla is a very beautiful and active 16-year-old girl. She is captain of her high school cheerleading team, has played the lead role in three of the school's plays this year, and is taking classes for a future career in modeling. Sharla takes exceptionally good care of her body and skin from the inside out, so it was quite disturbing for her when one day she noticed that her slight acne had begun to worsen.

During her teenage years, Sharla has had periodic face and skin conditions resulting from sensitive skin. It turns out that she is very sensitive to detergents, soaps, lotions, and perfumes. It is very difficult for her to keep the rashes under control when she breaks the rules and wears perfume for special occasions such as school dances.

Sharla has received prescriptions from the compounding pharmacy for all types of perfume-free creams over the years. Almost all have helped, and she uses this pharmacy exclusively for all new formulations she is prescribed. She has received some prescriptions in heavy jars or small tubes depending on the area to be treated.

1. When Sharla had a round, mild rash on her bottom left cheek, she was prescribed listfal 34 g and palfite 16 g combined. How many mg is this?

_____

_____

_____

2. When her legs were covered in a rash, Sharla was prescribed 12 pounds of crexopen cream. How much is this in ounces?

_____

_____

_____

3. For the mild hypersensitive reaction just under her ear, she was prescribed junisten 1.2 kilograms. How many ounces is this?

_____

_____

_____

_____

CHAPTER 15

Concentrations and Dilutions

After completing Chapter 15 from the textbook, you should be able to:	Related Activity in the Workbook/Lab Manual
1. Calculate weight/weight concentrations.	Review Questions Pharmacy Calculation Problems PTCB Exam Practice Questions
2. Calculate weight/volume concentrations.	Review Questions Pharmacy Calculation Problems PTCB Exam Practice Questions Activity 15-1, Activity 15-2, Lab 15-1
3. Calculate volume/volume concentrations.	Review Questions Pharmacy Calculation Problems PTCB Exam Practice Questions Activity 15-1
4. Calculate dilutions of stock solutions.	Review Questions Pharmacy Calculation Problems PTCB Exam Practice Questions Lab 15-1

INTRODUCTION

Concentrations and dilutions, which can feel overwhelming and intimidating, are really no more than a series of simple ratios and proportions. Concentrations of many pharmaceutical preparations are expressed as a percent strength. Percent strength represents how many grams of active ingredient are in 100 mL. In the case of solids such as ointments, percent strength represents the number of grams of active ingredient contained in 100 g. Percent strength can be reduced to a fraction or to a decimal, which may be useful in solving these calculations. It is best to convert any ratio strengths to a percent. As a pharmacy technician, you will use concentrations and dilutions in a variety of pharmacy practice settings, so it is important that you master this skill.

208   CHAPTER 15 *Concentrations and Dilutions*   © 2009 Pearson Education, Inc.

REVIEW QUESTIONS

Match the following.

1. _____ concentration
2. _____ diluent
3. _____ percent strength
4. _____ % volume/volume
5. _____ % weight/volume
6. _____ % weight/weight

a. percent strength concentration of a liquid active ingredient contained within a liquid base

b. percent strength concentration of a solid active ingredient contained within a solid base

c. percent strength concentration of a solid active ingredient contained within a liquid base

d. refers to the strength of active pharmaceutical ingredient in a medication.

e. representation of the number of grams of active ingredient contained in 100 mL

f. a substance used to dilute another substance

True or False?

7. Grams and milliliters are used interchangeably in concentration problems, depending on whether you are working with solids in grams or liquids in milliliters, as they are considered equivalent measures.

    T   F

8. To accurately perform w/v concentration calculations, the proportion must be set up as grams over mL.

    T   F

9. When mixing powders with liquids, the liquid (base) quantity is considered the total quantity, as the powder will either dissolve or suspend within the base liquid.

    T   F

Choose the best answer.

10. To prevent errors while documenting quantities, what is the rule when it comes to decimals?
    a. Never use a fraction stated as a decimal.
    b. Be sure to have the product in stock.
    c. Always use the number 0 before any fraction.
    d. Only use whole numbers.

11. How many 500 mg metronidazole tablets will be needed to compound the following prescription for a patient? "Metronidazole 3%, suspending agent 30%, simple syrup 40% qsad H_2O to 150 mL."
    a. 9
    b. 7
    c. 10
    d. 18

12. You get in a prescription for "Amoxil 400 mg po tid × 10 days." Your pharmacy has in stock an Amoxil® oral suspension 250 mg/5 mL. What is the exact volume of medication you will need to correctly and completely fill the prescription for the patient?
    a. 150 mL
    b. 168 mL
    c. 240 mL
    d. 200 mL

13. How many grams of 2% silver nitrate ointment will deliver 1 gram of the active ingredient?
    a. 25 g   c. 50 g
    b. 4 g   d. 20 g

14. What volume of 5% aluminum acetate solution will be needed if 120 mL of 0.05% solution are extemporaneously compounded for patient use?
    a. 12 mL   c. 8.3 mL
    b. 1.2 mL   d. 0.83 mL

15. Calculate the flow rate in drops per minute if a physician orders D5W/NS 1,400 mL over 12 hours using an administration set that delivers 40 gtts/mL.
    a. 87 gtts/min   c. 117 gtts/min
    b. 68 gtts/min   d. 78 gtts/min

16. 325 mg could also be written as:
    a. 2 gr.   c. 10 gr.
    b. 5 gr.   d. 1/2 gr.

17. From the following formula, calculate in kilograms the quantity of miconazole needed to prepare 12 kg of powder.

    zinc oxide 1 part

    calamine 2 parts

    miconazole 1.5 parts

    bismuth subgallate 3 parts

    talcum 8 parts
    a. 15.5   c. 1.16
    b. 0.097   d. 1.5

18. Calculate the flow rate for an IV of 1,000 mL to run in over 8 hours with a set calibrated at 20 gtt/mL.
    a. 41.6 gtt/min   c. 125.1 gtt/min
    b. 17.36 gtt/min   d. 50 gtt/min

PHARMACY CALCULATION PROBLEMS

Calculate the following.

1. How many grams of drug are contained in 500 mL of a 20% solution?

2. A technician needs to compound metoclopramide suspension 5 mg/5 mL, qsad 100 mL. Metoclopramide is available in 10 mg tablets. How many tablets will you need to triturate for this compound?

3. What is the percent strength of a solution that is made by adding 200 mL of sterile water to 600 mL of a 25% solution?

4. If a technician is compounding a 5% hydrocortisone emulsion in 120 g of aquaphilic ointment, how many grams of hydrocortisone powder will she need?

5. How many grams of active ingredient are in 500 milliliters of a 1:20 solution?

PTCB EXAM PRACTICE QUESTIONS

1. You have 200 mL of a 30% solution. You dilute the solution to 600 mL. What is the percent strength of the final solution?
   a. 60
   b. 30
   c. 12
   d. 10

2. A solution of ampicillin contains 250 mg/mL. What is the percent strength of the solution?
   a. 2.5
   b. 25
   c. 12.5
   d. 15.2

3. How many grams of amino acid are in 500 mL of 8.5% solution?
   a. 64.3
   b. 42.5
   c. 16
   d. 8.5

4. Neostigmine is available in a 1:1000 concentration in a 20 mL vial. You have a prescription for 16 mg. How many mL are required?
   a. 1.6
   b. 16
   c. 12.5
   d. 1.2

5. Epinephrine is available as a 1:1000 w/v solution. If the patient dose is 0.2 mg IM, how many mL are needed?
   a. 2
   b. 1
   c. 0.2
   d. 0.1

ACTIVITY 15-1: Case Study—Dosing

Instructions: Read the following scenario and then answer the critical thinking questions.

Wintertime brings a barrage of colds throughout the Hudson family. They are a very active family of Dad, Mom, two boys (11 and 14) and two girls (8 and 12). Each child participates in at least one winter sport, keeping them on the go. The children spend a lot of time riding to games with other families and their parents think this makes it easier to pick up infections. Although they manage to avoid most ailments year round, three weeks in January of each year seem to bring an assortment of infection bugs to this household. This past winter was no exception.

When January rolled around, the infections hit this family like dominoes. The pattern is almost the same every year. Once everyone was sick at the same time and everyone received treatments for different bacterial infections.

1. Dad received cefotetan in either 1 g or 2 g for IM injection. The 1 g vial would be mixed with 2 mL sterile water and the 2 g would be mixed with 3 mL of sterile water. What is the concentration of the 1 g and the 2 g cefotetan with these diluent amounts?

   _____

   _____

   _____

   _____

2. Mom is going to receive a Zithromax® suspension 500 mg per day for 1 day, then 250 mg per day for 4 days. The concentration available to you is 200 mg/5 mL. How many teaspoonfuls does Mom receive per dose on day 1? How many on day 2?

   _____

   _____

   _____

   _____

3. The 8-year-old girl weighs 42 lbs. and will receive Unasyn® at 300 mg/kg/day. How much is her dose per day?

   _____

   _____

   _____

4. The 14-year-old boy is going to receive ceftriaxone 2 g IV daily for 3 days, to be infused over 30 minutes. For a 2 g dose, 19.2 mL of sterile water were added to the vial and the medication was then injected into a 100 mL bag of NS. How many mL/min are infused if the total volume of the piggyback has to empty out over 30 minutes?

   _____

   _____

   _____

   _____

ACTIVITY 15-2: Case Study—Reconstitution

Instructions: Read the following scenario and then answer the critical thinking questions.

Jeremy is a 24-year-old recent graduate of the pharmacy technician program at the community college. This is his first job in pharmacy and within 6 months he is already being trained to make small preparations in the sterile preparation area of the home infusion pharmacy where he is employed. Training in this area begins with practicing reconstitution techniques for a while and then moving up to larger volumes.

In the course of the workday, Jeremy makes a lot of low-volume products that are less than 50 mL. Jeremy enjoys his work and is especially happy with the fact that he gets to apply the knowledge he obtained in school. For the most part, the medications he works with in this pharmacy use sterile water as the main diluent. Jeremy works with any number of powder medications in vials, all of which he needs to reconstitute.

1. Jeremy has a 1 g vial of vancomycin and adds 10 mL of sterile water. What is the final concentration of the vancomycin?

   _____

   _____

   _____

   _____

2. If Jeremy were to add 20 mL sterile water to this vancomycin, what would be the final concentration?

   _____

   _____

   _____

   _____

3. What is the final concentration if Jeremy had 2 g of vancomycin and he added 20 mL sterile water to this vial?

   _____

   _____

   _____

   _____

ACTIVITY 15-3: Case Study—Concentration

Instructions: Read the following scenario and then answer the critical thinking questions.

Note: False medication names are used in this case study.

Renee is a clinical pharmacy technician at a mid-sized hospital with about 120 patient beds. This bed count includes a small 20-bed unit that is for patients who require a little longer stay for rehabilitation purposes. Typically these patients are a little older and less mobile than patients who are in the hospital for routine surgical needs. Many of these patients move on to some sort of assisted living situation, such as community apartment homes where part-time nursing care is available.

Part of the care the nurses provide to these patients is the administration of medications such as IV infusions, insulin shots (for the squeamish), and other types of injections (such as cyanocobalamin). Other nurses occasionally have to do careful calculation and administration of pain medications in suspension or injectable forms.

Part of Renee's job is to help provide the medications to nursing for patient administration; this includes mixing of unit-dose preparations such as injectables or oral liquids. In addition, Renee helps double-check all the calculations, as part of a safety check. Because she works in pharmacy, Renee also knows what drug forms and strengths are immediately available.

1. Bascoletine is available as 30 mg/mL in a 15 mL vial. How many total mg are available in this vial?

2. If the nurse withdrew one-quarter of the vial contents for a dose, how many mgs would be in that dose?

3. The doctor prescribes the entire vial of medication from question #1, divided into 5 equal doses. How many mg and mL would each dose have?

4. Using the medication information from question #1, how many mg are in 5 mL?

LAB 15-1: Concentrations in the Kitchen

Objective:

Demonstrate the ability to measure liquids and work with solutions of differing concentrations.

Pre-Lab Information:

- Review Chapter 15 in the textbook.
- Gather the following materials:
  - 20, 50, and 100 mL graduated cylinders
  - bottle of chilled cranberry juice
  - bottle of chilled apple juice
  - bottle of chilled drinking water
  - paper cups to contain the liquid "medication"

Explanation:

It is important for pharmacy technicians to understand how to calculate the percent strength of solutions of varying concentrations. This exercise will give you the opportunity to experience working with solutions of different concentrations and the calculations involving dilutions.

Activity:

Use the materials in the preceding list to prepare the solutions as instructed; then answer the following questions about the resulting concentrations.

Assumptions:

- The chilled apple juice should be considered a 100% solution (100 g/100 mL)
- The chilled cranberry juice should be considered a 100% solution (100 g/100 mL)
- The chilled water should be considered a 0% solution

1. Measure 20 mL of the 100% cranberry juice solution. Dilute the solution to 80 mL with water. What is the percent strength of the final solution?

   _____

   _____

2. Measure 55 mL of the 100% apple juice solution and mix it with 35 mL of the 100% cranberry juice solution. What is the final percent strength of the apple juice in the new cranapple solution?

   _____

   _____

3. Using the solution from question #2, what is the final percent strength of the cranberry juice in the new cranapple solution?

   _____

   _____

4. Measure 60 mL of the 100% cranberry juice and dilute it to 100 mL with water. What is the percent strength of the resulting solution?

_____

_____

5. Make a 50% solution of cranberry juice by mixing 25 mL of the cranberry juice with 25 mL of drinking water. Take 30 mL of the diluted cranberry juice (50%) and mix it with 20 mL apple juice. How many grams of cranberry are in the new mixture?

_____

_____

6. What is the percent strength of the diluted cranberry juice in the solution from question #5?

_____

_____

Student Name: _____

Lab Partner: _____

Grade/Comments: _____

_____

_____

Student Comments: _____

_____

_____

CHAPTER 16
Alligations

After completing Chapter 16 from the textbook, you should be able to:	Related Activity in the Workbook/Lab Manual
1. Understand when to use the alligation principle for calculations.	Review Questions Pharmacy Calculation Problems PTCB Exam Practice Questions Activity 16-1, Activity 16-2, Activity 16-3, Lab 16-1
2. Calculate and solve a variety of alligation-related problems.	Review Questions Pharmacy Calculation Problems PTCB Exam Practice Questions Activity 16-1, Activity 16-2, Activity 16-3, Lab 16-1

INTRODUCTION

The alligation method is used in the pharmacy when it is necessary to mix two products that have different percent strengths of the same active ingredient. The strength of the final product will fall between the strengths of each original product. Although these calculations can be confusing at first, once you master the alligation grid, you should be able to perform these calculations easily.

REVIEW QUESTIONS

Fill in the blanks.

1. Solvents and diluents such as water, vanishing cream base, and white petrolatum are considered a percent strength of _____.

2. Liquids, including solutions, syrups, elixirs, and even lotions, are expressed in _____.

3. Solids are expressed in _____. These include powders, creams, and ointments.

4. The alligation formula requires that you express the strength as a _____ when setting up the problem.

5. When writing percents or using decimals, always use a leading _____.

6. 1 fl. oz. is commonly rounded to _____ mL.

7. 1 avoirdupois oz. is commonly rounded to _____ g.

8. The _____ strength goes in the top left box of an alligation grid.

9. The _____ strength goes in the bottom left box of an alligation grid.

10. The _____ goes in the center box of an alligation grid.

Use alligations to answer the following questions.

You have one gallon of silver nitrate 1% stock solution, which you can dilute with distilled water. How many milliliters of each will you need to make 1 L of silver nitrate 0.25% solution?

11. _____ mL of the 1% stock solution

12. _____ mL of distilled water

You have hydrocortisone 10% ointment and hydrocortisone 2% ointment. How many grams of each will you use to prepare hydrocortisone 5% ointment 120 g?

13. _____ g of the 10% ointment

14. _____ g of the 2% ointment

Prepare 480 mL of a 1:30 solution using a 1:10 solution and a 1:50 solution.

15. _____ mL of the 1:50 solution

16. _____ mL of the 1:10 solution

17. How many grams of 10% ointment should you add to 20 g of 2% ointment to make 5% ointment? _____ g

18. How many milliliters of water should you add to 50 mL of betadine 0.25% solution to prepare betadine 1:1000 solution? _____ mL

19. How many grams of lidocaine 2% ointment should you mix with 22.5 g of lidocaine 10% ointment to prepare lidocaine 5% ointment 2 oz.? _____ g

20. Convert 25% to a ratio strength. _____

21. 1:2 is what percentage strength? _____

Fill in the blanks.

22. 1:2   50%   0.50   _____

23. _____   33%   0.33 $\frac{1}{3}$

24. 3:4   _____   0.75 $\frac{3}{4}$

25. 1:1   100%   _____   1

PHARMACY CALCULATION PROBLEMS

Calculate the following.

1. A technician is compounding 16 ounces of zinc oxide 7.5% ointment. In stock, there is zinc oxide 20% ointment and petroleum jelly. How many ounces of each will the technician need to make the final product?

2. You have to compound 1 liter of a 4% solution. The pharmacy has a 12% solution and a 2% solution in stock. How many milliliters of each will be needed to make the final product?

3. You need to prepare a 2% solution from the 10% solution and sterile water that is in stock. Four fluid ounces are required for the prescription. How many milliliters of each (the 10% solution and water) will you need to make the final product?

4. You need 0.5 L of a 2.5% solution for a prescription. The pharmacy has on hand a 1:5 solution and a 1:100 solution. How many milliliters of each will be needed for this compound?

5. A prescription calls for 32 fl. oz. of a 1:1000 solution that is to be compounded. The pharmacy stocks a 1:20 solution and sterile water. How many milliliters of each will be required for this compound?

PTCB EXAM PRACTICE QUESTIONS

1. Calculate how many mL of 50% dextrose solution and how many mL of water are needed to prepare 4.5 L of a 1% solution.
   a. 4,410 mL dextrose and 90 mL water
   b. 500 mL dextrose and 4,000 mL water
   c. 90 mL dextrose and 4,410 mL water
   d. 95 mL dextrose and 4,405 mL water

2. How many mL of a 15% solution of sodium chloride and how many mL of water should be used to prepare 1 liter of a 0.9% solution of sodium chloride?
   a. 60 mL 15% and 940 mL water
   b. 940 mL 15% and 60 mL water
   c. 500 mL 15% and 500 mL water
   d. 200 mL 15% and 800 mL water

3. How many grams of 10% boric acid ointment should be mixed with petrolatum (0%) to prepare 700 g of a 5% boric acid ointment?
   a. 300 g petrolatum and 400 g 10%
   b. 200 g petrolatum and 500 g 10%
   c. 300 g 10% and 400 g petrolatum
   d. 350 g 10% and 400 g petrolatum

4. You are asked to prepare 2.5 liters of a 1:20 solution from a 30% solution and water. How many mL of the 30% solution and how many mL of water are needed?
   a. 500 mL water and 2,000 mL 30% solution
   b. 417 mL 30% solution and 2,083 mL water
   c. 417 mL water and 2,083 mL 30% solution
   d. 2,000 mL water and 500 mL 30% solution

5. Calculate how many mL of 50% dextrose solution and how many mL of 10% dextrose solution are needed to prepare 4.5 L of a 1% solution.
   a. 3,802 mL 50% solution and 698 mL 10% solution
   b. 3,802 mL 10% solution and 698 mL 50% solution
   c. 3.8 mL 50% solution and 0.7 mL 10% solution
   d. 3.8 mL 10% solution and 0.7 mL 50% solution

ACTIVITY 16-1: Case Study—Cream

Instructions: Read the following scenario and then answer the critical thinking questions.

Jerry Rands is hypersensitive to numerous substances, and frequently develops a small rash somewhere on his body. He is not even sure of all the things he is sensitive to! All he knows is that over the course of his lifetime he has had a skin rash at least once a month somewhere on his body. He has been to the pharmacy to purchase anti-itch cream in many different brands and strengths. Jerry's doctor usually advises him to purchase the OTC or prescription-strength product known as hydrocortisone cream.

The time has come again when Jerry develops a small rash and asks the doctor which strength he will need to treat this one. Just like anybody else, Jerry has a small collection of these creams in his medicine cabinet that are still in date and available for use. The problem, however, lies in getting the correct strength when he has only certain amounts of certain strengths. It seems that he does not have enough of the strength the doctor ordered this time, so he wonders if he can mix them.

1. Jerry is to use hydrocortisone 1% cream. All he has available is 2.5% and 0.25%. How many grams of 2.5% hydrocortisone cream should be mixed with 240 g of 0.25% hydrocortisone cream to make 1% hydrocortisone cream?

   _____

   _____

   _____

   _____

2. The doctor tells Jerry to divide the total amount of cream calculated in question #1 into 6 even doses for application. How many grams are in each dose?

   _____

   _____

   _____

   _____

3. What is the total amount of 1% hydrocortisone cream Jerry mixed?

   _____

   _____

   _____

   _____

4. Jerry decides to divide the total amount of 1% hydrocortisone cream he has mixed into 2 ounce jars. How many jars does he need?

_____

_____

_____

_____

ACTIVITY 16-2: Case Study—Gelcaps

Instructions: Read the following scenario and then answer the critical thinking questions.

Maryann works in a mid-sized veterinarian compounding pharmacy. Each day brings something new and creative. She may receive an order for suppositories for medium-size rodents or syringes filled with antibiotics for baby birds. Maryann's job requires her to have solid math skills and excellent aseptic technique.

Compounding is used to formulate prescriptions when no commercial strength is available—and animal pharmaceuticals are a very narrow field. Compounding medications for animals fills a void in a world where little is known about what works on a grand scale for a general species. More and more information appears every week for new formulations and animal behavior. With these updates occurring constantly, Maryann must stay on top of her education and training to remain an asset to her chosen field.

A major part of Maryann's compounding is the creation of various gelcaps for various medications. It is a very convenient form for most animals, and flavoring is easily added to this drug form under most conditions.

1. The following formula is to make a total of 50 gelcaps. How much of each ingredient is needed to make only 10 gelcaps?

FORMULA

caffeine	0.6 g
aspirin	2.0 g
inert ingredient	0.25 g

_____

_____

_____

_____

2. How much is needed to make 15 capsules?

_____

_____

_____

_____

3. What is the total number of grams of all 3 ingredients for 20 capsules?

_____

_____

_____

_____

ACTIVITY 16-3: Case Study—Bulk

Instructions: Read the following scenario and then answer the critical thinking questions.

Note: False names are used for the homeopathic substances in this case study.

Part of the day at the homeopathic manufacturing pharmacy where Lynette works is spent mixing large batches of specialty gels for patients who require these large amounts to fill their prescriptions. A variety of herbs is available to Lynette here, and it always smells like a fresh meadow of grass and trees. Lynette has to wear all the appropriate gear, such as gloves and gowns, because the strength of some of these compounds can cause hypersensitivity skin reactions.

As her employer is a small facility, part of Lynette's duties includes the purchasing of the larger-size containers, lids, and packaging tools. It is not uncommon for Lynette to make a 2,000 g jar full of homeopathic gel for muscle aches. All the compounds in this facility come in at least four different strengths.

1. Lynette is making histkatel crucious gel for muscle fatigue. She needs to have a 6% final concentration. How many grams of 10% histkatel crucious gel should be mixed with 1,800 g of 5% histkatel crucious gel to make the 6% gel?

_____

_____

_____

_____

2. How much is the total amount of histkatel crucious gel compounded?

_____

_____

_____

_____

3. How many pounds does this total add up to?

_____

_____

_____

_____

4. Lynette is to package the bulk gel into as few 8 ounce sealed jars as she can. How many jars does she need?

_____

_____

_____

_____

LAB 6-1: Alligation in the Kitchen

Objective:

Calculate and measure using the alligation method to gain experience measuring liquids and visualizing the relationship between different concentrations.

Pre-Lab Information:

- Review Chapter 16, "Alligations," in the textbook.
- Gather the following materials:
  - 20, 50, and 100 mL graduated cylinders
  - bottle of chilled soda, such as ginger ale or Sprite®
  - chocolate, cherry, or strawberry syrup
  - paper cups to contain the liquid "medication"

Explanation:

As a pharmacy technician, you may use the alligation method when you need to mix together two products that have different percent strengths of the same active ingredient. This exercise gives you the opportunity to experience working with liquids of differing concentrations using the alligation method.

Activity:

Use the materials in the preceding list to prepare the following "prescriptions" using the alligation method. You may use the alligation table below as a guide.

Remember, to find the mL needed for each %, you take the parts high ÷ TOTAL parts × the mL you want.

Note: The % for each "soda/syrup" is fictitious; obviously, you will be using 100% soda and 100% syrup.

Sample Alligation Table

% High:		Parts High:
	% Desired:	
% Low:		Parts Low: Total Parts:

You may round your answers to the nearest whole number.

1. You are asked to prepare 150 mL of a 50% soda/syrup solution. You have on hand a 90% soda solution and syrup (0%). Using the alligation method, calculate the mL of each solution and prepare the "Rx."

   a. mL 90% soda: _____

   b. mL syrup: _____

2. You are asked to prepare 200 mL of a 30% syrup/soda solution. You have on hand a 70% syrup solution and a 50% soda solution. Using the alligation method, calculate the mL of each solution and prepare the "Rx."

   a. mL 50% soda: _____

   b. mL 70% syrup: _____

3. You are asked to prepare 120 mL of a 1:8 soda solution. You have on hand a 50% soda solution and a 1:100 syrup solution. *Note:* You must convert the ratio to % to use the alligation table. Calculate the mL of each solution and prepare the "Rx."

   a. mL soda: _____

   b. mL syrup: _____

Student Name: _____

Lab Partner: _____

Grade/Comments: _____

_____

_____

Student Comments: _____

_____

_____

CHAPTER 17
Parenteral Calculations

After completing Chapter 17 from the textbook, you should be able to:	Related Activity in the Workbook/Lab Manual
1. Illustrate the principle of basic dimensional analysis.	Review Questions Pharmacy Calculation Problems PTCB Exam Practice Questions Activity 17-1, Activity 17-3, Activity 17-4, Lab 17-1
2. Calculate flow duration for parenteral products.	Review Questions Pharmacy Calculation Problems PTCB Exam Practice Questions Activity 17-1, Lab 17-1
3. Calculate the volume per hour for parenteral orders.	Review Questions Pharmacy Calculation Problems PTCB Exam Practice Questions Activity 17-2, Activity 17-3, Activity 17-4, Lab 17-1
4. Calculate the drug per hour for parenteral products.	Review Questions Pharmacy Calculation Problems PTCB Exam Practice Questions Activity 17-2, Activity 17-3, Activity 17-4, Lab 17-1
5. Calculate drip rates in both drops/minute and milliliters/hour.	Review Questions Pharmacy Calculation Problems PTCB Exam Practice Questions Activity 17-2, Activity 17-3, Activity 17-4, Lab 17-1
6. Calculate TPN milliequivalents.	Review Questions Pharmacy Calculation Problems PTCB Exam Practice Questions Lab 17-1

INTRODUCTION

The preparation and administration of parenteral products, such as IVs, infusions, TPN, and chemotherapy, require the performance of specific calculations. It is common for individuals to become overwhelmed and confused when approaching complex pharmacy calculations. The truth is, however, that although many pharmacy calculations appear to be complex, they are in actuality very simple. Often described as the most difficult and challenging calculations used in pharmacy, parenteral calculations, drip rates and TPN milliequivalents are all solved with basic, fundamental math and arithmetic skills. The use of proportions, cross-multiplication, and dimensional analysis will aid you in performing virtually all parenteral calculations that you will need to solve as a pharmacy technician.

REVIEW QUESTIONS

Match the following.

1. drop factor

2. drops per minute

3. mg/hr

4. flow rates

5. flow rate duration

6. hypertonic solutions

7. isotonic solutions

8. hypotonic solutions

9. IV infusion

10. micro drip

11. TPN

12. mL/hr

a. solutions that have osmotic pressure equal to that of cell contents

b. length of time over which an IV will be administered

c. amount of fluid to be administered intravenously per hour

d. term describing a number of pharmacy calculations used in the preparation of IV infusions

e. dose that will be administered per hour of infusion

f. solution made to replenish many of the body's basic nutritional needs via parenteral administration

g. compounded solution that provides fluids, specific medications, nutrients, electrolytes, and minerals

h. volume of medication to be administered per minute

i. solutions that have greater osmotic pressure than cell contents

j. solutions that have a lower osmotic pressure than cell contents

k. abbreviated listing referring to a specific drip rate

l. most commonly used drip rate; 60 gtts/mL

Solve the following problems.

13. A 2 L IV bag is being administered at a rate of 400 mL per hour. How long will this IV bag last?
_____

14. A 2 L IV is to be administered at 500 mL/hr. How long will the IV last? _____

15. A patient is set to start a 250 mL infusion of amoxicillin in lactated Ringers 5% at noon. The bag is to be administered at a rate of 125 mL per hour. At what time will the infusion be complete?
_____

16. Three 500 mL IV bags are to be infused at a rate of 150 mL per hour. How long will these three bags last? _____

17. Three 2 L IV bags containing ciprofloxacin and NS are set to be administered at a rate of 250 mL per hour at 1:00 p.m. When will all three bags be completely administered? _____

18. A patient is to receive 500 mL infused over 2 hours. What is the rate of infusion in mL per hour?
_____

19. A 500 mL IV, containing 2 mg of Toradol®, is to be given over 100 minutes. What is the rate of infusion in mL per hour? _____

20. 500 mL of D5W containing 1 g of lidocaine hydrochloride is to be given over 250 minutes. What is the infusion rate in mL per hour? _____

PHARMACY CALCULATION QUESTIONS

Calculate the following.

1. How many hours will a 2 L bag of TPN last if it is scheduled to run at 90 mL/hr?

2. A bag of heparin IV with a concentration of 25,000 units/250 mL is to be hung for a patient. How many units per hour will the patient receive if the solution is infusing at 50 mL/hr?

3. What is the flow rate in mL/hr for vancomycin 1 g/250 mL IV, if it is to infuse over 90 minutes?

4. What is the flow rate in gtts/min for 100 mL of an antifungal to be administered over 60 minutes? The tubing is calibrated at 60 gtts/mL.

5. If a 1 L bag of D5NS with 20 KCl is hung at 0700, when will the new bag be due if it is running at 125 mL/hr?

PTCB EXAM PRACTICE QUESTIONS

1. If a 1 liter bag of D5W is run through an IV into a patient's arm over 8 hours, what is the rate of infusion in mL/hr?
   a. 100
   b. 10
   c. 12.5
   d. 125

2. If a 1,000 mL bag of normal saline is run at 100 mL/hr, how long will the bag last?
   a. 8   c. 12
   b. 10   d. 6

3. If the infusion rate for an IV is 80 mL/hr and it is run for $4\frac{1}{2}$ hours, how many mL has the patient received?
   a. 300   c. 360
   b. 320   d. 380

4. How many drops per minute will a patient receive if an IV of 1,000 mL of 5% dextrose injection is run in over 8 hours? The drip factor is 15 drops/mL.
   a. 8   c. 32
   b. 16   d. 43

5. You receive an order for heparin IV to infuse at 1,000 units per hour. What will be the flow rate in mL/hr for a 500 mL bag of D5W with 25,000 units of heparin?
   a. 5   c. 2
   b. 10   d. 1

ACTIVITY 17-1: Case Study—Iron Dextran

Instructions: Read the following scenario and then answer the critical thinking questions.

After arguing with his then-girlfriend of whom his family did not approve, Philip drove away from the house in an angry state. He is certain now that he was not in the right frame of mind to be driving that night. The car spun out of control on a fairly isolated road and hit a tree. Eventually, Philip made it out alive, but he spent 12 weeks in the hospital recuperating. He did not call his family as he probably should have, because the last time he spoke to them, things ended on bad terms. It has now been 8 months since the accident, and Philip has not seen his family during that time. He is reuniting with them now to discuss the accident because he had decided that it would help him heal emotionally.

Philip was lucky to have made it back to health. He suffered a concussion, a fractured arm, and multiple bruises. The doctors told him he lost a lot of blood, but he is not exactly sure from what part of his body or how much. Philip received excellent care at the major medical center, where he recalls being on numerous medications. Now all his family members are sharing stories of various hospital stays, and the discussion turns to the medications they recall getting, especially the IVs that hung on the poles while they were inpatients. Philip recalls one, called iron dextran, being "really black."

1. The first dose of iron dextran that Philip received was a test dose of 25 mg in 100 mL NS infused over 20 minutes. What was the concentration of this piggyback?

   _____

   _____

   _____

   _____

2. What was the infusion rate per minute for this test dose of iron dextran?

   _____

   _____

   _____

   _____

3. Philip's total daily dose of iron dextran became 1 g, mixed in a 1 L bag of NS and infused over 8 hours. What was the rate per hour?

_____

_____

_____

_____

4. Using the same information as in question #3, how much iron dextran did Philip receive per hour?

_____

_____

_____

_____

ACTIVITY 17-2: The Delicate Art of TPN Compounding

TPN stands for total parenteral nutrition. It may also be referred to as central parenteral nutrition (CPN), parenteral nutrition, or hyperalimentation. Regardless of what it is called in different parts of the country a TPN is an intravenous infusion containing dextrose (carbohydrates), amino acids (protein), water, and sometimes lipids (fats). TPN provides nutrients to patients with medical conditions that prevent them from physically eating, absorbing nutrients via their gastrointestinal systems, or absorbing enough calories through normal eating. Special TPNs are also used for premature infants who have undeveloped digestive systems. Other additives can be mixed into a TPN, such as famotidine, insulin, multivitamins, and a variety of electrolytes.

TPNs can be complex and require adherence to certain protocols throughout the entire process, from when a physician writes an order to when a technician compounds the product. Compounding a TPN manually the first few times can be nerve-racking, but after a while it becomes an art.

Compounding a TPN

Proper procedures must be strictly followed when preparing a TPN. After the pharmacy receives the TPN order, the pharmacist needs to calculate the correct percentages of dextrose, amino acids, water, and occasionally lipids. The lipids are often given separately, mostly because of an increased risk of precipitation and other problems that can occur when the additives in a TPN are not completely compatible. The pharmacist also calculates the amount of additional electrolytes to be added, making sure that the patient is not getting too much or too little of a mineral. Examples of some electrolytes are trace elements, potassium chloride, potassium phosphate, calcium gluconate, sodium acetate, and sodium phosphate. Certain medications such as insulin or ranitidine, can also be added. Multiple vitamins and vitamins such as folic acid or thiamine may be added to the admixture as well.

Automated TPN Compounding

If a hospital or home infusion pharmacy compounds a high volume of TPNs every day, it may take advantage of automated compounding equipment to assist in the workflow. A pharmacist puts the TPN order into the compounder's computer, and then a technician sets up the compounder with a special tubing set that connects all the solutions to the compounder. The compounder is operated in a horizontal laminar airflow hood using aseptic technique. One type of compounding machine measures all the main components (dextrose, water, and the amino acids), while another type measures out the electrolytes, vitamins, and other additives. The technician attaches a special tube from the bag to the compounder and hangs the bag on a scale. Through the series of tubes and pumps, this sophisticated technology slowly fills the bag with the correct amount of each additive based on the specific gravity of each component. After it is finished, the TPN can be removed and labeled appropriately.

Compounding machines have many advantages. Only minimal handling of the fluids and additives is needed (except to change out empty bottles), so aseptic technique can easily be maintained. The machines are very fast, and an entire custom TPN can be compounded in a few minutes. Most compounding software has safety features to alert the pharmacist if there is too much of an additive, or alerts the technician when a stock bottle has to be changed.

However, there are a few disadvantages. Automated compounding equipment is expensive. It also takes up a lot of space, and a special airflow hood may be dedicated just to TPN compounding. Compounders are very sensitive. Each fluid is measured by specific gravity; thus, you must be careful not to bump the bag that is being filled. If the scale accidentally gets bumped during the filling cycle, the compounder will usually stop in mid-fill. If this happens, the rest of the fill will have to be reprogrammed by a pharmacist, or you may have to start over from the beginning.

Some pharmacies use a combination of automated and manual systems. The bulk fluids, such as dextrose and amino acids, may be run on a compounder, but all the electrolytes may be drawn up separately. It all depends on the volume of TPNs that the pharmacy routinely compounds each day.

Manual Compounding of TPNs

In a smaller pharmacy where TPN usage is too low to warrant expensive automated equipment, other options may be chosen. The pharmacy may incorporate "ready-to-use" TPN solutions that are pre-made by the manufacturer. These come with varying amounts of amino acids, dextrose, water, and sometimes electrolytes. With this type of system, it is difficult to make the truly custom TPNs that are easily compounded with an automated system. If the pharmacy does not use premixed TPNs, dextrose and amino acids can also be purchased separately in different concentrations and different-size bags. Depending on the order, various amounts of each can be manually transferred into one larger bag to create the TPN. In either case, additives such as electrolytes and vitamins must be drawn up by hand in syringes and injected into the TPN. This method can be time-consuming, especially when you are trying to do a custom TPN manually with a dozen more additives in syringes. A key point to remember when compounding TPNs by hand is that TPNs take special care. The more manipulations that are done on a TPN, the harder it is to maintain aseptic technique. As more products are added, the more likely it is that some of them will develop compatibility issues with other ingredients. It is a good idea to gently shake the TPN bag in between additives to encourage a more uniform solution. This also discourages any precipitation from forming; precipitation will, of course, render the TPN unusable. Two types of additives should always be added as far apart from one another as possible. Any electrolyte with a phosphate base can easily form precipitates when it comes in direct contact with a calcium additive. One good method is to add all the phosphates first (such as potassium phosphate or sodium phosphate), then add the other non-calcium additives (such as multivitamins, insulin, or trace elements), and then add the calcium last (like calcium gluconate). Even when using this order of operations, it is a good idea to shake the bag gently in between additives.

Asepsis

Most people who are on TPN are very sick and their immune systems are functioning poorly, so aseptic technique must be strictly followed. With so many additives and fluid transfers, it is vital that you do your best to keep the TPN as free from contaminants as possible. If after compounding a TPN, you notice little white flakes in the TPN, like snow, a cloudy haze, or anything else unusual, notify the pharmacist. Precipitates may occasionally form, even when the greatest care has been taken, and a TPN should not be dispensed if these conditions are present. When lipids are directly added to the TPN, the likelihood of these problems increases, so be attentive and learn what to look for. However, prevention is the best method for creating perfect TPNs. If you are using good aseptic technique, shaking gently between additives, and keeping the phosphates away from the calcium, you will succeed in this delicate art of compounding TPNs.

Activity:

Now that you have learned more about total parenteral nutrition, answer the following questions.

1. What are some advantages of using automated compounding equipment to prepare TPNs?

_____

_____

_____

_____

2. What are some disadvantages of using automated compounding equipment to prepare TPNs?

_____

_____

_____

_____

3. Which two electrolytes should be added apart from each other to avoid possible precipitation in a TPN?

_____

_____

_____

_____

4. Why is it harder to maintain aseptic technique when compounding a custom manual TPN versus one compounded by automation?

_____

_____

_____

_____

5. Search the Internet to find news stories about automated compounding equipment for preparing TPNs and describe what information you find. Based on your research, discuss the importance of the role the pharmacy technician plays in preparing TPNs.

_____

_____

_____

_____

6. Research the electrolytes commonly used in a TPN. List each one and its average dose.

_____

_____

_____

_____

ACTIVITY 17-3: Case Study—IV Lipids

Instructions: Read the following scenario and then answer the critical thinking questions.

Melanie is an experienced pharmacy technician who has worked in a variety of hospital pharmacy settings. Her favorite area, and one in which she is quite proficient, is the IV sterile preparation realm. Over her 24-year career in pharmacy, she has worked in 3 different hospitals mixing IV preparations. She notices that although they all follow good aseptic technique guidelines, each facility may have different ways to go about getting the end result.

For Melanie, this has actually been a real benefit, as she gets to see a variety of ways to perform her craft and can choose the best of each system. For example, the last hospital she worked at made its main TPNs with the lipids added—a mix known as the "three in one" bag. This made the final product very heavy and milky white. Where she works now, the lipids are piggybacked during TPN infusion. The average patient receives 250 mL–500 mL of 10% or 20% lipids solution one to three times a week.

1. What are lipids?

    _____

    _____

    _____

    _____

2. To run a 20% 500 mL bottle of lipids over 12 hours would require what drip rate?

    _____

    _____

    _____

3. Refer to the lipid scenario in question #2. After 3 hours, another piggyback IV is run into the patient and the lipids are slowed down to a 14-hour rate. How much longer would the lipids run with what is left?

    _____

    _____

    _____

    _____

4. Is it necessary to use filter needles when infusing lipids in non-TPN preparations?

    _____

    _____

    _____

    _____

ACTIVITY 17-4: Case Study—IV Solution (TPN)

Instructions: Read the following scenario and then answer the critical thinking questions.

Madeleine is a TPN pharmacy technician at the 600-bed University Hospital. Working in such a large facility, she could easily prepare a total of up to 30 TPNs in any given day. The hospital deals with a lot of specialty cases; they see patients with all kinds of reasons for being on TPN. For example, some patients are in comas, others have swollen throats, and many others are in situations Madeleine might not get to see if she worked in a smaller pharmacy. Madeleine has learned a lot during her four years at this facility. The pharmacists and other pharmacy technicians are eager to share their knowledge whenever they discover a new technique or new medication.

TPNs are a specialty because they provide nutrition for patients who cannot receive it otherwise. This hospital is lucky enough to have a designated area in the pharmacy that is sufficiently sized for preparing TPNs. Ample storage in this area keeps all of the necessary ingredients close at hand, which helps cut down on the time it takes to prepare so many TPNs.

1. Once made and taken to the nursing area to await infusion, how is the TPN stored?
   _____
   _____
   _____
   _____

2. Is a filter needle required for infusion of a TPN, or just during preparation? What size needle would be used?
   _____
   _____
   _____
   _____

3. How long is a TPN good for at room temperature?
   _____
   _____
   _____
   _____

4. What are the key components of a TPN?
   _____
   _____
   _____
   _____

5. Madeleine carefully examines each TPN when she is finished. What is she looking for?
   _____
   _____
   _____
   _____

6. What are electrolytes and why are they important?
   _____
   _____
   _____
   _____

LAB 17-1: Calculating a TPN

Objective:

Calculate the milliliters of electrolytes and additives needed to prepare a TPN.

Pre-Lab Information:

- Review Chapter 17, "Parenteral Calculations," in your textbook.
- Review the information on TPNs contained in Activity 17-2, "The Delicate Art of TPN Compounding."
- Visit legitimate websites that will give you reliable information about TPN compounding, such as www.uspharmacist.com and www.ashp.org.

Explanation:

Depending on the career path you choose to take as a pharmacy technician, you may need to perform the calculations required to make a TPN. There is absolutely no room for error in TPN compounding, so all calculations are checked by at least one pharmacist; some hospitals require two different pharmacists to check calculations before a TPN is compounded.

Activity:

Part One

In the following exercise, you will be given several electrolytes and additives that must be added manually to a TPN. Calculate the milliliters needed to be drawn up in syringes for each additive and an appropriate order in which to insert the additives (to avoid precipitation) into the TPN bag. Round to the nearest tenth if necessary.

Additive	Concentration in Stock	Amount Needed for Order	Milliliters Needed
MVI (multiple vitamins, IV)	Not applicable	10 mL	
calcium gluconate	4.65 mEq/mL	45 mEq	
potassium phosphate	45 mmol/15 mL	30 mmol	
insulin R	100 units/mL	10 units	
magnesium sulfate	0.5 g/mL	5 g	
famotidine	10 mg/mL	20 mg	

Part Two

Visit an infusion pharmacy to witness firsthand how TPN compounding is done. This process is complex, but a demonstration may clear up some confusion.

Student Name: _____

Lab Partner: _____

Grade/Comments: _____

_____

_____

Student Comments: _____

_____

_____

CHAPTER 18
Dosage Formulations and Administration

After completing Chapter 18 from the textbook, you should be able to:	Related Activity in the Workbook/Lab Manual
1. Explain drug nomenclature.	Review Questions Lab 18-1
2. Define medication error.	Review Questions Activity 18-1, Lab 18-2
3. List and explain the rights of medication administration.	Review Questions Activity 18-2, Lab 18-2
4. Identify various dosage formulations.	Review Questions, PTCB Exam Practice Questions Activity 18-2, Activity 18-3, Activity 18-4
5. Identify the advantages and disadvantages of solid and liquid medication dosage formulations.	Review Questions, PTCB Exam Practice Questions Activity 18-4
6. Explain the differences between solutions, emulsions, and suspensions.	Review Questions, PTCB Exam Practice Questions Activity 18-4
7. Explain the difference between ointments and creams.	Review Questions, PTCB Exam Practice Questions Activity 18-4
8. Identify the various routes of administration and give examples of each.	Review Questions, PTCB Exam Practice Questions Activity 18-2, Activity 18-4
9. Give examples of common medications for various routes of administration.	Review Questions Activity 18-1, Activity 18-4, Lab 18-1
10. Identify the advantages and disadvantages of each route of administration.	Review Questions Activity 18-4
11. Identify the parenteral routes of administration.	Review Questions, PTCB Exam Practice Questions Activity 18-4
12. Explain the difference between transdermal and topical routes of administration.	Review Questions, PTCB Exam Practice Questions Activity 18-4
13. Explain the difference between sublingual and buccal routes of administration.	Review Questions, PTCB Exam Practice Questions Activity 18-4
14. Identify the abbreviations for the common routes of administration and dosage formulations.	Review Questions Activity 18-4

INTRODUCTION

As a pharmacy technician, one of your many responsibilities is to work with the pharmacist to prepare and dispense medications to patients. You need to know that drugs can come from one of three sources: natural, synthetic, or genetically engineered.

You also need to understand the concept of drug nomenclature and how to recognize a drug's chemical, generic, and trade/brand names. Finally, you must be familiar with the meaning of and use for each dosage form and route. Most of the dosage forms do imply a certain route that is to be used. However, many dosage forms may be administered via several different routes. For example, a tablet is commonly administered orally, but it can be administered vaginally as well. Liquid medications can also be administered in a variety of ways. If the prescription order is not clear as to the dosage form and route, the pharmacy staff and medical staff must work together to determine what is best for the patient and to avoid medication errors.

REVIEW QUESTIONS

Match the following.

1._____ anhydrous
2._____ aromatic
3._____ aqueous
4._____ dosage form
5._____ emollient
6._____ emulsion
7._____ formulary
8._____ HMO
9._____ homogenous
10._____ hydrophobic
11._____ nomenclature
12._____ occlusive
13._____ oleaginous
14._____ route of administration
15._____ synthesized
16._____ semi-synthetic
17._____ synthetic
18._____ viscous
19._____ volatile

a. actual form of the drug
b. listing of drugs approved for use
c. a group having all the same qualities
d. evaporates rapidly
e. set of names; way of naming
f. without water
g. thick; almost jelly-like
h. containing oil; has oil-like properties
i. having a fragrant aroma
j. a naturally occurring compound that has been chemically altered
k. drug produced in a laboratory to imitate a naturally occurring compound
l. contains water
m. health maintenance organization
n. liquid mixture of water and oil
o. how a drug is introduced into or on the body
p. closes off; keeps air away
q. repels water
r. softening and soothing to the skin
s. drugs that are not naturally occurring in the body

Choose the best answer.

20. Which is not one of the classifications of sources of drugs?
a. genetically engineered
b. synthetic
c. natural
d. manufactured

21. An advantage of solid-dose medications is:
    a. longer shelf life before expiration.
    b. dosing is more accurate.
    c. patients are able to self-administer.
    d. all of the above.

22. Ointments are:
    a. semisolid.
    b. solid.
    c. semiliquid.
    d. jellyfied.

Match the following drugs with their sources.

23. _____ digoxin   a. periwinkle
24. _____ aspirin   b. foxglove
25. _____ human growth hormone   c. synthetic opium
26. _____ vincristine   d. white willow bark
27. _____ OxyContin   e. pituitary gland

Fill in the blanks.

28. _____ are solid medications that are compacted into small, formed shapes.

29. _____ release carbon dioxide when they come into contact with liquid.

30. Also called pastilles or troches, _____ are a hard, disk-shaped, solid dosage form that contain a sugar base.

31. Oleaginous ointments are _____ used to soothe and cool the skin or mucous membranes.

32. _____ are liquid solutions that may be either alcoholic or hydroalcoholic.

PHARMACY CALCULATION PROBLEMS

Calculate the following.

1. Levetiracetam is usually initiated at 20 mg/kg/day in 2 divided doses for a pediatric patient. Determine the dose in milligrams for a boy who weighs 50 pounds.

2. Levetiracetam comes in a 100 mg/mL oral solution. How many milliliters will you need per dose for the patient in question #1?

3. If a patient is receiving ondansetron 4 mg IVP tid prn, what is the maximum daily dosage the patient will receive in milligrams?

4. If an acetaminophen 80 mg suppository is prescribed q4–6 hr prn, what is the maximum number of suppositories the patient can receive in a day?

PTCB EXAM PRACTICE QUESTIONS

1. The best known example of a sublingual tablet formulation is:
   a. hydrochlorothiazide.
   b. nitroglycerin.
   c. digoxin.
   d. codeine.

2. Which would *not* be caused by particulate material in an intravenous injection?
   a. air emboli
   b. thrombus
   c. phlebitis
   d. necrosis

3. Ointments are likely to be used in which route of administration?
   a. oral
   b. buccal
   c. topical
   d. sublingual

4. Which ophthalmic formulation will maintain the drug in contact with the eye the longest?
   a. solution
   b. suspension
   c. gel
   d. ointment

5. What is the term for an injection directly into a joint?
   a. intracardiac
   b. intrapleural
   c. intravitreal
   d. intra-articular

ACTIVITY 18-1: Case Study—Pain and Therapy

Instructions: Read the following scenario and then answer the critical thinking questions.

Mrs. Harris, a mother of four children (all of whom are under 12 years of age), still has a fair amount of pain after her car accident nearly four months ago. She hurt her shoulder and has experienced radiating pain around the upper back, shoulder, and neck for months now. However, the doctors say that nothing major is wrong, and she does not need surgery.

Initially Mrs. Harris was prescribed a strong painkiller, along with ibuprofen for the inflammation; then she was taken off the painkiller. However, her pain continued even weeks after the accident, and she was prescribed Vicodin one to two tablets two to three times daily as needed. Mrs. Harris is in so much pain that if she does not take the Vicodin in time, she is unable to move for a while after ingesting the dose. Whenever she exerts herself, she finds that the pain intensifies, and she can barely make it to the next timed dose. If she takes the Vicodin on time, she is relaxed so much that the pain is just a memory.

In addition to the pain medication, her doctor is going to order physical therapy for Mrs. Harris, in an attempt to help with mobility. The doctor has the nurse phone the therapy center and arrange for a recurring appointment for Mrs. Harris to begin physical therapy.

1. What are some considerations regarding therapy scheduling for Mrs. Harris?

_____

_____

_____

2. Even though Mrs. Harris blames all of her pain on the car accident, do you think the fact that she has four children at home contributes to her condition? Why or why not?

_____

_____

_____

3. Can you think of other side effects that Mrs. Harris might experience from the pain medicine when the physical therapy begins?

_____

_____

_____

ACTIVITY 18-2: Case Study—The Elderly and Medicine

Instructions: Read the following scenario and then answer the critical thinking questions.

Mrs. Wheaten is a lovely 87-year-old woman who reminds you of your grandmother. When she was in her 50s, she was diagnosed with bipolar depression; she has been coming to the retail pharmacy where you work for more than 22 years. Over the years, she has slowed down a bit and has had a few medical conditions arise. For example, she has high blood pressure that is hard to control, and sometimes has trouble breathing. She is also being treated with lithium for her bipolar condition. Other than that, she is much healthier than many people 10 years younger.

Today she presents at the pharmacy with a cough, stuffy nose, and slight headache. As with most people in the winter, Mrs. Wheaten has developed a cold with cough. She requests a box of pseudoephedrine, which is behind the counter. She also requests a recommendation from the pharmacist as to which cough medicine to take, how often, for how long, and how much. Mrs. Harris has an aspirin allergy and would like to stay away from drugs containing aspirin.

1. What does the pharmacist take into consideration about Mrs. Wheaten before recommending a drug selection and dose?

_____

_____

_____

2. How do you handle her request for pseudoephedrine?

_____

_____

_____

3. Mrs. Harris would also like to know how much ibuprofen she can take to make her headache go away. How much should be given in this situation?

_____

_____

_____

ACTIVITY 18-3: Case Study—Long-Acting Option

Instructions: Read the following scenario and then answer the critical thinking questions.

Matthew is a 45-year-old male who has been battling depression for a very long time. At your pharmacy, his medication history is a catalogue of one depression medicine after another, with each one seeming to fail only to be replaced by a prescription for another. Because he usually takes his medicine two to three times a day, the number of tablets dispensed to Matthew over the last year alone totals about 1,000.

You feel sorry for this patient because he visits so much—approximately every two to three weeks—for a new medication. Sometimes his mood is pleasant and he can carry on a conversation, but during some visits he seems disorganized and lost, and talks to himself. Some of the pharmacy staff refer to him as "The Ghost of Mr. Matt." You think at first that Matthew seems scattered at times because his medicine is changed so often.

During one of the conversations you had with Matthew, he told you that a friend comes by at seven in the morning and cooks him a nice breakfast, complete with a glass of milk. The rest of the day he either sleeps or gets busy. He says that his thoughts get so scattered as the day progresses that he becomes forgetful and cannot remember a thing.

Today Matthew has come to the pharmacy to pick up yet another new medicine for his depression: bupropion 75 mg twice a day. While at the intake window, you ask if he needs anything else and he says he sure doesn't think so, that he has enough medicine to supply an army.

1. Why do you think Matthew has an overstock of medication?

_____

_____

_____

2. Can you see any medication option for Matthew's situation today?

_____

_____

_____

3. What is the advantage of the option you selected over what he has been prescribed over the past year?

_____

_____

_____

ACTIVITY 18-4: Dosage Forms

Correct interpretation of standard pharmacy abbreviations found on prescriptions and medical orders is critical in your role as a pharmacy technician. Equally important is your ability to determine the appropriate route of administration for the dosage form given.

Activity:

The three scenarios that follow document each patient's current medical condition or history. After reading each scenario, use your knowledge of that patient's unique situation to determine which dosage form would be most beneficial to her or him.

Scenario 1

Anka, a 37-year-old woman, has just been hospitalized. She has a stomach virus and has been experiencing vomiting and diarrhea for three days. The doctor wants to give her ondansetron 4 mg tid prn for the nausea. He has also ordered IV fluids to help with her dehydration.

Scenario 2

Jared, a 7-year-old boy, has been admitted to the hospital. His mother brought him in because he had a bad seizure an hour and a half ago. He was diagnosed with a seizure disorder the year before. Jared seems coherent, and has no other medical issues. His physician would like to start him on a different medication, levetiracetam 200 mg bid.

Scenario 3

Jaime, a 3-year-old boy, has been complaining of a sore throat and is having trouble swallowing. He also has a mild fever. His mother called his pediatrician, who said to give him acetaminophen 80 mg every 4–6 hours until the doctor could see him the next morning.

Questions:

1. What is the best dosage form of ondansetron for Anka, based on her current medical condition?

   _____

   _____

   _____

   _____

2. What is the best dosage form of levetiracetam for Jared?

   _____

   _____

   _____

   _____

3. Which dosage form would you choose to give to Jaime for his fever and sore throat?

   _____

   _____

   _____

   _____

4. Why do you think there are so many different kinds of dosage formulations?

_____

_____

_____

_____

5. What is the difference between transdermal and topical routes of administration?

_____

_____

_____

_____

6. What is the difference between sublingual and buccal routes of administration?

_____

_____

_____

_____

7. See how well you remember the abbreviations for the common routes of administration and dosage formulations by completing the following table.

	Route of Administration	Abbreviation
a.	buccal	
b.	by mouth	
c.	external	
d.	inhalation	
e.	injection	
f.	intradermal	
g.	intramuscular	
h.	intravenous	
i.	intravenous push	
j.	mouth/throat	
k.	nasal	
l.	ophthalmic	
m.	oral	
n.	otic	
o.	rectally	
p.	subcutaneous	
q.	sublingual	
r.	transdermal	

LAB 18-1: Identifying Chemical, Generic, and Brand Names of Drugs

Objectives:

Recognize and describe the differences between chemical, generic (nonproprietary), and brand/trade (proprietary) drug names.

Explain which types of names are commonly used and the purpose of the United States Adopted Names Council (USAN).

Pre-Lab Information:

- Review Chapter 18, "Dosage Formulations and Administration," in your textbook.
- Search on the Internet for the United States Adopted Names Council. One webpage you might try is http://www.ama-assn.org/ama/pub/category/2956.html. Research the USAN's main purpose, scope of practice, and approved drug-name stems.

Explanation:

When a drug company develops a new drug, it has to name it. Three different names are assigned to the drug. The chemical name, which is based on the chemical formula of the medication, is rarely used in pharmacy practice. For example, the full chemical name of Tylenol® is N-acetyl-p-aminophenol. (You can see why it is used by only a handful of people, generally scientists or chemists.)

A generic name or nonproprietary name is also assigned to each drug. Generic drug names are not usually capitalized. If the medication is in the same class as another medication, it may have a similar suffix or stem. For example, most beta blockers have an "-olol" ending, like aten*olol* or metopr*olol*. The drug manufacturer may enlist the help of the USAN to give a unique generic name to the new drug. USAN's primary goal is to create a name that will not look or sound like that of another drug already in existence.

The proprietary name (brand/trade name) is always capitalized, and symbols may indicate that the name is trademarked. This usually also indicates that the company has a patent on the medication. While under patent protection, the drug will be marketed exclusively under the brand name. A drug patent is good for 20 years, but after research, development, and animal and clinical trials, only a few years may actually be left on the patent. After the patent expires, other companies can manufacture the drug under its generic name.

Activity:

Part One

In each of the following questions there are three drug names. You must determine which are the chemical, generic, and trade names. In addition, you must search USAN's approved stems on the Internet, and determine the appropriate category for each drug based on its generic name.

> Hint:
> Look at the suffix. For example, for candesartan, look for "-sartan" on the USAN stems page; you will find that it is an angiotensin II receptor antagonist.

1. (S)-1-[N2-(1-carboxy-3-phenylpropyl)-L-lysyl]-L-proline dehydrate _____

   lisinopril _____

   Zestril _____

   Category: _____

2. famciclovir _____

   Famvir _____

   2-[2-(2-amino-9H-purin-9-yl)ethyl]-1,3-propanediol diacetate _____

   Category: _____

3. Zantac _____

   N[2-[[[5-[(dimethylamino)methyl]-2-furanyl]methyl]thio]ethyl]-N′-methyl-2-nitro-1,1-ethenediamine HCl _____

   ranitidine _____

   Category: _____

4. 3-[2-(dimethylamino)ethyl]-N-methyl-indole-5-methanesulfonamide succinate (1:1) _____

   Imitrex _____

   sumatriptan succinate _____

   Category: _____

5. celecoxib _____

   Celebrex _____

   4-[5-(4-methylphenyl)-3-(trifluoromethyl)-1H-pyrazol-1-yl] benzenesulfonamide _____

   Category: _____

Part Two

Review the following list of drug names, and note for each whether it is a brand (B) or generic (G) name. Then, determine the route of administration of each drug. Note that all drug names in the list appear in lower case so as not to give you any clues.

Drug	Brand or Generic?	Route of Administration?
nicoderm		
pulmicort respules		
miconazole		
tetrahydrozoline		
cortisporin		
insulin		
benzylpenicillin		
atorvastatin		
elidel		
zolpidem		
enbrel		
monistat		
oxycodone		
spiriva		
duragesic		
flonase		
rhinocort aqua		
benzaclin		

Student Name: _____

Lab Partner: _____

Grade/Comments: _____

_____

_____

Student Comments: _____

_____

_____

_____

LAB 18-2: Reporting Medication Errors and Adverse Reactions

Objectives:

Explain the importance of reporting medication errors and adverse drug reactions to your employer and the FDA.

Demonstrate a procedure used to report adverse drug reactions (ADRs) to MedWatch.

Pre-Lab Information:

- Review Chapter 18, "Dosage Formulations and Administration," in your textbook.
- Visit the website www. medwatch. gov. Research the different methods for reporting adverse reactions and drug errors. Learn which products can be reported and which products are exempt. Locate Form 3500 and its instructions.

Explanation:

Thousands of ADRs occur annually. These ADRs include patients' unusual reactions to drugs, as well as medication dosing errors. These reactions and errors can lead to hospitalization and medical intervention, permanent disability, and even death. MedWatch is a national reporting program through the U.S. Department of Health and Human Services, which is overseen by the FDA. Such occurrences should be reported through your pharmacy's internal ADR system, typically by telephone, e-mail, or fax. In addition, ADRs should be reported to MedWatch. You can do this online or by downloading Form 3500. By compiling data related to medication errors or adverse reactions via MedWatch, the FDA is better able to determine if a product is unsafe or if medical practices at a hospital are irresponsible. It is our responsibility as healthcare professionals to report these instances, which will help maintain a safe and comfortable environment for our patients.

Activity:

Download and print Form 3500 from the MedWatch website. Then, read the following mock scenario that describes an ADR. Using the information given, fill out Form 3500 as if it were a real adverse reaction. The following information has been dramatized and does not represent a real, identifiable individual or drug. *Do not* mail the form to MedWatch or complete the form online, as this would be considered fraudulent reporting.

Scenario

On 6/9/08, Mr. Jones started a new medication, Diaglitazone 10 mg, once daily. Diaglitazone is a new medication produced by FarmTek for the treatment of diabetes. Six hours later, at approximately 1:00 p.m., Mr. Jones presented to the emergency room with abdominal complaints. By 9:00 p.m., his liver and kidneys had completely shut down, and he then suffered cardiac failure. He was pronounced dead at 1:50 a.m. on 6/10/08. His wife indicated that he was 54 years old and weighed about 190 lb. Although he had been diabetic for 10 years, he had no previous history of liver or kidney problems. He did not require insulin injections, but had been taking lipystatin 50 mg once daily for slightly elevated cholesterol. He had been taking another diabetes medication, glucozide 7 mg, but he had stopped taking it on 6/8/08 in order to start the new medication. Other than the cholesterol, he had no previous heart or blood pressure issues. He was Caucasian, a nonsmoker, and walked every day for exercise. Lab tests confirmed that there was no existing kidney, liver, or heart disease. The doctors suspected an adverse reaction to the new drug, Diaglitazone.

1. You are a pharmacy technician on duty in the emergency room satellite pharmacy the night Mr. Jones is brought to the hospital. Complete Form 3500 to the best of your ability with the information given in the scenario.

2. Why do you think the doctors suspect an adverse reaction, when Mr. Jones had taken only one dose?

_____

_____

_____

_____

3. What do you think could happen if this type of incident were reported to MedWatch?

_____

_____

_____

_____

4. Could this type of incident be prevented? Explain.

_____

_____

_____

_____

Student Name: _____

Lab Partner: _____

Grade/Comments: _____

_____

_____

Student Comments: _____

_____

_____

CHAPTER 19
The Body and Drugs

After completing Chapter 19 from the textbook, you should be able to:	Related Activity in the Workbook/Lab Manual
1. Explain the differences between pharmacodynamics and pharmacokinetics.	Review Questions, PTCB Exam Practice Questions Activity 19-1, Activity 19-2
2. Understand the ways in which cell receptors react to drugs.	Review Questions Lab 19-1, Lab 19-2
3. Describe mechanism of action and identify and understand its key factor.	Review Questions Activity 19-3, Lab 19-2
4. Explain how drugs are absorbed, distributed, metabolized, and cleared by the body.	Review Questions, PTCB Exam Practice Questions Activity 19-1, Activity 19-2, Activity 19-3, Lab 19-1, Lab 19-2
5. Explain the difference between fat-soluble and water-soluble drugs and give examples of each.	Review Questions Lab 19-3
6. Identify and explain the effect of bioavailability and its relationship to drug effectiveness.	Review Questions Activity 19-3, Activity 19-4, Activity 19-5
7. Understand addiction and addictive behavior.	Review Questions, PTCB Exam Practice Questions Lab 19-1
8. Describe the role of the pharmacy technician in identifying drug-abusing patients.	Review Questions Lab 19-1
9. List and identify some drugs that interact with alcohol.	Review Questions Lab 19-1

INTRODUCTION

Pharmacology is the study of drugs, including their composition, uses, application, and effects. Although the pharmacist is responsible for using his or her specialized knowledge to provide pharmaceutical care to patients, pharmacy technicians too must understand the basics of pharmacology. *Pharmacodynamics* is the study of how drugs produce their effects on the desired cells and how the drug is then processed by the body. *Pharmacokinetics* is the study of how the body handles drugs, how drugs are changed from their original form into something that the body can use, and how they are eliminated from the body.

REVIEW QUESTIONS

Match the following.

1._____ absorption
2._____ agonist
3._____ bioavailability
4._____ clearance
5._____ dependency
6._____ excretion
7._____ metabolism
8._____ addiction
9._____ tolerance
10._____ metabolites
11._____ half-life
12._____ distribution
13._____ antagonist

a. physical need
b. a drug that prevents receptor activation
c. a drug that activates a receptor
d. how a drug moves from the blood to the site of action
e. how drugs are eliminated
f. compulsive craving or need
g. substance produced by metabolization
h. time required for serum level to decrease by half
i. process of transforming a drug
j. requires larger dose to achieve the same effect
k. the amount of a drug that becomes available
l. how a drug moves from the introduction site to the bloodstream
m. time it takes a drug to be eliminated

Choose the best answer.

14. Pharmacodynamics can be described as the study of:
    a. receptors producing a specific effect.
    b. what the body does to a drug.
    c. the process of drug interactions.
    d. how drugs are made.

15. How a drug works is called:
    a. effective distribution.
    b. chemical process.
    c. mechanism of action.
    d. potency.

16. An antagonist:
    a. is very annoying.
    b. produces certain predicted actions.
    c. stops a drug from working.
    d. neutralizes the effects of narcotics.

17. ED50 refers to the:
    a. amount of a drug that produces half the normal response.
    b. binding medium used in compounding.
    c. effective drug at 50%.
    d. top 50 most effective drugs.

18. Once a drug is at a serum concentration of less than 3%, it is considered:
    a. nontoxic.
    b. out of range.
    c. eliminated.
    d. ineffective.

19. Which is not a form of excretion?
    a. breath
    b. sweat
    c. urine
    d. odor

20. Pinocytosis is a:
    a. form of transportation of drugs into cells.
    b. a medicinally powerful plant.
    c. a rare type of gum disease.
    d. none of the above.

21. Which of the following is not a route of absorption?
    a. stomach lining
    b. blood
    c. urine
    d. cell membranes

22. The rate of administration of a drug is determined by the:
    a. prescriber.
    b. research and development process.
    c. chemical nature of the drug.
    d. health of the patient.

23. Denial is a sign of:
    a. addiction.
    b. dependence.
    c. truth avoidance.
    d. psychological unbalance.

24. Which of these drugs may produce increased heart rate when mixed with alcohol?
    a. hydrocodone
    b. alprazolam
    c. metformin
    d. warfarin

25. Pharmacokinetics is a term for the study of:
    a. receptors producing a specific effect.
    b. the time course of a drug in the body.
    c. the process of drug interactions.
    d. how drugs are made.

True or False?

26. Salts do not matter if the active ingredient is the same.

    T   F

27. The absorption of a drug governs the bioavailability of that drug.

    T   F

28. Addiction is the same as dependence.

    T   F

29. Withdrawal is not difficult if a patient is merely dependent on a drug.

    T   F

30. When a person constantly needs a higher dose of a drug, it is a sure sign that the patient is an addict.

    T   F

PHARMACY CALCULATION PROBLEMS

Calculate the following.

1. On Wednesdays, a pharmacy offers a 10% discount for senior citizens on all their prescription and over-the-counter medications. How much would a person save if she purchased $219 worth of medications?

2. A man has brought in a prescription for ranitidine 300 mg. The physician did not indicate DAW on the prescription, but the customer insists on getting the brand-name drug. The insurance company will charge him the price of the co-pay, plus the difference in price between the generic and the brand. This is known as *difference pricing*. Calculate the cost to the customer if the generic price is $11.25 and the brand price is $27.95. His usual co-pay is $10.

   Hint: co-pay + (brand price − generic price) = cost

3. A customer wants to pay difference pricing for a prescription for nabumetone 500 mg. The price of the brand-name drug is $85.49 and the price of the generic drug is $17.99. Her usual co-pay is $15. What will the insurance company charge the customer using difference pricing?

4. A pharmacy sets its retail prices as a 30% markup of cost. If a 100-count bottle of acetaminophen 325 mg costs the pharmacy $1.49, what will the retail price be for this item?

PTCB EXAM PRACTICE QUESTIONS

1. What is a drug called that binds to a receptor but does not produce a response?
   a. agonist
   b. antagonist
   c. hormone
   d. neurotransmitter

2. Which organ is responsible for drug metabolism?
   a. kidney
   b. intestines
   c. lungs
   d. liver

3. All of the following drugs may be used to assist patients with smoking cessation *except*:
   a. nicotine patch.
   b. Chantix®.
   c. Dilantin®.
   d. Wellbutrin®.

4. Which organ is responsible for the majority of drug excretion?
   a. kidney
   c. lungs
   b. intestines
   d. liver

5. Drug tolerance usually only involves which of the following components?
   a. physiological factors
   c. the immune system
   b. psychological factors
   d. obsessive compulsive behavior

ACTIVITY 19-1: Common Drug Interactions

Look up http://www.mayoclinic.com/health/serotonin-syndrome/DS00860 on the Web. This problem—serotonin syndrome—occurs most frequently with combinations of drugs or herbal supplements that affect serotonin.

Perform a general Internet search on the phrase "herbal interactions." You should find many legitimate papers and documents regarding this specific type of interaction.

Although monitoring drug interactions is primarily the pharmacist's job, pharmacy technicians need to be aware of possible interactions and responsible when they encounter or learn of such possibilities. Many drug interactions tend to occur in older patients, as this population may have many different medical treatments for various maladies. As a person takes more and more medications for various illnesses (many take five or more different medications every day), the potential for drug-drug interaction increases. However, interactions do not occur only in the elderly.

With more medications being made available over the counter, and the recent boom in herbal supplementation, many people treat themselves for various conditions without consulting a physician or a pharmacist. This factor increases the potential for serious drug-drug and drug-herb interactions. Most people are under the impression that herbal supplements are "natural" and that they have no side effects. This is not necessarily true, as you will learn. Certain herbal supplements can indeed cause interactions, and many also have side effects. St. John's wort, supposed to be a natural antidepressant, can interact badly if the patient is also taking prescription antidepressant medication. Those taking St. John's wort also experience photosensitivity and are easily sunburned. Dietary supplements, such as herbal remedies, are not regulated by the FDA as medications are. Therefore, different brands of the same supplement may not have the same potency or quality. For example, a customer who has not had a reaction to a drug changes to a higher-potency supplement and thereby unknowingly triggers a drug-herb interaction.

Diet can also play a role in interactions. Patients taking warfarin as a blood thinner are advised to avoid green, leafy vegetables and other foods that contain high amounts of vitamin K, because it is a natural coagulant. Because it has the opposite effect of warfarin, vitamin K will interfere with the blood-thinning properties of the warfarin. As you can see, it is important to be vigilant about possible interactions by educating yourself so that you can be responsive when you observe a potential for these interactions.

In pharmacy practice, computers are programmed with alerts that display when a potential drug interaction is found. This warning system is invaluable to pharmacy professionals and their customers. Nevertheless, pharmacy is a dynamic and changing environment. New drugs are introduced every year and updated information regarding current medications is not always available, so there may be times when the warning system does not have the information necessary to issue potential alerts. In addition, if a patient goes to multiple pharmacies, it is difficult to track likely drug interactions for all of the patient's medications.

Activity:

The following table lists some common drug-herb and drug-drug interactions, plus a simplified explanation of the effects of their interactions. Review the table, then use it to answer the questions that follow.

Drug or Drug Class	Interacting Drug, Class, or Herb	Interaction
antidepressants (ex.: SSRIs, MAOIs)	St. John's wort	Increased risk of serotonin syndrome
antiplatelets (ex.: aspirin, warfarin, clopidogrel)	gingko biloba	Increased risk of bleeding
benzodiazepine hypnotics (ex.: alprazolam, diazepam)	antifungal agents ending in -azole (ex.: fluconazole)	Increased benzodiazepine serum concentrations, resulting in excessive sedation
benzodiazepines, antipsychotics, alcohol	kava kava	Increased sedation, lethargy, disorientation
digoxin	clarithromycin and erythromycin	Increased digoxin levels, resulting in digoxin toxicity
fluoroquinolones (ex.: ciprofloxacin, levofloxacin)	antacids containing aluminum or magnesium compounds	Decreased absorption of fluoroquinolones
MAO inhibitors (ex.: phenylzine, tranylcypromine)	anorexiants (ex.: phentermine, dextroamphetamine), decongestants (ex.: pseudoephedrine, phenylephrine), vasopressors (ex.: dopamine, ephedrine)	Increased risk of serotonin syndrome or hypertensive event due to increased norepinephrine levels
nitrates (ex.: nitroglycerin, isosorbide)	sildenafil, tadalafil, vardenafil	Increased risk of hypotension
oral contraceptives (estrogen-progestin combinations)	most antibiotics, rifampin	Increased risk of contraceptive failure
SSRIs (ex.: escitalopram, fluoxetine, paroxetine)	MAO inhibitors	Increased risk of serotonin syndrome
tetracyclines	penicillins, antacids, compounds containing iron	Reduced absorption of tetracyclines
theophylline	fluoroquinolone antibiotics (ex.: ciprofloxacin, levofloxacin, fluvoxamine)	Increased theophylline levels, resulting in theophylline toxicity
warfarin	aspirin, NSAIDs, antihyperlipidemics-fibric type (ex.: fenofibrate, gemfibrozil), thyroid hormones	Increased risk of bleeding
warfarin	barbiturates (ex.: butalbital, phenobarbital), Vitamin K (phytonadione), vegetables containing vitamin K	Decreased anticoagulant effect

Questions:

1. What type of reaction might occur if a patient was taking paroxetine and St. John's wort?
   a. increased risk of bleeding
   b. increased risk of serotonin syndrome
   c. decreased absorption of paroxetine
   d. decreased absorption of St. John's wort

2. Which of the following can cause a drug-diet interaction?
   a. consuming antacids with ciprofloxacin
   b. taking antibiotics with oral birth control
   c. eating spinach while taking warfarin
   d. taking an iron supplement with tetracycline

3. What reaction might occur if a patient was taking nitroglycerin capsules and sildenafil?
   a. increased risk of hypotension
   b. increased risk of bleeding
   c. increased risk of contraceptive failure
   d. increased risk of serotonin syndrome

4. Many people feel that it is unnecessary to disclose to their physician all the dietary supplements they take. Could this common practice jeopardize their health? Explain your answer.

   _____

   _____

   _____

   _____

5. Go to the following website: http://www.mayoclinic.com/health/serotonin-syndrome/DS00860

   a. When does serotonin syndrome occur most frequently?

   _____

   _____

   b. What are the signs and symptoms of serotonin syndrome?

   _____

   _____

   c. Name five drugs that can lead to serotonin syndrome.

   _____

   _____

   d. What are ways to prevent serotonin syndrome?

   _____

   _____

6. What popular herbs or OTC products do you or your family use on a regular basis? Choose one and research common drug interactions with that herbal or OTC product.

_____

_____

_____

_____

ACTIVITY 19-2: Case Study—Identifying Drug Interactions

Instructions: Read the following scenario and then answer the critical thinking questions.

An elderly woman brings four new prescriptions to the pharmacy, two from one physician and two from another. The first prescription is for ciprofloxacin 500 mg tablets and fluconazole 100 mg tablets. The second prescription is for theophylline 200 mg tablets and warfarin 2 mg. The 82-year-old woman seems a little confused as the technician confirms her personal information. She goes to sit down while the technician starts entering the prescriptions into the computer. While entering the new prescriptions, the technician notices that this customer has many different medications on her profile. Upon further examination, the technician discovers that many of the medications are also from different doctors. For example, the woman recently had prescriptions filled for clonazepam, fenofibrate, magnesium oxide, levothyroxine, and sertraline. Multiple drug-drug interactions alerts appear on the monitor. The technician asks her supervising pharmacist to review the alerts.

1. Using this customer's profile, list all the potential interactions between her existing medications and her new prescriptions.

_____

_____

_____

_____

2. If you were the technician, how would you handle this situation?

_____

_____

_____

_____

3. Do you think the customer's age could play a factor in potential drug-drug interactions? Explain.

_____

_____

_____

_____

ACTIVITY 19-3: Case Study—Calcium Bioavailability

Instructions: Read the following scenario and then answer the critical thinking questions.

Christina is a 48-year-old premenopausal woman with a busy lifestyle. She pops a vitamin every now and then, but she gleans most of her daily vitamins from eating a wide variety of foods. Although she is not a health nut, she has many female friends who are in tune with the nutritional needs of women as they age. One thing she knows for sure is that she needs to look at supplementing her diet with calcium for healthy bones as she ages.

Christina finds that many products claim to have better bioavailability than others. It is much too confusing because, as she discovers, each person you ask may give a different answer. Each of her friends seems to be taking a different type of calcium, and the products they use have a wide variety of pricing and claims.

Christina finally decides to research this on her own and make her own decision on which calcium supplement she will begin taking. The choices she encounters go by different names, and she does not know what this means. She finds calcium acetate, calcium citrate, calcium carbonate, calcium gluconate, calcium phosphate, calcium lactate, and eggshell calcium.

1. What is meant by the term *bioavailability*?

2. What are the differences between the calcium forms listed?

3. Which of these is a "better" calcium supplement? Which one has the best bioavailability?

4. Are there any special considerations when taking calcium supplements?

5. What information in this scenario makes you agree that now is a good time for Christina to begin taking a calcium supplement?

6. What substances interfere with calcium absorption?

ACTIVITY 19-4: Case Study—Fastest Response

Instructions: Read the following scenario and then answer the critical thinking questions.

Charlie is a 72-year-old widower who leads a fairly sedentary lifestyle and smokes two packs of cigarette a day. He takes occasional daily walks and trips to the grocery store. Almost every morning Charlie take his fox terrier mix for a five-block walk to meet some other friends at the local donut shop. In the earl morning hours, the men talk and tell tales of what life was like when they were growing up. This all take place over some delicious home-baked pastries and several cups of questionable-tasting coffee.

Charlie's medication profile resembles that of any man his age who has not lived a healthy life: some bloo pressure problems, shortness of breath, and a heart condition or two. Charlie has seen some pretty scar times, medically speaking, in his life. For example, he has been the recipient of nitroglycerin many time He has received it in a buccal extended-release tablet form, a sublingual tablet form, and an ointment form

1. Describe an example of when Charlie would have received nitroglycerin buccal extended-release tablets. How long did the tablet take to work?

    _____

    _____

    _____

2. Describe an example of when Charlie would have used sublingual nitroglycerin tablets. How long did it take before Charlie felt the effects of the medication and then what was the duration of its effectiveness?

    _____

    _____

    _____

3. Describe an example of when Charlie would have used a nitroglycerin ointment.

    _____

    _____

    _____

4. How does nitroglycerin work?

    _____

    _____

    _____

ACTIVITY 19-5: Case Study—Time for Some Help

Instructions: Read the following scenario and then answer the critical thinking questions.

Marilyn Strader is a 38-year-old, happily married housewife and mother. She has a wonderful husband named Kenneth, two beautiful children, and a small circle of friends she meets with on Saturday to shop or go on outings. She and her husband own a mid-sized auto repair shop that does moderately well. The shop specializes in Ford vehicles and has a staff of about 15 mechanics and office people.

In addition to owning the shop, Kenneth has volunteered through the national reserves since coming out of military service about 11 years ago. Unfortunately, the military has now called Kenneth up for active service, and he is to be deployed to a foreign country for an undetermined amount of time. The family goes into a tailspin emotionally. Marilyn is very upset, but knows she must support her husband, who feels it is his duty to serve.

As the date of Kenneth's deployment comes closer, Marilyn is consumed with the thought of being alone. She feels as if a death is coming to the family, and is overwhelmed with the idea of running the shop and taking care of her children without her husband. Kenneth tries to train her in all the things he does in the shop (outside of auto repair) to prepare her for his absence. To accommodate this extra time requirement, Marilyn no longer visits with her friends on the weekends. She is so sad that she cannot even take their calls, because she is tired of them asking if she is all right. No, she is not all right, she wants to scream—but instead she trudges along almost like she is in a bad dream.

When Kenneth is a week away from deployment. Marilyn has reached a new low. She barely gets dressed, never visits anyone, and seems to cry at the drop of a hat. She is tense and irritable, and complains of body aches. Kenneth forces her to see her doctor, who examines her and prescribes nortriptyline.

1. Given the facts in this scenario, what do you think Marilyn is suffering from?

   _____

   _____

2. What is nortriptyline?

   _____

   _____

   _____

3. What are some precautions with nortriptyline regarding dosage and use?

   _____

   _____

   _____

4. How long does it take for nortriptyline to take effect?

   _____

   _____

   _____

LAB 19-1: Web Research Activity—Understanding Addiction

Objective:

Learn about drug addiction by researching the topic at the Mayo Clinic website.

Pre-Lab Information:

- Review Chapter 19 in the textbook.
- Explore the following website: http://www.mayoclinic.com/health/drug-addiction/DS00183

Explanation:

This exercise will give you the opportunity to research and better understand drug addiction. As a pharmacy technician, you may encounter patients with drug addictions, and it is important to understand this disease.

Activity:

Using the Mayo Clinic website (http://www.mayoclinic.com/health/drug-addiction/DS00183), answer the following questions.

1. What are the six general characteristics that you might find with any drug addiction?

   _____

   _____

   _____

   _____

   _____

   _____

2. What are the five risk factors for developing an addiction?

   _____

   _____

   _____

   _____

3. What are the seven major complications associated with addiction?

   _____

   _____

   _____

   _____

   _____

   _____

4. After withdrawal treatment (detoxification), what are the three major categories of continued addiction treatment?

_____

_____

_____

5. What are the four steps listed in this article that parents can take to help children avoid addiction?

_____

_____

_____

_____

Student Name: _____

Lab Partner: _____

Grade/Comments: _____

_____

_____

Student Comments: _____

_____

_____

LAB 19-2: Web Research Activity: Agonists Versus Antagonists

Objective:

Learn about drug agonists and antagonists by researching the topic using the Merck Manual website.

Pre-Lab Information:

- Review Chapter 19 in the textbook.
- Visit the website: http://www.merck.com/mmhe/sec02/ch012/ch012b.html

Explanation:

This exercise gives you the opportunity to explore the differences in how agonist and antagonist drugs affect the body. The following is a summary of the information you should study.

Drugs that target receptors are classified as either agonists or antagonists. *Agonist* drugs activate, or stimulate, their receptors, triggering a response that increases or decreases the cell's activity. *Antagonist* drugs block access by or attachment of the body's natural agonists, usually neurotransmitters, to receptors and thereby prevent or reduce cell responses to natural agonists.

Agonist and antagonist drugs can be used together in patients with asthma. For example, albuterol (Proventil® or Ventolin®) can be used with ipratropium (Atrovent®). Albuterol, an agonist, attaches to specific (adrenergic) receptors on cells in the respiratory tract, causing relaxation of smooth muscle cells and thus widening of the airways (*bronchodilation*). Ipratropium, an antagonist, attaches to other (cholinergic) receptors, blocking the attachment of acetylcholine, a neurotransmitter that causes contraction of smooth muscle cells and thus narrowing of the airways (*bronchoconstriction*). Both drugs work to widen the airways, and thus make breathing easier, but they do so in different ways.

Beta blockers, such as propranolol (Inderal®), are a widely used group of antagonists. These drugs are used to treat high blood pressure, angina (chest pain caused by an inadequate blood supply to the heart muscle), and certain abnormal heart rhythms, as well as to prevent migraines. They block or reduce stimulation of the heart by the agonist hormones epinephrine (adrenaline) and norepinephrine (noradrenaline), which are released during stress. Antagonists such as beta blockers are most effective when the concentration of the agonist is high in a specific part of the body. A roadblock stops more vehicles during the 5:00 p.m. rush hour than at 3:00 a.m.; similarly, beta blockers, given in doses that have little effect on normal heart function, may have a greater effect during sudden surges of hormones released during stress, and thereby protect the heart from excess stimulation.

Activity:

Using the Merck Manual website (http://www.merck.com/mmhe/sec02/ch012/ch012b.html) and the preceding summary, answer the following questions.

1. What effect does an agonist drug have on its respective receptor?

   _____

   _____

   _____

2. What effect does an antagonist drug have on its respective receptor?

   _____

   _____

   _____

3. Beta blockers are antagonist drugs. What effect do they have on the heart?

   _____

   _____

   _____

4. Albuterol is an agonist drug. What effect does it have on the respiratory system?

   _____

   _____

   _____

Student Name: _____

Lab Partner: _____

Grade/Comments: _____

_____

_____

Student Comments: _____

_____

_____

LAB 19-3: Fat-Soluble and Water-Soluble Drugs

Objective:

Explore the differences between fat-soluble and water-soluble drugs by researching the topic using the Merck Manual website.

Pre-Lab Information:

- Review Chapter 19 in the textbook.
- Explore the website at http://www.merck.com/mmhe/sec02/ch011/ch011d.html
- Review the following summary of the website material.

Drug distribution refers to the movement of drug to and from the blood and various tissues of the body (for example, fat, muscle, and brain tissue) and the relative proportions of drug in the tissues.

After a drug is absorbed into the bloodstream, it rapidly circulates through the body. The average circulation time of blood is 1 minute. As the blood recirculates, the drug moves from the bloodstream into the body's tissues.

Once absorbed, most drugs do not spread evenly throughout the body. Drugs that dissolve in water (water-soluble drugs), such as the antihypertensive drug atenolol (Tenormin®), tend to stay within the blood and the fluid that surrounds cells (interstitial space). Drugs that dissolve in fat (fat-soluble drugs), such as the anesthetic drug halothane, tend to concentrate in fatty tissues. Other drugs concentrate mainly in only one small part of the body (for example, iodine concentrates mainly in the thyroid gland), because the tissues there have a special attraction for (affinity) and ability to retain the drug.

Drugs penetrate different tissues at different speeds, depending on the drug's ability to cross membranes. For example, the anesthetic thiopental (Pentothal®), a highly fat-soluble drug, rapidly enters the brain, but the antibiotic penicillin, a water-soluble drug, does not. In general, fat-soluble drugs can cross cell membranes more quickly than water-soluble drugs can. For some drugs, transport mechanisms aid movement into or out of the tissues.

Some drugs leave the bloodstream very slowly, because they bind tightly to proteins circulating in the blood. Others quickly leave the bloodstream and enter other tissues, because they are less tightly bound to blood proteins. Some or virtually all molecules of a drug in the blood may be bound to blood proteins. The protein-bound part is generally inactive. As unbound drug is distributed to tissues and its level in the bloodstream decreases, blood proteins gradually release the drug bound to them. Thus, the bound drug in the bloodstream may act as a reservoir of the drug.

Some drugs accumulate in certain tissues, which can also act as reservoirs of extra drug. These tissues slowly release the drug into the bloodstream, keeping blood levels of the drug from decreasing rapidly and thereby prolonging the effect of the drug. Some drugs, such as those that accumulate in fatty tissues, leave the tissues so slowly that they circulate in the bloodstream for days after a person has stopped taking the drug.

Distribution of a given drug may also vary from person to person. For instance, obese people may store large amounts of fat-soluble drugs, whereas very thin people may store relatively little. Older people, even when thin, may store large amounts of fat-soluble drugs because the proportion of body fat increases with age.

Explanation:

This exercise gives you the opportunity to explore how the characteristics of drugs differ depending on whether the compound is water- or fat-soluble.

Activity:

Using the Merck Manual website (http://www.merck.com/mmhe/sec02/ch011/ch011d.html) and the preceding summary, answer the following questions.

1. What are the implications for a drug that is fat-soluble?

   _____

   _____

   _____

   _____

2. In what organs is a fat-soluble drug likely to accumulate?

   _____

   _____

   _____

3. What are the implications for a drug that is water-soluble?

   _____

   _____

   _____

   _____

Student Name: _____

Lab Partner: _____

Grade/Comments: _____

_____

_____

Student Comments: _____

_____

_____

CHAPTER 20
Drug Classifications

After completing Chapter 20 from the textbook, you should be able to:	Related Activity in the Workbook/Lab Manual
1. List and explain a variety of drug classifications.	Review Questions, PTCB Exam Practice Questions Activity 20-1, Activity 20-2, Activity 20-3, Activity 20-4, Lab 20-1
2. Understand the five pregnancy categories and how they affect drug classifications.	Review Questions, PTCB Exam Practice Questions Lab 20-1, Lab 20-2
3. List and describe the five schedules of controlled substances and identify drugs assigned to each schedule.	Review Questions, PTCB Exam Practice Questions Activity 20-2, Lab 20-1, Lab 20-3

INTRODUCTION

Pharmacology is a complex, diversified, and intriguing science. To be successful as a pharmacy technician, you need to understand the basics of how drugs are classified, what the classifications mean, and what conditions or diseases the drugs in each class treat. Drugs are classified into categories according to their chemical ingredients, the method by which they are used, and by the body organ they affect. They are further designated by separate classes and groups. Two of the most common classifications are therapeutic usefulness, such as analgesics (used to relieve pain), and pharmacological activity, such as diuretics (used to promote the excretion of urine). Two other important classifications of drugs are: pregnancy categories, which are used to determine the potential harm to the fetus if the drug is taken by a pregnant woman; and controlled substances classes, which are used to indicate the potential for abuse or the addictive nature of the drug.

Many drugs are also available over the counter (OTC). It is an important pharmacy technician duty to understand drug classifications and which drug products are available to patients OTC. This will ensure that the patient receives the best possible care, as properly educated and well-informed pharmacy technicians are much more helpful to both patients and pharmacists.

REVIEW QUESTIONS

Match the following.

1._____ edema   **a.** apprehension, uneasiness

2._____ anxiety   **b.** loss of connection to reality

3._____ teratogenetic   **c.** swelling

4._____ psychosis   **d.** lack of energy, despair, guilt

5._____ depression   **e.** birth defect

Match the brand-name drug with its generic name.

6. meperidine	**a.** Inderal®
7. clonidine	**b.** Flagy®
8. metronidazole	**c.** Nizoral®
9. mebendazole	**d.** Thorazine®
10. ketoconazole	**e.** Norvasc®
11. acyclovir	**f.** Zithromax®
12. cefdinir	**g.** Lunesta®
13. clarithromycin	**h.** Demerol®
14. enalapril	**i.** Vasotec®
15. propranolol	**j.** Dilantin®
16. amlodipine	**k.** Ativan™
17. lorazepam	**l.** Vermox®
18. phenytoin	**m.** Restoril®
19. chlorpromazine	**n.** Biaxin®
20. temazepam	**o.** Omnicef®
21. eszopiclone	**p.** Catapres®

Choose the best answer.

22. An example of a calcium channel blocker medication is:
    a. felodipine.
    b. gemfibrozil.
    c. labetolol.
    d. hydralazine.

23. Loop diuretics are indicated for:
    a. osteoporosis.
    b. gout.
    c. infection.
    d. edema.

24. Antiemetics are indicated for:
    a. diarrhea.
    b. nausea and vomiting.
    c. constipation.
    d. acid reflux.

25. A hemostatic drug is used to:
    a. increase blood plasma.
    b. stop bleeding.

    c. prevent blood clots.
    d. break down blood clots.

26. An example of a C-III drug is:
    a. codeine with acetaminophen.
    b. fentanyl.

    c. phenobarbital.
    d. THC.

27. The class of drug that has the highest potential for addiction and abuse is:
    a. C-I.
    b. C-II.

    c. C-III.
    d. C-IV.

28. Which is an OTC antipyretic?
    a. Benadryl®
    b. Pepcid®

    c. Dramamine®
    d. Tylenol®

29. Of the following pregnancy categories, which indicates the lowest risk?
    a. A
    b. B

    c. C
    d. D

30. NSAIDs are used to treat:
    a. inflammation and pain.
    b. fever.

    c. none of the above.
    d. both a and b.

PHARMACY CALCULATION QUESTIONS

1. A medication is to be dosed at 10 mg/kg/day in 3 divided doses. The patient weighs 79 kg. How many milligrams will the patient get in each dose?

2. A patient weighing 182 pounds requires 0.25 mg/kg bolus dose of abciximab. Abciximab comes in a concentration of 2 mg/mL. How many mL will the technician need to draw up for the bolus?

3. Ziprasidone for injection yields a 20 mg/mL concentration after reconstitution. How many mL would be required for a 10 mg dose?

4. 40 units of insulin R must be added to a TPN. If the concentration of insulin R is 100 units/mL, how many mL should be added to the TPN?

PTCB EXAM PRACTICE QUESTIONS

1. Diflucan® (fluconazole) belongs to which of the following drug classifications?
   a. aminoglycoside
   b. antiviral
   c. cephalosporin
   d. antifungal

2. Inderal® (propranolol) belongs to which of the following drug classifications?
   a. calcium channel blocker
   b. beta-adrenergic blocker
   c. ACE inhibitor
   d. antihyperlipidemic

3. Paxil® (paroxetine) belongs to which of the following drug classifications?
   a. antidepressant
   b. antipsychotic
   c. anticonvulsant
   d. antiparkinson

4. Plavix® (clopidogrel) belongs to which of the following drug classifications?
   a. anticoagulant
   b. antiemetic
   c. antiplatelet
   d. thrombolytic

5. Prevacid® (lansoprazole) belongs to which of the following drug classifications?
   a. H2 antagonist
   b. laxative
   c. antidiarrheal
   d. proton pump inhibitor (PPI)

ACTIVITY 20-1: Case Study—Inhalers

Instructions: Read the following scenario and then answer the critical thinking questions.

Harold is a 57-year-old man who has a multitude of health problems, including asthma that is getting worse as he ages. He is on many inhalers and his healthcare provider often adds or changes them as Harold's disease progresses. For the most part, Harold is compliant with his inhaler regime, although sometimes when he has an asthma attack he will take extra puffs with any number of the inhalers he has. Sometimes it just happens to be the one he is closest to at the time. In short, Harold uses the inhalers inappropriately at times when he feels he is not breathing well. Lately Harold is using them more and more, especially after walking his dog around the block or while gardening.

Harold's medication profile consists of the following inhalers for his asthma: Flovent®, Atrovent®, Foradil®, and Proventil®. Today he brings a prescription for Aerobid® to the retail pharmacy where you work to have it filled. Harold believes that this inhaler is for the asthma attacks he has been having after he walks the dog.

1. Looking at Harold's profile, which inhaler is in the same class as the newly prescribed Aerobid®?
   _____
   _____
   _____
   _____

2. What precautions would the pharmacist warn about while counseling this patient, especially given the preceding information?

_____

_____

_____

_____

3. What medical conditions could interact with the new inhaler?

_____

_____

_____

_____

4. How should the new drug be used?

_____

_____

_____

_____

ACTIVITY 20-2: Case Study—New Drug Approval

Instructions: Read the following scenario and then answer the critical thinking questions.

The United States Food and Drug Administration (FDA) is the agency that approves drugs (for specified indications). Numerous drugs are reviewed each year after a lengthy process involving an application and submission of clinical trial results. The FDA, under the Controlled Substances Act, classifies medications, including pain medications, in one of five schedules according to certain criteria.

A new drug has recently come up for review and the manufacturers are hoping to receive approval soon for an indication of mild to moderate pain relief. All the proper paperwork and positive clinical trial information is complete. It appears as if this medication is going to make a huge difference to many people for pain management.

This new drug has a low potential for abuse relative to the other substances in a higher abuse potential schedule classification than this rating; also, abuse of this drug may lead to only limited physical dependence or psychological dependence relative to the drugs in a higher abuse potential schedule classification than this rating. The new drug has a currently accepted medical use in treatment in the United States.

1. Another pain medication in this schedule is pregabalin. What is the controlled substance classification for pregabalin?

_____

_____

2. What other medication in this same classification is used for diarrhea?

_____

_____

3. Which two federal departments determine which drugs are added to or removed from the various schedules?

_____

_____

ACTIVITY 20-3: Case Study—Multiple Sedatives

Instructions: Read the following scenario and then answer the critical thinking questions.

Doug is a 27-year-old male and quite the party animal. Doug has a problem with drugs. Ever since he was a teenager, Doug has experimented with just about anything he could get his hands on.

After a night of partying with alcohol and drugs, Doug crashed his car into a brick wall and somehow survived, although to this day he has a lot of back, neck, and shoulder pain. His doctor prescribes Vicodin®, as the pain is severe at times, and Doug manages quite well with this therapy. This pain does not affect Doug's drug addiction, however, as he still uses any medicine he can get for any reason. For example, if he has a headache, he takes a Vicodin® and three acetaminophen because, as he says, "Three must be better than two!"

Doug once again went to a party. He took his Vicodin at 8:00 p.m. and his pain subsided by 8:45 p.m. At the party one hour later, Doug had about two alcoholic drinks. Someone at the party offered Doug a Valium® and he gladly ingested it. Doug grew tired and when he arrived home at 11:30 p.m. all he wanted to do was sleep, so he fell into bed. By morning Doug could barely breathe or move. Somehow he managed to call an ambulance and was taken to the hospital.

1. Why couldn't Doug breathe the next morning?

_____

_____

_____

2. Are there any special concerns regarding Doug's use of both Vicodin® and acetaminophen?

_____

_____

_____

3. If Doug were to overdose on the Vicodin® and acetaminophen, what treatment might the hospital provide?

_____

_____

_____

ACTIVITY 20-4: Matching the Disease State/Symptom to the Drug Classification

As a pharmacy technician, you need to be familiar with which drug classifications are used to treat specific disease states or symptoms.

Activity:

The following exercise presents a list of symptoms and disease states and a second list of drug classifications. Review the symptoms and diseases in the first list, then choose the best treatment for each from the second list. Write the letter of the drug classification on the line next to the corresponding symptom/disease state.

Symptoms and Disease States

1. _____ allergic reaction due to exposure to cats
2. _____ chronic gastric reflux
3. _____ exercise-induced asthma
4. _____ athlete's foot
5. _____ herpes simplex II
6. _____ strep throat infection
7. _____ high blood pressure
8. _____ nausea
9. _____ depression
10. _____ back spasms due to recent injury
11. _____ high cholesterol
12. _____ mild sprained ankle
13. _____ seizure disorder
14. _____ schizophrenia
15. _____ edema and hypertension

Drug Classifications

a. proton pump inhibitors
b. macrolides
c. antihistamines
d. antihyperlipidemics
e. antifungals
f. antiemetics
g. antivirals
h. muscle relaxants
i. NSAIDs
j. ACE inhibitors
k. anticonvulsants
l. bronchodilators
m. antipsychotics
n. diuretics
o. SSRIs

LAB 20-1: Memorizing the Top 200 Drugs

Objective:

To memorize the names and uses of the 200 most-prescribed ("top 200") drugs.

Pre-Lab Information:

Review Chapter 20, "Drug Classifications," and the top 200 drug list in Appendix A of the textbook.

Explanation:

It is important for you to know the brand and generic names of the most commonly prescribed drugs, as well as their primary uses.

Activity:

Use the following 12 exercises to help you learn the top 200 drugs.

1. Commonly Used Drugs, Part 1
2. Commonly Used Drugs, Part 2
3. Commonly Used Drugs, Part 3
4. Commonly Used Drugs, Part 4
5. Commonly Used Drugs, Part 5
6. Commonly Used Drugs, Part 6
7. Commonly Used Drugs, Part 7
8. Commonly Used Drugs, Part 8
9. Commonly Used Drugs, Part 9
10. Commonly Used Drugs, Part 10
11. Commonly Used Drugs, Part 11
12. Commonly Used Drugs, Part 12

Note: Duplicate drugs in the top 200 list have *not* been included.

Exercise 1: Commonly Used Drugs, Part 1

Select the generic name of the drug and place the corresponding letter next to the brand name.

Brand Name

1. _____ Advil, Motrin®
2. _____ Ambien®
3. _____ Darvocet-N®
4. _____ Glucophage®
5. _____ HydroDIURIL, Microzide®
6. _____ Keflex®
7. _____ Lasix®
8. _____ Lexapro®
9. _____ Lipitor®
10. _____ Lortab, Vicodin®
11. _____ Maxzide, Dyazide®
12. _____ Nexium®
13. _____ Norvasc®
14. _____ Prelone/Deltasone®
15. _____ Prinivil, Zestril®
16. _____ Proventil, Ventolin®
17. _____ Singulair®
18. _____ Synthroid/Levoxyl®
19. _____ Tenormin®
20. _____ Toprol-XL®
21. _____ Trimox/Amoxil®
22. _____ Xanax®
23. _____ Zithromax®
24. _____ Zocor®
25. _____ Zoloft®

Generic Name

a. albuterol inhaler
b. alprazolam
c. amlodipine
d. amoxicillin
e. atenolol
f. atorvastatin
g. azithromycin
h. cephalexin
i. escitalopram
j. esomeprazole
k. furosemide
l. hydrochlorothiazide
m. hydrocodone w/APAP
n. ibuprofen
o. levothyroxine
p. lisinopril
q. metformin
r. metoprolol ER
s. montelukast
t. prednisone
u. propoxyphene/APAP
v. sertraline
w. simvastatin
x. triamterene/HCTZ
y. zolpidem

Exercise 2: Commonly Used Drugs, Part 2

Select the correct drug use and place the corresponding letter next to the drug name.

Drug Name

1. _____ Advil, Motrin®
2. _____ Ambien®
3. _____ Darvocet-N®
4. _____ Glucophage®
5. _____ HydroDIURIL, Microzide®
6. _____ Keflex®
7. _____ Lasix®
8. _____ Lexapro®
9. _____ Lipitor®
10. _____ Lortab, Vicodin®
11. _____ Maxzide, Dyazide®
12. _____ Nexium®
13. _____ Norvasc®
14. _____ Prelone/Deltasone®
15. _____ Prinivil, Zestril®
16. _____ Proventil, Ventolin®
17. _____ Singulair®
18. _____ Synthroid/Levoxyl®
19. _____ Tenormin®
20. _____ Toprol-XL®
21. _____ Trimox/Amoxil®
22. _____ Xanax®
23. _____ Zithromax®
24. _____ Zocor®
25. _____ Zoloft®

Drug Use

a. anti-anxiety (benzodiazepine)
b. antibiotic
c. antidepressant
d. antihyperglycemic (diabetes)
e. antihypertensive (blood pressure and heart)
f. gastric acid inhibitor
g. lipid-lowering agent
h. narcotic analgesic
i. non-benzodiazepine hypnotic
j. NSAID (inflammation and pain)
k. respiratory (asthma and COPD)
l. steroid (inflammation)
m. synthetic thyroid hormone
n. diuretic

Exercise 3: Commonly Used Drugs, Part 3

Select the brand name of the drug and place the corresponding letter next to the generic name.

Generic Name	Brand Name
1. _____ acetaminophen-codeine	a. Prevacid
2. _____ alendronate	b. Lopressor
3. _____ amitriptyline	c. Prozac
4. _____ amoxicillin clavulanate	d. Ativan
5. _____ cetirizine	e. Plavix
6. _____ clonazepam	f. Endocet/Roxicet/Percocet
7. _____ clopidogrel	g. Augmentin
8. _____ conjugated estrogen	h. Advair Diskus
9. _____ cyclobenzaprine	i. Fosamax
10. _____ fluoxetine	j. Effexor XR
11. _____ fluticasone	k. Coumadin
12. _____ fluticasone/salmeterol	l. Paxil
13. _____ gabapentin	m. Klonopin
14. _____ lansoprazole	n. Zyrtec
15. _____ levofloxacin	o. Protonix
16. _____ lorazepam	p. K-Dur/Klor-Con
17. _____ metoprolol	q. Tylenol/Codeine No. 3
18. _____ oxycodone/APAP	r. Cotrim, Septra, Bactrim
19. _____ pantoprazole	s. Neurontin
20. _____ paroxetine	t. Premarin
21. _____ potassium chloride	u. Flonase
22. _____ sulfamethoxazole/trimethoprim	v. Desyrel
23. _____ trazodone	w. Flexeril
24. _____ venlafaxine	x. Elavil
25. _____ warfarin	y. Levaquin

Exercise 4: Commonly Used Drugs, Part 4

Select the correct drug use and place the corresponding letter next to the brand name.

Brand Name

1. _____ Prevacid
2. _____ Lopressor
3. _____ Prozac
4. _____ Ativan
5. _____ Plavix
6. _____ Endocet/Roxicet/Percocet
7. _____ Augmentin
8. _____ Advair Diskus
9. _____ Fosamax
10. _____ Effexor XR
11. _____ Coumadin
12. _____ Paxil
13. _____ Klonopin
14. _____ Zyrtec
15. _____ Protonix
16. _____ K-Dur/Klor-Con
17. _____ Tylenol/Codeine No. 3
18. _____ Cotrim, Septra, Bactrim
19. _____ Neurontin
20. _____ Premarin
21. _____ Flonase
22. _____ Desyrel
23. _____ Flexeril
24. _____ Elavil
25. _____ Levaquin

Drug Use

a. anti-anxiety (benzodiazepine)
b. antibiotic
c. antibiotic (sulfa derivative)
d. anticoagulant
e. anticonvulsant (neuropathic pain)
f. antidepressant
g. antihistamine (allergy)
h. antihypertensive (blood pressure and heart)
i. antiplatelet and clot inhibitor
j. gastric acid inhibitor
k. C-II narcotic analgesic
l. narcotic analgesic w/Tylenol
m. osteoporosis
n. potassium replacement
o. respiratory inhaler
p. skeletal muscle relaxant
q. steroid inhaler
r. synthetic estrogen hormone

Exercise 5: Commonly Used Drugs, Part 5

Select the generic name of the drug and place the corresponding letter next to the brand name.

Brand Name	Generic Name
1. _____ Zyloprim	a. valsartan/HCTZ
2. _____ Lotrel	b. diazepam
3. _____ Wellbutrin SR	c. fexofenadine
4. _____ Soma	d. tramadol
5. _____ Celebrex	e. ranitidine HCl
6. _____ Cipro	f. ciprofloxacin
7. _____ Clonidine	g. ezetimibe
8. _____ Valium	h. rosiglitazone
9. _____ Vibramycin	i. bupropion HCl
10. _____ Vasotec	j. naproxen
11. _____ Zetia	k. valsartan
12. _____ Allegra	l. amlodipine/benazepril
13. _____ Diflucan	m. celecoxib
14. _____ Prinzide/Zestoretic	n. methylprednisolone
15. _____ Mevacor	o. allopurinol
16. _____ Medrol	p. clonidine
17. _____ Naprosyn/Aleve	q. enalapril
18. _____ Altace	r. lisinopril/HCTZ
19. _____ Zantac	s. lovastatin
20. _____ Avandia	t. ramipril
21. _____ Viagra	u. carisoprodol
22. _____ Ultram	v. doxycycline
23. _____ Diovan	w. fluconazole
24. _____ Diovan HCT	x. sildenafil

Exercise 6: Commonly Used Drugs, Part 6

Select the correct drug use and place the corresponding letter next to the drug name.

Drug Name

1. _____ Zyloprim
2. _____ Lotrel
3. _____ Wellbutrin SR
4. _____ Soma
5. _____ Celebrex
6. _____ Cipro
7. _____ Clonidine
8. _____ Valium
9. _____ Vibramycin
10. _____ Vasotec
11. _____ Zetia
12. _____ Allegra
13. _____ Diflucan
14. _____ Prinzide/Zestoretic
15. _____ Mevacor
16. _____ Medrol
17. _____ Naprosyn/Aleve
18. _____ Altace
19. _____ Zantac
20. _____ Avandia
21. _____ Viagra
22. _____ Ultram
23. _____ Diovan
24. _____ Diovan HCT

Drug Use

a. anti-anxiety (benzodiazepine)
b. antibiotic
c. antidepressant
d. antifungal
e. anti-gout
f. antihistamine (allergy)
g. antihyperglycemic (diabetes)
h. antihypertensive (blood pressure and heart)
i. erectile dysfunction
j. gastric acid inhibitor
k. lipid-lowering agent (cholesterol)
l. non-narcotic analgesic
m. NSAID (inflammation and pain)
n. skeletal muscle relaxant
o. steroid

Exercise 7: Commonly Used Drugs, Part 7

Select the generic name of the drug and place the corresponding letter next to the brand name.

Brand Name	Generic Name
1. _____ Vytorin	a. amphetamine
2. _____ Veetids	b. carvedilol
3. _____ TriCor	c. citalopram
4. _____ Seroquel	d. digoxin
5. _____ Pravachol	e. ezetimibe and simvastatin
6. _____ Phenergan	f. fenofibrate
7. _____ Nasonex	g. folic acid
8. _____ Mobic	h. glipizide ER
9. _____ Lantus	i. glyburide
10. _____ Lanoxin	j. insulin glargine
11. _____ Isordil	k. isosorbide dinitrate
12. _____ Glucotrol XL	l. losartan
13. _____ Folvite	m. meloxicam
14. _____ Flomax	n. methylphenidate XR
15. _____ DiaBeta, Micronase, Glynase	o. mometasone
16. _____ Crestor	p. penicillin VK
17. _____ Cozaar	q. pioglitazone
18. _____ Coreg	r. pravastatin
19. _____ Concerta	s. promethazine
20. _____ Celexa	t. quetiapine
21. _____ Calan	u. risedronate
22. _____ Adderall XR	v. rosuvastatin
23. _____ Actos	w. tamsulosin
24. _____ Actonel	x. verapamil

Exercise 8: Commonly Used Drugs, Part 8

Select the correct drug use and place the corresponding letter next to the drug name.

Drug Name

1. _____ Vytorin
2. _____ Veetids
3. _____ TriCor
4. _____ Seroquel
5. _____ Pravachol
6. _____ Phenergan
7. _____ Nasonex
8. _____ Mobic
9. _____ Lantus
10. _____ Lanoxin
11. _____ Isordil
12. _____ Glucotrol XL
13. _____ Folvite
14. _____ Flomax
15. _____ DiaBeta, Micronase, Glynase
16. _____ Crestor
17. _____ Cozaar
18. _____ Coreg
19. _____ Concerta
20. _____ Celexa
21. _____ Calan
22. _____ Adderall XR
23. _____ Actos
24. _____ Actonel

Drug Use

a. angina/heart
b. antibiotic
c. antidepressant
d. antihistamine/nausea
e. antihyperglycemic (diabetes)
f. antihypertensive (blood pressure and heart)
g. cardiac glycoside (heart)
h. CNS stimulant (ADHD)
i. enlarged prostate (BPH)
j. lipid-lowering agent (cholesterol)
k. nasal anti-inflammatory agent
l. NSAID (inflammation and pain)
m. osteoporosis
n. psychotropic (antipsychotic)
o. vitamin supplement

Exercise 9: Commonly Used Drugs, Part 9

Select the generic name of the drug and place the corresponding letter next to the brand name.

Brand Name	Generic Name
1. _____ Accupril	a. benazepril
2. _____ Aciphex	b. cefdinir
3. _____ Aldactone	c. clindamycin
4. _____ Amaryl	d. digoxin
5. _____ Atarax/Vistaril	e. estradiol
6. _____ Avapro	f. gemfibrozil
7. _____ Cleocin	g. glimepiride
8. _____ Climara/Estraderm	h. hydroxyzine
9. _____ Combivent	i. ipratropium/albuterol inhaler
10. _____ Digitek	j. irbesartan
11. _____ Flagyl	k. latanoprost
12. _____ Glucophage XR	l. losartan/HCTZ
13. _____ Hyzaar	m. metformin ER
14. _____ Kenalog	n. metronidazole
15. _____ Lopid	o. omeprazole
16. _____ Lotensin	p. quinapril
17. _____ Omnicef	q. rabeprazole
18. _____ Prilosec	r. risperidone
19. _____ Restoril	s. spironolactone
20. _____ Risperdal	t. temazepam
21. _____ Topamax	u. topiramate
22. _____ Valtrex	v. triamcinolone
23. _____ Xalatan	w. valacyclovir

Exercise 10: Commonly Used Drugs, Part 10

Select the correct drug use and place the corresponding letter next to the drug name.

Brand Name

1. _____ Accupril
2. _____ Aciphex
3. _____ Aldactone
4. _____ Amaryl
5. _____ Atarax/Vistaril
6. _____ Avapro
7. _____ Cleocin
8. _____ Climara/Estraderm
9. _____ Combivent
10. _____ Digitek
11. _____ Flagyl
12. _____ Glucophage XR
13. _____ Hyzaar
14. _____ Kenalog
15. _____ Lopid
16. _____ Lotensin
17. _____ Omnicef
18. _____ Prilosec
19. _____ Restoril
20. _____ Risperdal
21. _____ Topamax
22. _____ Valtrex
23. _____ Xalatan

Drug Use

a. hypnotic (sleep)
b. gastric acid inhibitor
c. antibiotic
d. respiratory agent
e. psychotropic (antipsychotic)
f. cardiac glycoside (heart)
g. diuretic (blood pressure)
h. antiviral
i. prostaglandin (glaucoma)
j. antihyperglycemic (diabetes)
k. antihypertensive (blood pressure and heart)
l. steroid
m. anticonvulsant
n. lipid-lowering agent (cholesterol)
o. estrogen patch
p. antihistamine

Exercise 11: Commonly Used Drugs, Part 11

Select the generic name of the drug and place the corresponding letter next to the brand name.

Brand Name

1. _____ Allegra-D
2. _____ Antivert
3. _____ Benicar
4. _____ Cardizem CD
5. _____ Cardura
6. _____ Clarinex
7. _____ Cymbalta
8. _____ Detrol LA
9. _____ Evista
10. _____ Glucotrol
11. _____ Glucovance
12. _____ Imitrex
13. _____ Lamictal
14. _____ Macrobid/Macrodantin
15. _____ Minocin
16. _____ OxyContin
17. _____ Phenergan w/codeine
18. _____ Reglan
19. _____ Relafen
20. _____ Remeron
21. _____ Strattera
22. _____ Voltaren
23. _____ Ziac
24. _____ Zyprexa
25. _____ Zyrtec Syrup

Generic Name

a. atomoxetine
b. bisoprolol/HCTZ
c. cetirizine syrup
d. desloratadine
e. diclofenac
f. diltiazem CD
g. doxazosin
h. duloxetine
i. fexofenadine/pseudoephedrine
j. glipizide
k. glyburide/metformin
l. lamotrigine
m. meclizine
n. metoclopramide
o. minocycline
p. mirtazapine
q. nabumetone
r. nitrofurantoin
s. olanzapine
t. olmesartan
u. oxycodone
v. promethazine w/codeine
w. raloxifene
x. sumatriptan
y. tolterodine

Exercise 12: Commonly Used Drugs, Part 12

Select the correct drug use and place the corresponding letter next to the drug name.

Brand Name	Drug Use
1. _____ Allegra-D	**a.** antibiotic
2. _____ Antivert	**b.** antidepressant
3. _____ Benicar	**c.** antihistamine (allergy)
4. _____ Cardizem CD	**d.** antihistamine (dizziness)
5. _____ Cardura	**e.** antihyperglycemic (diabetes)
6. _____ Clarinex	**f.** antihypertensive (blood pressure and heart)
7. _____ Cymbalta	**g.** antitussive (cough)
8. _____ Detrol LA	**h.** CNS stimulant (ADHD)
9. _____ Evista	**i.** gastrointestinal (nausea)
10. _____ Glucotrol	**j.** NSAID (inflammation and pain)
11. _____ Glucovance	**k.** osteoporosis
12. _____ Imitrex	**l.** urinary antispasmodic
13. _____ Lamictal	**m.** narcotic analgesic
14. _____ Macrobid/Macrodantin	**n.** antimigraine
15. _____ Minocin	**o.** psychotropic (antipsychotic)
16. _____ OxyContin	**p.** anticonvulsant (seizures)
17. _____ Phenergan w/codeine	
18. _____ Reglan	
19. _____ Relafen	
20. _____ Remeron	
21. _____ Strattera	
22. _____ Voltaren	
23. _____ Ziac	
24. _____ Zyprexa	
25. _____ Zyrtec Syrup	

Student Name: _____

Lab Partner: _____

Grade/Comments: _____

_____

_____

Student Comments: _____

_____

_____

LAB 20-2: Understanding Pregnancy Categories

Objective:

Understand the importance of caution when pregnant women use prescription drugs.

Pre-Lab Information:

- Review the pregnancy categories discussed in Chapter 20 of the textbook.
- Visit the following FDA Web site: http://www.4women.gov/faq/pregmed.htm

Explanation:

Pregnancy categories are determined on the basis of the potential harm a drug may cause to the fetus. The five pregnancy categories of safety are A, B, C, D, and X, with A being the lowest risk and X being the highest. As a pharmacy technician, it is important for you to understand the concept of risk versus benefit—especially as it applies to drugs taken during pregnancy.

Activity:

Visit the following FDA Web site and use the information there to answer the questions related to drugs used in pregnancy: http://www.4women.gov/faq/pregmed.htm

1. Write the definition of Pregnancy Category A as it applies to *human studies only.*

_____

_____

_____

_____

2. Write the definition of Pregnancy Category B as it applies to *human studies only.*

_____

_____

_____

_____

3. Write the definition of Pregnancy Category C as it applies to *human studies only.*

_____

_____

_____

_____

4. Write the definition of Pregnancy Category D as it applies to *human studies only.*

_____

_____

_____

_____

5. Write the definition of Pregnancy Category X as it applies to *human studies only*.

   _____

   _____

   _____

   _____

6. To which pregnancy category does the drug phenytoin (Dilantin®) belong?

   _____

   _____

7. To which pregnancy category does the drug isotretinoin (Accutane®) belong?

   _____

   _____

8. To which pregnancy category does the drug fluconazole (Diflucan®) belong?

   _____

   _____

9. To which pregnancy category does the drug levothyroxine (Synthroid®) belong?

   _____

   _____

10. To which pregnancy category does the drug ondansetron (Zofran®) belong?

   _____

   _____

Student Name: _____

Lab Partner: _____

Grade/Comments: _____

_____

_____

Student Comments: _____

_____

_____

LAB 20-3: Recognizing Controlled Drugs

Objective:

To recognize which drugs are in Schedule II and understand how these drugs and prescriptions for them are handled.

Pre-Lab Information:

Review the Controlled Drug Categories in Chapter 20 of the textbook.

Explanation:

Because federal and state laws dictate that Schedule II drugs are maintained and dispensed with greater scrutiny, it is important for you to be able to recognize which drugs fall in this category.

Activity:

Visit the DEA online at: http://www.deadiversion.usdoj.gov/schedules/schedules.htm

Then complete the following exercise designed to help you match brand to generic names for Schedule II controlled drugs.

Controlled Drug Exercise:

Select the generic name of the drug and place the corresponding letter next to the brand name, then list the Schedule (I–V) for that particular drug.

Brand Name	Generic Name	Schedule
1. _____ Ambien	a. zolpidem	_____
2. _____ Ativan	b. triazolam	_____
3. _____ Cocaine	c. thiopental	_____
4. _____ Darvon, Darvocet	d. temazepam	_____
5. _____ Demerol	e. secobarbital	_____
6. _____ Dexedrine	f. propoxyphene	_____
7. _____ Dilaudid	g. phentermine	_____
8. _____ Dolophine	h. pentobarbital	_____
9. _____ Duragesic	i. oxycodone	_____
10. _____ Fastin	j. oxazepam	_____
11. _____ Halcion	k. morphine	_____
12. _____ Klonopin	l. midazolam	_____
13. _____ Librium	m. methylphenidate	_____
14. _____ Lorcet, Lortab, Vicodin	n. methadone	_____
15. _____ MS Contin, Oramorph	o. meperidine	_____
16. _____ Nembutal	p. lorazepam	_____
17. _____ OxyContin, Percocet	q. hydromorphone	_____
18. _____ Pentothal	r. hydrocodone/APAP	_____

19. _____ ProSom   s. fentanyl   _____
20. _____ Restoril   t. estazolam   _____
21. _____ Ritalin, Concerta u. diazepam   _____
22. _____ Seconal   v. cocaine   _____
23. _____ Serax   w. clonazepam   _____
24. _____ Valium   x. chlordiazepoxide   _____
25. _____ Versed   y. amphetamine   _____
26. _____ Xanax   z. alprazolam   _____

Student Name: _____

Lab Partner: _____

Grade/Comments: _____

_____

_____

Student Comments: _____

_____

_____

CHAPTER 21
The Skin

After completing Chapter 21 from the textbook, you should be able to:	Related Activity in the Workbook/Lab Manual
1. List, identify, and diagram the basic anatomical structure of the skin.	Review Questions, PTCB Exam Practice Questions Activity 21-1
2. Explain the function or physiology of the skin.	Review Questions, PTCB Exam Practice Questions Activity 21-3, Activity 21-5
3. List and define common diseases affecting the skin and understand the causes, symptoms, and pharmaceutical treatments associated with each disease.	Review Questions, PTCB Exam Practice Questions Activity 21-2, Activity 21-3, Activity 21-4, Activity 21-5
4. Define the following skin diseases and list common drugs used in their treatment: psoriasis, eczema, impetigo, athlete's foot, acne, and lice.	Review Questions, PTCB Exam Practice Questions
5. Discuss the significance of the development of the newest FDA- approved drugs for the treatment of psoriasis.	Review Questions, PTCB Exam Practice Questions

INTRODUCTION

The skin is the largest organ of the body. It consists of three main layers: the epidermis, the dermis, and the subcutaneous layer. Important functions of the skin include serving as a barrier to foreign organisms and debris, managing the regulation of body temperature, excreting salts and excess water, and acting as a "shock absorber" to protect the underlying organs. Unfortunately, the skin plays host to a wide variety of more than 1,000 medical conditions and diseases, ranging from minor irritations to severe infections. Although creams and ointments are widely used to treat skin conditions, treatment options also include oral and injectable medications. As a pharmacy technician, it is important for you to understand the basic anatomy and physiology of the skin and the conditions that affect it, so that you have greater insight into how the drugs used to treat these conditions work.

REVIEW QUESTIONS

Match the following.

1. _____ acne
2. _____ sebum
3. _____ carcinoma
4. _____ pathogenic
5. _____ rosacea
6. _____ mitigation
7. _____ eczema
8. _____ bacteriostatic
9. _____ infection
10. _____ pigmentation
11. _____ bactericidal
12. _____ psoriasis
13. _____ rash
14. _____ parasite

a. oily substance produced by glands
b. an organism living in or on another organism
c. condition of red, inflamed skin
d. disease-causing
e. kills microorganisms
f. inhibits growth of microorganisms
g. inflammatory condition with itch, redness, blisters, and oozing
h. infection plus sebum overproduction
i. invasion of pathogens
j. malignant tumor
k. lessening of severity
l. chronic facial skin disorder accompanied by chronic redness and inflammation
m. coloring of skin
n. noncontagious chronic disease characterized by thick, red, scaly skin

True or False?

15. The skin is the largest organ of the body.

    T   F

16. The outermost layer of the skin is the dermis.

    T   F

17. Eczema is a chronic immune disorder.

    T   F

18. Ringworm is an example of a bacterial infection.

    T   F

19. Greasy foods or chocolate may cause acne.

    T   F

Choose the best answer.

20. Normal body temperature regulated by the skin is:
    a. 98.6 degrees Fahrenheit.
    b. 89.6 degrees Fahrenheit.
    c. 69.8 degrees Celsius.
    d. 98.6 degrees Celsius.

21. Skin infections are not caused by which of the following?
    a. bacteria
    b. cancer
    c. fungi
    d. viruses

22. The most severe burn would be classified as:
    a. first degree.
    c. third degree.
    b. second degree.
    d. fourth degree.

23. The second most common skin cancer is:
    a. malignant melanoma.
    c. basal cell carcinoma.
    b. actinic keratosis.
    d. squamous cell cancer.

Fill in the blanks.

24. An acute, deep infection of the connective tissue is called _____.

25. Small red bumps and intense itching caused by mites is known as _____.

26. A chronic disorder of unknown cause, with symptoms including pimples, lesions, and redness, is _____.

27. The color of the skin is caused by the amount of _____.

28. If a person sustained burns to the leg, groin, and abdomen, he would be burned over _____% of his body.

Match the following ulcer descriptions with their classifications.

29. _____ Stage I   a. lesion extending through skin to the bone
30. _____ Stage II   b. crater-like lesion extending through tissue
31. _____ Stage III   c. reddening of unbroken skin
32. _____ Stage IV   d. abrasion or blister

PHARMACY CALCULATION PROBLEMS

Calculate the following.

1. A prescription reads: "Clindamycin 2% in aquaphilic ointment; 60 g. Apply to affected body part twice daily." The pharmacy stocks clindamycin 150 mg capsules. How many capsules will be needed to prepare this compound?

2. A physician has requested a compound for lidocaine 3% in 120 mL calamine lotion. How many milligrams of lidocaine powder must be added to the calamine lotion for the compound?

3. A compound is to contain equal parts nystatin cream, clotrimazole 1% cream, and triamcinolone 0.05% cream. How many grams of each product will be required to make 4 ounces?

4. A physician wants to dilute 100 mL of a 10% topical solution to a 4% solution with sterile water. How many mL of sterile water will you need?

PTCB EXAM PRACTICE QUESTIONS

1. Which is the middle layer of the skin?
   a. subcutaneous
   b. epidermis
   c. dermis
   d. adipose

2. What is an acute, deep infection of the skin and connective tissue accompanied by inflammation?
   a. basal cell carcinoma
   b. eczema
   c. psoriasis
   d. cellulitis

3. Which drug is used to treat psoriasis?
   a. Enbrel®
   b. clofibrate
   c. Restasis®
   d. Silvadene®

4. What disease is caused by bacteria and an overproduction of sebum?
   a. eczema
   b. acne
   c. psoriasis
   d. cellulitis

5. What kind of skin infection is described as a mycosis?
   a. fungal
   b. bacterial
   c. viral
   d. parasitic

ACTIVITY 21-1: Anatomy Worksheet—The Skin

Label the following illustration of the skin.

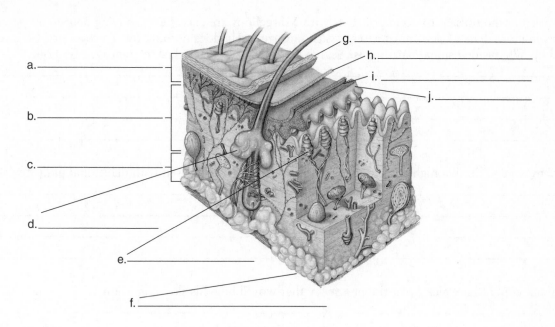

a._____

b._____

c._____

d._____

e._____

f._____

g._____

h._____

i._____

j._____

ACTIVITY 21-2: Case Study—Morgellons

Instructions: Read the following scenario and then answer the critical thinking questions.

Note: Based in part on a true situation.

Mark and his wife Carol built a home in the suburbs three years ago and have been very happy. One day, however, when Mark is working in the den, he begins screaming out his wife's name. Carol runs to him and Mark keeps saying that it feels as if little "bugs" are crawling all over him. He is itching uncontrollably and has a burning sensation. Carol takes Mark to the doctor, who finds nothing, but advises Mark to use an OTC anti-itching cream.

These symptoms continue for weeks, with the addition of constant fatigue. Convinced that the doctor's diagnosis was correct, Mark tries every type of cream and anti-itch product available trying to get control of his symptoms.

Like something out of a science fiction movie, soon Mark develops painful sores all over his body, which ooze blue fibers, white threads, and black specks of sand-like material. Frightened by this, Mike and Carol head to the emergency room. Upon examination, Mike is diagnosed with delusional parasitosis. Mike is convinced that his body has been invaded by some type of parasitic bug, but cannot convince the doctor, who has found no such evidence of parasites. The doctor ignores the small bundles of fibers oozing from the sores and advises Mark to use an OTC antifungal cream.

A few days later, Mark is watching a popular morning news show that discusses a strange skin condition with symptoms exactly like Mark's. They name this condition *Morgellons*. The program states that there are a few cases in the United States, and that the Centers for Disease Control and Prevention is currently investigating. It is not yet known what it is or what might cure it. Healthcare providers have seen a higher incidence of Morgellons patients who also have fibromyalgia, attention deficit/hyperactivity disorder (ADHD), and chronic fatigue syndrome.

Mark makes an appointment with a dermatologist after viewing the TV program and has a sample of his fibers taken and sent to a forensic lab. Results show that the fibers are not related to anything in the national database; it is determined that the fibers are not manmade and do not come from a plant.

1. Patients who present to dermatologists with Morgellons are classified as having delusional parasitosis in more than 95 percent of cases, which unfortunately does nothing for the sores or fiber extrusion. What is delusional parasitosis? Search the Internet or use other references to find out.

_____

_____

_____

_____

2. Why do you think a high percentage of these patients are diagnosed with delusional parasitosis?

_____

_____

_____

_____

3. What could Mark pick up at the pharmacy that would help his skin condition?

_____

_____

_____

_____

4. What do you think is the likely psychological impact of this condition on Mark and his family?

_____

_____

_____

_____

ACTIVITY 21-3: Case Study—A Skin Infection

Instructions: Read the following scenario and then answer the critical thinking questions.

Mr. Tuttle has been coming to the retail pharmacy where you work for four years, ever since his daughter, Laura, was born. You have seen Laura grow from birth to a preschooler. Mr. Tuttle brings Laura, now 4 years old, with him to the pharmacy today and asks for any type of cream that would help heal her skin rash. The pharmacist talks to Mr. Tuttle, who repeats his request for a recommendation and lifts Laura's sleeve to reveal the rash. There are no lesions anywhere else on her body. Laura has several reddish, round lesions on her arm that are slightly raised and scaling. Pinpoint pustules around the edges of the lesions accompany these. Laura has no fever or any other symptoms. The pharmacist refers Mr. Tuttle to a doctor.

1. What was the rash on Laura's arm?

   _____

   _____

2. What is the treatment for Laura's rash?

   _____

   _____

3. Is Laura's condition considered contagious? If so, where might she have contracted it?

   _____

   _____

ACTIVITY 21-4: Case Study—A Skin Condition

Instructions: Read the following scenario and then answer the critical thinking questions.

Mrs. Cortez, a Hispanic woman, brings her 13-year-old daughter, Sarah, with her to the retail pharmacy where you work. She purchases a variety of skin care creams from the cosmetic section. Sarah has what appears to be uneven skin coloring on her face, particularly close to her nose. It is nothing significant, but Sarah is getting to an age at which she is more concerned about her appearance.

Mrs. Cortez returns after a week and asks to talk to the pharmacist about Sarah's skin spots. She explains to the pharmacist that Sarah has been using cold cream, but has noticed that the spots are changing in size. She is wondering if the cold cream is the cause of the change, or if Sarah might have cancer. Mrs. Cortez continues, saying that Sarah has a few of these symmetrical spots on her body, but the condition is now appearing on her face and she thinks it is spreading. Mrs. Cortez also adds that Sarah has become extremely sensitive to the sun.

No one else in the family has this condition. Sarah is referred to her doctor.

1. What is the name of the skin condition Sarah has?

   _____

   _____

2. Is there a cream in the pharmacy that could help with this condition?

   _____

   _____

3. What are some treatments for Sarah's condition?

   _____

   _____

4. How would the emotional impact of this condition be different for Sarah than for an adult?

   _____

   _____

   _____

   _____

ACTIVITY 21-5: What is Chemical Photosensitivity?

As you have learned, drugs sometimes interact with each other to cause unwanted consequences. Sometimes drugs or other chemical substances can interact with sunlight in a condition called *chemical photosensitivity*. Go online to learn more about chemical photosensitivity, then answer the following questions.

1. What are photosensitizers? Give five examples of substances that might contain photosensitizers.

   _____

   _____

   _____

   _____

   _____

2. Name five short-term effects of exposure to photosensitizers:

   _____

   _____

   _____

   _____

   _____

3. Name five long-term effects of exposure to photosensitizers:

   _____

   _____

   _____

   _____

   _____

4. Describe the difference between a photoallergic reaction and a phototoxic reaction. Which type of reaction is more common? Which type of reaction is harder to diagnose, and why?

   _____

   _____

   _____

   _____

5. Will using a sunscreen protect a person who is photosensitive?

   _____

   _____

   _____

   _____

6. Name five common OTC drugs and five prescription drugs that are known to cause chemical photosensitivity in some patients.

_____

_____

_____

_____

_____

7. Did anything you learned about chemical photosensitivity surprise you? If so, what?

_____

_____

_____

_____

CHAPTER 22
Eyes and Ears

After completing Chapter 22 from the textbook, you should be able to:	Related Activity in the Workbook/Lab Manual
1. List, identify, and diagram the basic anatomical structure and parts of the eye and ear.	Review Questions, PTCB Exam Practice Questions Activity 22-1
2. Describe the function or physiology of the ears and eyes.	Review Questions, PTCB Exam Practice Questions
3. List and define common diseases affecting the eyes and ears.	Review Questions, PTCB Exam Practice Questions Activity 22-2, Activity 22-3, Activity 22-5
4. Demonstrate a comprehensive understanding of the causes, symptoms, and pharmaceutical treatments associated with the common diseases affecting the eyes and ears.	Review Questions, PTCB Exam Practice Questions Activity 22-1, Activity 22-4

INTRODUCTION

Seeing and hearing are two of our basic senses. Although both the eyes and the ears are susceptible to a variety of disorders, these maladies can normally be prevented, controlled, or reversed with treatment, except in rare cases. A wide variety of treatment modalities is available to treat eye disorders. However, it is important that ophthalmic products be used safely and properly, because they are sterile. One of your most important responsibilities as a pharmacy technician is to thoroughly understand the basics of safe using of ophthalmic remedies. As a pharmacy technician, it is important for you to understand the basic anatomy and physiology of the eyes and ears and the conditions that affect them, so that you have greater insight into how the drugs used to treat these conditions work.

REVIEW QUESTIONS

Match the following.

1. _____ humor
2. _____ asymptomatic
3. _____ blepharitis
4. _____ hordeolum
5. _____ cataract
6. _____ cycloplegic
7. _____ conjunctivitis
8. _____ tinnitus
9. _____ glaucoma
10. _____ photoreceptors
11. _____ iridotomy
12. _____ retinopathy
13. _____ mucopurulent
14. _____ otitis media
15. _____ mydriatic
16. _____ ophthalmic
17. _____ eustachian tube

a. rods and cones
b. group of eye diseases
c. a noninflammatory disease of the retina
d. pertaining to the eye
e. a drug that causes paralysis of the eye
f. mucus or pus
g. chronic inflammation of the eye
h. showing no evidence of disease or abnormal condition
i. drug that dilates the eye
j. an obscurity of the lens
k. body fluid
l. inflammation of the eyelid
m. infection/inflammation of the middle ear
n. ringing or buzzing in the ear
o. an incision into the iris
p. an infection of the sebaceous gland of the eye
q. connects the ear with the throat

Choose the best answer.

18. The _____ is often referred to as the "film" of the camera.
    a. pupil
    b. cornea
    c. iris
    d. retina

19. The visual pathway for electrical impulses to the brain is the:
    a. cornea.
    b. sclera.
    c. iris.
    d. optic nerve.

20. Another name for stye is:
    a. hordeolum.
    b. humor.
    c. macula.
    d. conjunctiva.

21. Which of the following would not be appropriate for treating a stye?
    a. Augmentin® 500 mg po q8 hr
    b. dicloxacillin 250 mg po q6 hr
    c. erythromycin 250 mg po qid
    d. tetracycline 250 mg po qid

True or False?

22. Conjunctivitis is contagious.

   T   F

23. Most glaucoma is of the open-angle or wide-angle type.

   T   F

24. Oral medications that are used for hypertension can cause problems in patients with glaucoma.

   T   F

25. Cataracts are chronic and cannot be reversed.

   T   F

26. Looking directly into the sun may cause retinopathy.

   T   F

Fill in the blanks.

27. The snail-shaped part of the ear is called the _____.

28. _____ drops may be placed in the ear, but _____ may not be placed in the _____.

PHARMACY CALCULATION PROBLEMS

1. A 5 mL bottle of olopatadine, 0.1%, is dispensed for allergic conjunctivitis. If the patient uses 1 gtt ou q8 hr, how many days will the bottle last?

2. How many milligrams of pilocarpine are in a 10 mL bottle of pilocarpine 6% ophthalmic gel?

3. Azithromycin 100 mg/5 mL suspension is prescribed for a child's inner-ear infection. If the patient is to receive 100 mg on day 1 and 50 mg on days 2–5, how many mL will the patient need for the entire course?

4. If cephalexin 500 mg is prescribed qid × 10 days, how many grams will the patient receive over the entire course?

PTCB EXAM PRACTICE QUESTIONS

1. What disease of the eye is characterized by increased intraocular pressure?
   - a. conjunctivitis
   - b. cataract
   - c. glaucoma
   - d. macular degeneration

2. What is a condition of the eye in which the lens becomes opaque and interferes with clear vision?
   - a. conjunctivitis
   - b. cataract
   - c. glaucoma
   - d. macular degeneration

3. All of the following antibiotics must be monitored closely, to avoid damage to the ear and possible hearing loss, *except*:
   - a. gentamicin.
   - b. Amikacin®.
   - c. tobramycin.
   - d. Protonix®.

4. What eye ailment is often referred to as "pinkeye?"
   - a. conjunctivitis
   - b. cataract
   - c. glaucoma
   - d. macular degeneration

5. What is the medical term that describes ringing in the ears?
   - a. otitis media
   - b. tympanitis
   - c. tinnitus
   - d. vertigo

ACTIVITY 22-1: Anatomy Worksheet

The Eye

Label the following illustration of the eye.

a. _____

b. _____

c. _____

d. _____

e. _____

f. _____

g. _____

h. _____

i. _____

j. _____

k. _____

l. _____

m. _____

n. _____

o. _____

p. _____

q. _____

r. _____

s. _____

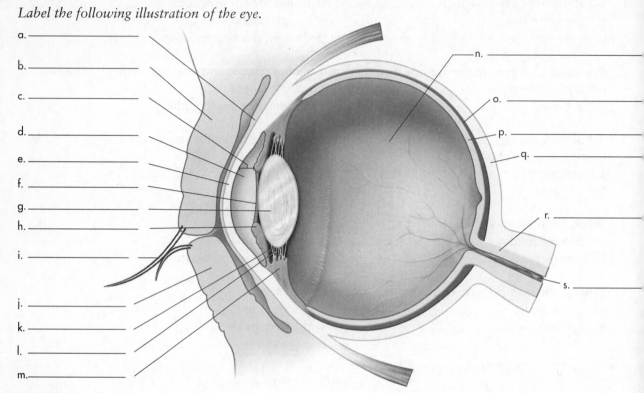

The Ear

Label the following illustration of the ear.

a. _____

b. _____

c. _____

d. _____

e. _____

f. _____

g. _____

h. _____

i. _____

j. _____

k. _____

To pharynx

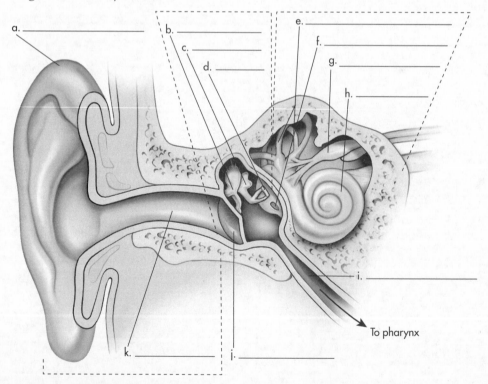

ACTIVITY 22-2: Case Study—An Unusual Prescription

Simon, a CPhT, received a questionable prescription in the pharmacy today. Something didn't seem right to him at first. Take a look at the prescription.

Dr. Jon Herring
Pediatric Outpatient Ear Clinic
2008 W. State St.
Rockford, IL
(815)555-1111

Name _Jessica Raley_____ Age_____

Address __678 Alpine Rd._____ Date _6/25/08_____

℞

Neomycin and Polymixin B Sulfates and
Gramicidin Ophthalmic Solution
5 ml
1-2 gtts AS TID X 7 days

No Refill _____ times   _Dr. J Herring_

_____
Signature

A generically equivalent drug product may be dispensed unless the practitioner hand writes the words
'Brand Necessary' or 'Brand Medically Necessary' on the face of the prescription.   6HUR133050

---

1. What did you find unusual about the prescription?

_____

_____

_____

2. Do you think there is an error in this prescription?

_____

_____

_____

3. Why would a physician write a prescription such as this?

_____

_____

_____

A Closer Look

We hope that you observed from the data on the prescription that it is acceptable to order ophthalmic drops for the ear. Ophthalmic products are gentle and safe enough for use in the ear. Still, if this physician did not work in a specialized ear clinic, the order could easily be questioned.

A physician may want to use a particular formula for a patient, but know that this formula is not available in an otic formulation. This may be due to patient allergies or other reasons. Although unusual, it is not uncommon to see eyedrops prescribed for the ear. However, it is *never* acceptable for an otic product to be prescribed for the eye. Otic formulations contain ingredients that can damage the eye, and otic drug inserts contain a specific warning not to use those products in the eyes.

ACTIVITY 22-3: Case Study—An Eye Condition

Instructions: Read the following scenario and then answer the critical thinking questions.

Mrs. Freeman takes her 6-year-old daughter to the doctor right from her day care, when she notices that her daughter's right eye is bright red. Now Mrs. Freeman remembers that her daughter has been scratching at this eye for a couple of days. When she looks closely at the eye, the mother notices that it is swollen and that a thick green discharge is oozing from the eye.

The doctor tells Mrs. Freeman that her daughter has a very common infection found in children, especially those who attend day-care centers. He takes a sample of the ooze from the eye and has it tested. He cautions Mrs. Freeman to keep the daughter out of school and day care until it clears up and orders eyedrops and eye ointment. He also tells Mrs. Freeman to wash in hot water any towels or clothes her daughter may have come into contact with.

1. What eye condition does the daughter seem to have?

_____

_____

2. Why did the doctor caution Mrs. Freeman to keep the daughter out of school and day care?

_____

_____

_____

_____

3. What is the proper way to instill eyedrops for this 6-year-old child?

_____

_____

_____

_____

4. What is the proper way to apply eye ointment for a 6-year-old child?

_____

_____

_____

_____

ACTIVITY 22-4: Case Study—An Ear Condition

Instructions: Read the following scenario and then answer the critical thinking questions.

Jarred is a strong, healthy 17-year-old senior, and a star of the swimming team at his high school. He has won many district competitions and college recruiters are monitoring his progress; Jarred thinks he may be able to obtain an athletic scholarship. He is in the water practicing seven days a week. In addition to swimming, Jarred also competes in track and tennis.

With the exception of a badly sprained ankle last year and some bouts with athlete's foot, Jarred has been in perfect health. On occasion, Jarred has moderate ear pain during swimming practice and experiences pressure in his ears. Often the pressure relieves itself within a few minutes. Sometimes, however, the pressure does not go away, and lately it has become quite painful. He asks his mother to look inside his ear because it has become increasingly itchy and hurts when he chews on the same side of his mouth as the sore ear. When his mother takes a look, she sees that it is swollen and red and appears to have pus oozing out of it.

Jarred's mother takes him to the doctor; the doctor also notices eczema-like skin surrounding the ear.

1. What condition might Jarred be experiencing?

_____

_____

2. Given the facts of the scenario, what is the probable cause of Jarred's problem?

_____

_____

_____

_____

3. What is the treatment for this type of condition?

_____

_____

_____

_____

4. Can Jarred still remain on the swimming team if he has this condition?

_____

_____

_____

_____

ACTIVITY 22-5: Case Study—Eye Trouble

Instructions: Read the following scenario and then answer the critical thinking questions.

Mr. Gaines is a 49-year-old African-American male who has been waking up every morning with a headache for more than a week. It has become so annoying that he is taking two aspirin before going to bed, in the hopes that he will not wake up with a headache the next morning. Sometimes he gets lucky.

Because he is nearly 50 years old, when Mr. Gaines begins having vision problems he shrugs it off, attributes them to middle age, and makes an appointment with his ophthalmologist. However, as the weeks and months go by, the problem gets much worse. His vision is blurry quite frequently and he sees "clouds" or "halos" most of the time. He also notices that his eyes become much more painful when doing ordinary things like reading or watching television. He realizes that his problem is not just a need for glasses, so he makes an appointment with his primary care physician.

In the meantime, Mr. Gaines sees his ophthalmologist again, who conducts a routine test that diagnoses the condition that is giving him so much trouble.

1. What diagnosis did Mr. Gaines's ophthalmologist make?

_____

_____

2. Is the routine test given by the ophthalmologist done for all patients, or only those who have symptoms similar to those experienced by Mr. Gaines?

_____

_____

_____

_____

3. What contributing factors put Mr. Gaines into a high-risk category for this condition?

_____

_____

_____

_____

4. What is the goal of treatment for this condition?

_____

_____

_____

_____

5. What pharmaceutical treatments are available for this condition?

_____

_____

_____

_____

6. Is this condition curable?

_____

_____

_____

_____

CHAPTER 23
The Gastrointestinal System

After completing Chapter 23 from the textbook, you should be able to:	Related Activity in the Workbook/Lab Manual
1. Identify the basic anatomical and structural parts of the digestive system.	Review Questions, PTCB Exam Practice Questions Activity 23-1
2. Describe the physiology of the digestive system.	Review Questions, PTCB Exam Practice Questions Activity 23-2, Activity 23-3, Activity 23-4
3. List and describe the three main categories of nutrients.	Review Questions, PTCB Exam Practice Questions Activity 23-2, Activity 23-3, Activity 23-4
4. Identify the functions and AMDR of the macronutrients.	Review Questions, PTCB Exam Practice Questions Activity 23-2, Activity 23-3, Activity 23-4
5. State the difference between essential and nonessential amino acids.	Review Questions Activity 23-2, Activity 23-3, Activity 23-4
6. Identify the functions, symptoms of deficiencies, and RDIs of the micronutrients.	Review Questions
7. Understand the importance of water to the body.	Review Questions Activity 23-2, Activity 23-3, Activity 23-4

INTRODUCTION

The gastrointestinal system manages digestion in the body. Food is broken down, absorbed, or chemically modified into substances that are required by the cells to survive and function properly. Waste products that the body cannot use are eliminated. The gastrointestinal system extends from the mouth to the anus.

Its six main parts are the mouth, esophagus, pharynx, stomach, and small and large intestines. Various supportive structures, accessory glands, and accessory organs also help to make up the complete digestive system. The main purpose of the digestive system is to fuel the body by taking in and metabolizing nutrients.

An estimated 70 million Americans suffer from one or more digestive disorders; this accounts for 13 percent of all hospitalizations. As a pharmacy technician, you should be aware of the most common digestive disorders that require pharmacological treatment, including conditions treated with OTC drugs.

REVIEW QUESTIONS

Match the following.

1. _____ chyme
2. _____ mastication
3. _____ protease
4. _____ lipid
5. _____ monosaccharide
6. _____ μg
7. _____ pepsinogen

a. fat
b. microgram
c. enzyme that begins protein breakdown
d. simplest form of carbohydrate
e. chewing
f. precursor to pepsin
g. liquid that food turns into before entering the small intestines

Choose the best answer.

8. Which of the following refers to LDL?
   a. bad cholesterol
   b. low-density lipoprotein
   c. a and b
   d. good cholesterol

9. Kilocalories (kcal) refers to:
   a. bad calories.
   b. food energy.
   c. good calories.
   d. a 1,000-calorie meal.

10. Good cholesterol is referred to as:
    a. high-density lipoprotein.
    b. DRI.
    c. HDL.
    d. a and c.

11. A good source of unsaturated fat is:
    a. canola oil.
    b. olive oil.
    c. both a and b.
    d. none of the above.

Fill in the blanks.

12. A precursor to pepsin is known as _____.
13. The liver produces _____, which is stored in the gallbladder.
14. As chyme enters the duodenum, it must be neutralized by bicarbonate; otherwise, a _____ ulcer will result.
15. _____ are nutrients needed by the body in larger quantities.
16. The only vitamin the body produces itself is vitamin _____.

Match the following.

17. _____ cecum   **a.** accessory organ
18. _____ tongue   **b.** small intestine
19. _____ pharynx   **c.** large intestine
20. _____ ileum   **d.** main digestive system

True or False?

21. GERD occurs because the lower esophageal sphincter relaxes when it should contract.
    T   F

22. Antihistamines work by boosting the action of H1 receptors.
    T   F

23. NSAIDs block the effect of the enzyme cyclooxygenase.
    T   F

24. Carbohydrates are bad for our health.
    T   F

Match the following drugs with a corresponding disease, condition, or treatment.

25. _____ Reglan®   **a.** therapy for *H. pylori* infection
26. _____ Transderm-scop®   **b.** postoperative vomiting drug
27. _____ CTZ   **c.** ulcer treatment
28. _____ Zofran®   **d.** antihistamine used as an antiemetic
29. _____ Compazine®   **e.** PPI drug
30. _____ Tagamet®   **f.** overproduction of acid
31. _____ double-drug theory   **g.** postemetogenic nausea
32. _____ Prilosec®   **h.** a type of laxative
33. _____ emollient   **i.** promotes proper sphincter function

Match the following vitamins with their names.

34. _____ vitamin A   **a.** niacin
35. _____ vitamin D   **b.** pantothenic acid
36. _____ vitamin C   **c.** thiamine
37. _____ vitamin K   **d.** folic acid
38. _____ vitamin B1   **e.** phytonadione
39. _____ vitamin B2   **f.** cyanocobalamin
40. _____ vitamin B3   **g.** retinol
41. _____ vitamin B5   **h.** pyridoxine
42. _____ vitamin B6   **i.** ascorbic acid
43. _____ vitamin B9   **j.** riboflavin
44. _____ vitamin B12   **k.** ergocalciferol

PHARMACY CALCULATION PROBLEMS

1. You need to compound lansoprazole suspension in a concentration of 3 mg/mL. In this suspension, you will need lansoprazole 30 mg capsules and sodium bicarbonate 8.4% solution. If you need to make 480 mL, how many capsules of lansoprazole will you need?

    $\frac{480\,mL}{}$ $\frac{3\,mg}{1\,mL}$ *48 capsules*

2. Sucralfate comes in a concentration of 1 g/10 mL. If a patient is receiving 10 mL qid, how many milligrams of sucralfate is the patient receiving daily?

    $\frac{1\,g}{10\,mL}$ $\frac{4000}{40\,mL}$ *4000 mg*

3. A 65-year-old woman weighing 156 lb. is to receive a midazolam IVP dosed at 0.02 mg/kg prior to her colonoscopy. If midazolam contains 1 mg/mL, how many mL will the patient receive?

    70.9 kg   1.42 mg $\frac{1\,mg}{mL}$

    1.42 mL

4. A standard pantoprazole drip at a hospital pharmacy contains 80 mg in 250 mL of 0.9% sodium chloride. If the patient is to receive 8 mg/hr, how many mL will be infused over each hour?

    8 mg/hr $\frac{80\,mg}{250\,mL}$ 25 mL/hr

PTCB EXAM PRACTICE QUESTIONS

1. Where in the gastrointestinal system are oral drugs absorbed?
    a. stomach
    b. small intestine
    c. large intestine
    d. mouth

2. What type of drug is omeprazole?
    a. proton pump inhibitor
    b. H2 blocker
    c. laxative
    d. antibiotic

3. A major cause of peptic ulcers is infection by which of the following bacteria?
    a. *Staphylococcus aureus*
    b. MRSA
    c. *E. coli*
    d. *H. pylori*

4. All of the following drugs are used to treat postemetogenic nausea *except*:
    a. Zofran®
    b. Colace®
    c. Kytril®
    d. Anzemet®

5. What type of laxative is Metamucil®?
    a. saline
    b. stimulant
    c. evacuant
    d. bulk-forming

ACTIVITY 23-1: Anatomy Worksheet—The Digestive System

Label the following illustration of the digestive system.

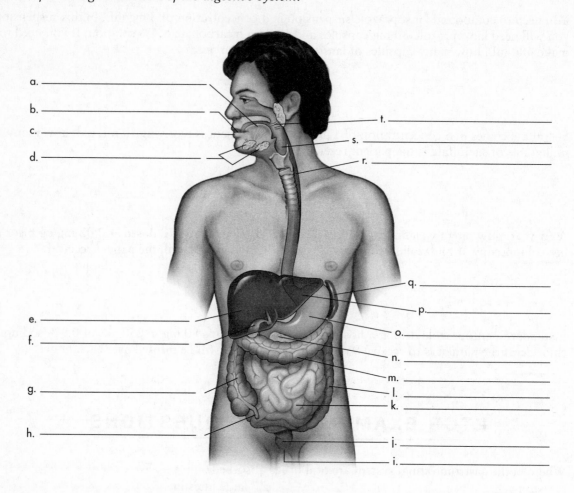

a. _____

b. _____

c. _____

d. _____

e. _____

f. _____

g. _____

h. _____

t. _____

s. _____

r. _____

q. _____

p. _____

o. _____

n. _____

m. _____

l. _____

k. _____

j. _____

i. _____

ACTIVITY 23-2: Case Study—Heartburn

Instructions: Read the following scenario and then answer the critical thinking questions.

Mr. Selescion is a 53-year-old executive who works out regularly. In addition to jogging, he swims, hikes, and lifts weights. Mr. Selescion does not always watch what he eats and has been known to indulge about once a week at a local Mexican restaurant. He loves their tamales, and sometimes buys enough to have leftovers for the next day. He drinks a lot of water and has wine on occasion with dinner.

The only problem he has ever encountered with his body has been stomach aches now and then, which he has had for years. Mr. Selescion began by taking OTC chewable tablets to help quell the "butterfly" feeling he had. He also remembers, a while back, buying a liquid antacid that tasted awful but seemed to work. Unfortunately, he did not think this was good, because he had to buy so much more than the chew tabs to get the same relief. He often drank way too much of the liquid antacid with no relief.

Mr. Selescion visits his doctor, who prescribes omeprazole to control the heartburn this patient experiences at least two to three times a week. As the weeks pass, the omeprazole does not seem to work. Mr. Selescion begins experiencing chest pain and tasting a very sour/bitter acid in the back of his throat. He also finds he cannot exercise within one hour after eating a meal. Concerned by this new development, he heads back to the doctor.

1. Based on the symptoms mentioned in this scenario, what do you think Mr. Selescion's affliction is?
   _____
   _____

2. Could Mr. Selescion have been using a better OTC medication to prevent this problem, other than chew tabs or liquid antacid?
   _____
   _____
   _____
   _____

3. Left untreated, what are some of the complications of Mr. Selescion's condition?
   _____
   _____
   _____
   _____

4. What tests are needed to evaluate GERD?
   _____
   _____
   _____
   _____

ACTIVITY 23-3: Case Study—Bowel Trouble

Instructions: Read the following scenario and then answer the critical thinking questions.

Jill is a 47-year-old, slightly overweight woman who has had periodic bouts of constipation for about the last eight years. They really have not been that much of an inconvenience and occur usually after Jill eats certain foods, such as bananas or cheese. Jill also drinks plenty of water, which seems to help reduce the incidences of constipation.

Jill then begins to experience intermittent diarrhea. This initially seems like a blessing to Jill, who would rather have diarrhea than constipation. Occasionally, she also experiences bloating and abdominal pain accompanying the diarrhea. Eventually, every time Jill eats—whether it is a snack or an entire meal—she has these symptoms. They seem to go away only when she is able to have a bowel movement.

Months later, Jill's situation has taken a turn for the worse. If she is not going to the bathroom, she certainly has the urge. The abdominal pain is constant, but much worse in the morning when she first wakes up. When the urge comes to relieve herself, Jill has mere minutes. Work or any activity lasting more than about 30 to 60 minutes creates the risk that she will not make it to the bathroom in time.

Jill makes an appointment with the doctor, who goes over her medical history. Jill takes Excedrin® for occasional headaches and used to use laxatives for the constipation she had in the past. Other than that, she is healthy. The doctor runs blood tests and orders a colonoscopy. Nothing is found.

1. Based on the information in this scenario, what condition is Jill most likely experiencing?
   _____
   _____

2. Why was the doctor not able to find anything?
   _____
   _____
   _____
   _____

3. Does eating certain foods, such as bananas or cheese, cause this condition?
   _____
   _____
   _____
   _____

4. Is there a cure for Jill's condition? Does her current condition lead to other, more serious conditions?
   _____
   _____
   _____
   _____

ACTIVITY 23-4: Case Study—A Liquid Diet

Instructions: Read the following scenario and then answer the critical thinking questions.

Ms. Ferrous is a mildly overweight, 33-year-old, Indian woman who had a baby two months ago. She is not happy with the fact that she is still a bit overweight, because she wants to fit into the clothes she wore before becoming pregnant. Ms. Ferrous feels that she needs to lose weight—fast. She decides to go on a liquid diet, one of those "meal in a can" types. There are lots of flavorful choices, and she does not find it dificult to stick to the plan, which includes three cans of fluid per day, lots of water, and an occasional low-calorie snack bar.

Ms. Ferrous starts having stomach pains, so she chews Tums® as if they are going out of style. When her friends tell her she takes too many of them, she replies that she needs the calcium.

On occasion, Ms. Ferrous's stomach pain becomes so intense that she needs to lie down for a little while and she also becomes nauseated. She begins to experience heartburn that increasingly worsens. It seems like every passing day she encounters a new pain: abdominal pain, shoulder pain, chest pain, and now the constant heartburn. Occasionally her stomach becomes so upset that she vomits. When she does vomit, she drinks another liquid meal because she is determined to lose the weight.

One morning, as she is bathing her baby, she has an excruciating, sharp pain in the chest area. It feels like intense heartburn, and she begins to beat on her chest. Convinced that she is experiencing a heart attack, she manages to call 911. When the ambulance arrives 45 minutes later, she is hunched over on the floor from the pain in her chest.

Once at the hospital, she vomits when they give her a liquid medicine to numb her throat. After the doctor asks about her symptoms, he orders an ultrasound and blood tests.

1. Why did the doctor order an ultrasound when he discovered that Ms. Ferrous was having chest pain?
   _____
   _____
   _____
   _____

2. Once the ultrasound results are read and the condition is confirmed, what is the treatment?
   _____
   _____
   _____
   _____

3. For severe cases of this condition, what can be done to help prevent future attacks?
   _____
   _____
   _____
   _____

CHAPTER 24
The Musculoskeletal System

After completing Chapter 24 from the textbook, you should be able to:	Related Activity in the Workbook/Lab Manual
1. List, identify, and diagram the basic anatomical structure and parts of the muscles and bones.	Review Questions, PTCB Exam Practice Questions Activity 24-1
2. Describe the functions of the muscles and bones and their physiology.	Review Questions, PTCB Exam Practice Questions Activity 24-1
3. List and define common diseases affecting the muscles and bones and demonstrate an understanding of the causes, symptoms, and pharmaceutical treatments associated with each disease.	Review Questions, PTCB Exam Practice Questions Activity 24-2, Activity 24-3, Activity 24-4, Lab 24-1
4. Describe the mechanisms and the complications of the following musculoskeletal diseases and comprehend how each class of drugs works: osteomyelitis, osteoarthritis, gout, inflammation, multiple sclerosis, and cerebral palsy.	Review Questions, PTCB Exam Practice Questions Activity 24-2, Activity 24-3, Activity 24-4, Lab 24-1
5. List the indications for use and mechanisms of action of ASA, NSAIDs, COX-2 inhibitors, antigout agents, calcitonin, bisphosphonates, SERMs, and skeletal muscle relaxants.	Review Questions, PTCB Exam Practice Questions Activity 24-2, Activity 24-3, Activity 24-4, Lab 24-1

INTRODUCTION

The musculoskeletal system, which consists of bones and skeletal muscles, provides the body with both form and movement. Its four main functions are to provide a framework or shape for the body, protect the internal organs, allow body movement, and provide storage for essential minerals. The musculoskeletal system is affected by numerous disorders, some of which cause only discomfort and pain, and some of which cause complete disability. Osteoporosis, the most prevalent bone disorder in the United States, affects approximately 20 million Americans, and is a major cause of bone fractures. Osteoarthritis, a progressive disease of the joints, affects up to 40 million Americans.

A wide range of pharmaceuticals is used for the treatment of diseases of the musculoskeletal system, although many provide only symptomatic relief. However, as a result of intensive research, new products aimed at the prevention or retardation of disease, particularly osteoporosis and osteoarthritis, may provide hope for the millions of Americans afflicted with these debilitating diseases. As a pharmacy technician, you should be aware of the most common musculoskeletal disorders that require pharmacological treatment, including conditions treated with OTC drugs.

REVIEW QUESTIONS

Match the following.

1. _____ bones
2. _____ marrow
3. _____ cartilage
4. _____ hematopoiesis
5. _____ joints
6. _____ ligaments
7. _____ muscle
8. _____ myocyte
9. _____ sarcomere
10. _____ synovial fluid
11. _____ tendons

a. tissue that gives shape to ears and nose
b. where bones are connected
c. contractile tissue
d. segment of striated muscle
e. bands holding joints together
f. calcified substance that provides shape and support
g. a muscle cell
h. attaches muscle to bone
i. spongy tissue found inside bone
j. fills the space between cartilage and bone
k. formation and development of blood cells

Choose the best answer.

12. Smooth muscles comprise or line all of the following except:
    a. stomach.
    b. lungs.
    c. neck.
    d. intestines.

13. Chemical and _____ interactions between actin and myosin cause muscles to react.
    a. electrical
    b. physical
    c. enzymatic
    d. synovial

14. Cranial and rib bones are classified as:
    a. long bones.
    b. short bones.
    c. flat bones.
    d. sesamoid bones.

15. Which of the following is included in injections as an antirheumatic agent?
    a. gold
    b. silver
    c. copper
    d. nickel

Match the following.

16. _____ osteoporosis
17. _____ bursitis
18. _____ myalgia
19. _____ anemia
20. _____ leukemia
21. _____ osteoarthritis
22. _____ rheumatoid arthritis
23. _____ gout
24. _____ osteomyelitis
25. _____ Paget's disease

a. autoimmune disease
b. when white blood cells experience DNA damage
c. bone brittleness due to lack of calcium
d. breakdown of joint cartilage
e. when bone breaks down more quickly than it rebuilds
f. failure of bone marrow to produce red blood cells
g. inflammation of small fluid pouches
h. caused by the deposit of uric acid in joints
i. muscle pain
j. bacterial infection of the bone

Match the following drugs with their classifications or indications.

26. _____ Dantrium®
27. _____ phenytoin
28. _____ Ridaura®
29. _____ colchicine
30. _____ Dolobid®
31. _____ diclofenac
32. _____ Zomig®

a. gout
b. salicylate
c. direct skeletal muscle relaxant
d. seizures
e. NSAID
f. antirheumatic agent
g. spasticity

PHARMACY CALCULATION PROBLEMS

Calculate the following.

1. If an employee gets paid $100/day and has to miss an average of 12 work days each year because of fibromyalgia, how much income is the employee losing each year due to illness?

2. Calculate the monthly medical (traditional and nontraditional) expenses for this fibromyalgia patient:

   medical insurance—$150/month

   medications—$89

   chiropractic and acupuncture—$119

   massage therapy—$45

   physician co-payments—$15

3. If an insurance company pays 60% of the retail price for medications, how much is the customer's co-pay if the total retail price is $223?

4. If a customer's co-payment is $57 and is 30% of the retail price, how much is the retail price?

PTCB EXAM PRACTICE QUESTIONS

1. Which of the following diseases is characterized by loss of bone density and makes the bones prone to fracture?
   a. osteoporosis
   b. osteomyelitis
   c. osteosarcoma
   d. osteoarthritis

2. Gout is a disorder involving the deposit of which of the following compounds in the joints and soft tissues, resulting in significant pain?
   a. potassium chloride
   b. hydrochloric acid
   c. uric acid
   d. calcium chloride

3. All of the following drugs are skeletal muscle relaxants *except*:
   a. Valium®.
   b. Flexeril®.
   c. Robaxin®.
   d. Celebrex®.

4. NSAIDs are a class of drugs used to treat:
   a. infection.
   b. inflammation.
   c. muscle weakness.
   d. bone loss.

5. All of the following are classifications of arthritis *except*:
   a. juvenile.
   b. osteo.
   c. rheumatoid.
   d. myoclonic.

ACTIVITY 24-1: Anatomy Worksheet

Types of Muscle

Label the following illustration of the different types of muscle.

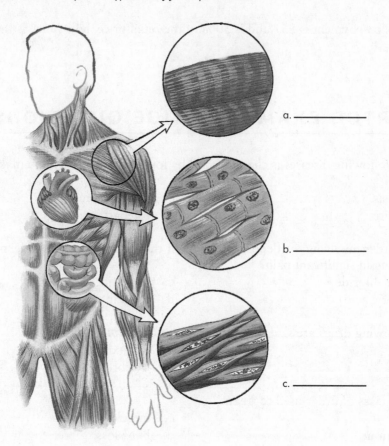

a. _____

b. _____

c. _____

The Long Bone

Label the following illustration of the long bone.

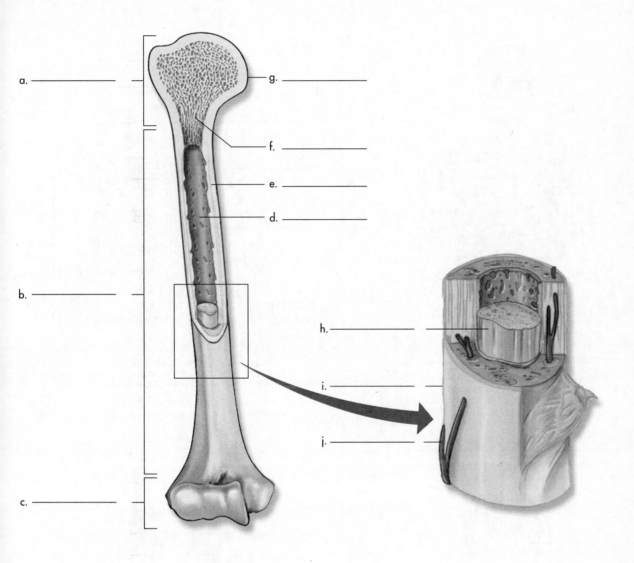

a. _____

b. _____

c. _____

g. _____

f. _____

e. _____

d. _____

h. _____

i. _____

j. _____

The Skeletal System

Label the following illustration of the skeletal system.

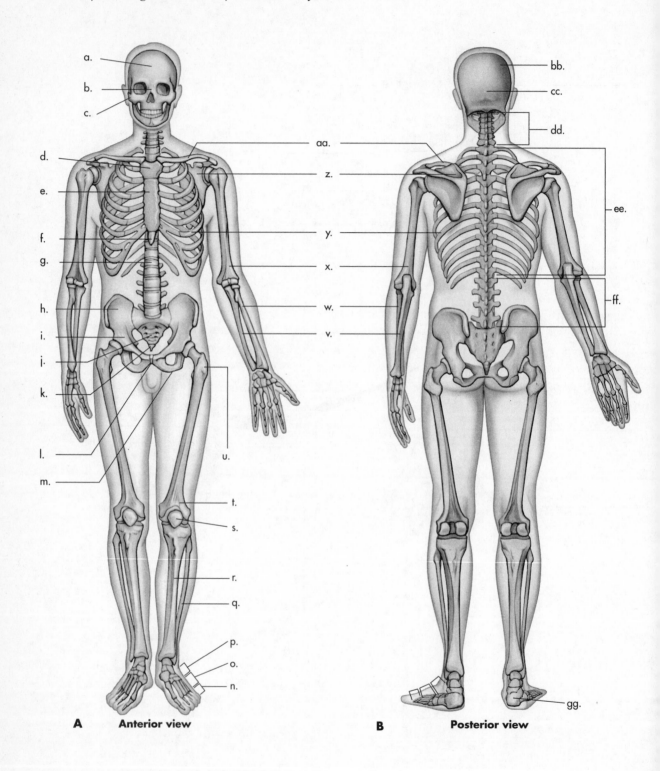

A   **Anterior view**

B   **Posterior view**

a. _____

b. _____

c. _____

d. _____

e. _____

f. _____

g. _____

h. _____

i. _____

j. _____

k. _____

l. _____

m. _____

n. _____

o. _____

p. _____

q. _____

r. _____

s. _____

t. _____

u. _____

v. _____

w. _____

x. _____

y. _____

z. _____

aa. _____

bb. _____

cc. _____

dd. _____

ee. _____

ff. _____

gg. _____

Questions:

1. Name four functions of the muscles.

   _____

   _____

   _____

   _____

2. Describe which parts of a muscle are responsible for its action and how they work together.

   _____

   _____

   _____

   _____

3. Name the three major muscle types and give an example of each.

   _____

   _____

   _____

4. Name five or more functions of bones.

   _____

   _____

   _____

   _____

   _____

5. Name the two types of bone marrow and the functions of each.

   _____

   _____

   _____

   _____

6. Research the changes that occur in the skeleton as we age. Start with an infant and end with an elderly adult. Create a timeline to track your findings.

ACTIVITY 24-2: Case Study—Arthritis and Inflammation

Instructions: Read the following scenario and then answer the critical thinking questions.

Arthur is a 57-year-old obese farmer who eats as much meat as he raises. He frequently experiences joint pain and inflammation and has for years. As the years go on, he finds it harder and harder each day to do simple things such as hitch a rope or even drive his tractor. Eventually he sees a doctor and is diagnosed with arthritis in both hands. He is prescribed NSAIDs, wears a copper bracelet, and seems to have the condition under control for now.

Early one morning, a constant throbbing pain on his hand awakens Arthur. He discovers a nodule that is red, swollen, and tender to the touch. When Arthur presses on it for relief, it moves around slightly, but it still is painful. Stubborn as he is and aware of his arthritis, he takes an NSAID and tries to go about his day. The NSAID does not work and the pain is too much, so Arthur heads in to see the doctor. For him, this is another day's work on the farm that he is losing. The doctor orders a blood and urine uric acid test but no X-ray of the bones.

1. What is this nodule on Arthur's hand? Is it arthritis?

   _____

   _____

2. What causes this condition in Arthur?

   _____

   _____

   _____

   _____

3. Based on the information given in the scenario, what might have contributed to this condition?

   _____

   _____

   _____

   _____

4. Initially, treatment includes timely pain relief, but how can Arthur help prevent this from happening again?

   _____

   _____

   _____

   _____

ACTIVITY 24-3: Case Study—Long Hours

Instructions: Read the following scenario and then answer the critical thinking questions.

All the pharmacy technicians at the PBM where you work put in long hours processing claims, including yourself. The hours were extended after picking up two more employer contracts, and you have all been working at this pace for more than a year now. Luckily, everyone seems to get along, for the most part, and everyone pulls their weight as far as workload is concerned. The majority of the work you all do is by computer and telephone. What was once an eight-hour day has turned into fourteen hours, including some Saturdays. The money is good, but you are not so sure it is a good trade-off for less family time.

Every once in a while your hands get tired and tingle a bit. You take a little rest, go to the bathroom, and by the time you come back, they do not tingle any more. One day, though, you are working at your computer and you find it hard to ignore the tingling, which has radiated to your wrist as well. You remember that when you were in bed last night you could hardly sleep because your hand was going numb and burning at the same time.

You take your break as usual, expecting the sensation to go away, but when you return to your computer you experience a sudden, sharp, piercing pain from your wrist radiating up your arm. It almost makes you cry, it hurts so badly. The pharmacy technician next to you asks what happened and you tell her. She tells you that she has been having the same problem and takes ibuprofen to make it go away.

1. Should you take the advice of your co-worker and try ibuprofen to relieve the pain?

   _____

   _____

   _____

   _____

2. What is the likely diagnosis in this case?

   _____

   _____

   _____

   _____

3. Drawing from the scenario, what factors contributed to causing this problem?

   _____

   _____

   _____

   _____

4. Do you believe the co-worker has the same diagnosis? What about the other pharmacy technicians where you work?

   _____

   _____

   _____

   _____

5. What can be done to prevent this condition from becoming too severe when you are hired to work in a similar position?

_____

_____

_____

_____

ACTIVITY 24-4: Case Study—Posture Changes

Instructions: Read the following scenario and then answer the critical thinking questions.

Mrs. Sweet is a 68-year-old, feeble, menopausal woman with a thyroid problem. She also suffers from frequent heartburn and constipation, but figures it is just a part of getting old.

Mrs. Sweet is extremely proud of the roses in her garden. Even at her age, she spends a large amount of time tending to them daily, pruning them and always planting new species. She also helps teach others how to grow wonderful roses through the community center in her town.

Mrs. Sweet has not noticed, but over the years her posture has changed. She appears to be hunched slightly forward when she goes for her next yearly checkup with the doctor. The doctor asks some questions and discovers that Mrs. Sweet has been experiencing lower back pain for a while ... but of course she is getting old. The doctor orders a bone mineral density assessment and an X-ray of the spine.

1. What do you think the doctor surmises is causing Mrs. Sweet's pain?

    _____

    _____

2. What factors in this case would contribute to Mrs. Sweet's problem?

    _____

    _____

    _____

    _____

3. What pharmaceutical treatment and prevention options are available for this condition?

    _____

    _____

    _____

    _____

4. Are there special considerations with taking calcium supplements for this condition?

    _____

    _____

    _____

    _____

5. Will Mrs. Sweet have to give up her favorite activities in order to control her condition?

    _____

    _____

    _____

    _____

LAB 24-1: Web Research—What Is Fibromyalgia?

Objective:

Familiarize yourself with fibromyalgia syndrome (FM), how it is diagnosed, and its symptoms and treatments.

Pre-Lab Information:

Use the website www.fibrohope.org to learn more about FM, its symptoms, and current treatment options. This site is sponsored in part by the National Fibromyalgia Association.

Explanation:

Fibromyalgia affects more than 6 million Americans, mostly women, but can affect persons of any age or gender. Until FM finally started gaining medical acceptance, most people with the syndrome were thought to be hypochondriacs. FM has many symptoms that mimic other diseases, such as lupus and chronic fatigue syndrome, so it can easily be misdiagnosed. For the past decade or so, it has been classified as a neuromuscular disorder and is usually treated by a rheumatologist or a physician specializing in arthritis. Currently, there are no blood tests or X-rays that can support a definitive diagnosis. However, there is a set of symptomatic criteria that one must meet to be diagnosed with FM. Most people with the disorder have an array of symptoms, including all-over muscle aches and pain (dull and stabbing), extreme fatigue, and insomnia or nonrestorative sleep. Those with FM also must have at least 11 of 18 common tender points that are located around the neck, shoulders, elbows, knees, hips, and lower back. Many people with FM also have additional disorders that tend to accompany the syndrome. A few of these associated disorders include irritable bowel syndrome (IBS), temporomandibular joint disorder (TMJ), Raynaud's syndrome, and depression.

Medical science is now theorizing that fibromyalgia is actually a central nervous system disorder, but the symptoms most people feel are in their muscles. Physicians usually treat FM patients with any one or a combination of medications, such as NSAIDs, pain relievers, muscle relaxants, antidepressants, and sedatives or hypnotics. However, few drugs give complete relief, and all of these are off-label uses. Many fibromyalgia sufferers find some relief with alternative therapies, such as acupuncture, massage therapy, or chiropractic care. Some find reduction of symptoms with mild exercise, careful nutrition, and relaxation exercises. Currently, there is one medication approved by the FDA to treat fibromyalgia, called pregabalin; however, other medications are under investigation as well. One hopeful contender, reboxetine, which is an antidepressant, is in clinical trials for its pain-relieving properties. There is no known cure at this time for fibromyalgia, but it is hoped that the public will become more aware of this debilitating syndrome, and research into treatment continues.

Activity:

Visit www.fibrohope.org and click on the main tabs on the left under the heading "Understanding Fibromyalgia." You will find information regarding diagnosis, symptoms, FAQs, and "10 Things You Should Know About Fibromyalgia." Also, read through some of the testimonials at the top of the home page. You will find the answers to the following questions on that website.

1. List four major symptoms of fibromyalgia.

   _____

   _____

   _____

   _____

2. Why would a physician prescribe a sleep medication for FM?

_____

_____

_____

_____

3. List five contributing symptoms/conditions associated with fibromyalgia.

_____

_____

_____

_____

_____

4. Who does fibromyalgia affect?

   a. women only

   b. women and men

   c. children

   d. anyone, regardless of race or gender

5. List three current treatments (traditional or nontraditional).

_____

_____

_____

Student Name: _____

Lab Partner: _____

Grade/Comments: _____

_____

_____

Student Comments: _____

_____

_____

CHAPTER 25
The Respiratory System

After completing Chapter 25 from the textbook, you should be able to:	Related Activity in the Workbook/Lab Manual
1. Identify and list the basic anatomical and structural parts of the respiratory tract.	Review Questions, PTCB Exam Practice Questions Activity 25-1
2. Describe the function or physiology of the individual parts of the respiratory system and the external exchange of oxygen and waste.	Review Questions, PTCB Exam Practice Questions Activity 25-1
3. List and define common diseases affecting the respiratory tract and understand the causes, symptoms, and pharmaceutical treatment associated with each disease.	Review Questions, PTCB Exam Practice Questions Activity 25-2, Activity 25-3, Activity 25-4, Lab 25-1
4. List the trade and generic names and identify the classification of various drugs used in treatment of diseases and conditions of the respiratory tract.	Review Questions, PTCB Exam Practice Questions Activity 25-2, Activity 25-3, Activity 25-4

INTRODUCTION

The respiratory system is responsible for providing all cells of the body with the oxygen necessary to perform their specific functions. It is the system involved in the intake of oxygen through inhalation, and the excretion of carbon monoxide through exhalation. The respiratory system is divided into two parts, the upper and lower respiratory tracts. The upper respiratory tract includes the nasal cavity, paranasal sinuses, pharynx, and larynx. The lower respiratory tract includes the trachea, two lungs, two main bronchi, secondary and tertiary bronchi, bronchioles, alveolar ducts, and alveoli.

The most common disease of the respiratory system is the common cold. Uncomplicated common colds are generally treated with OTC medications, including antihistamines, decongestants, cough suppressants, analgesics, antipyretics, and anti-inflammatories. The aim in treatment is to provide relief of symptoms. Naturally, the respiratory system is also prone to more serious diseases and conditions, such as asthma, which affects more than 15 million people and is responsible for as many as 1.5 million emergency room visits and 500,000 hospitalizations every year. If left uncontrolled, asthma can cause a long-term decline in lung function. Because many respiratory diseases are treated with some form of inhalation therapy, it is important for you, as a pharmacy technician, to be able to assist the pharmacist in educating clients as to the proper, safe use of inhalation products. You should also be aware of the most common respiratory disorders that require pharmacological treatment, including conditions treated with OTC drugs.

REVIEW QUESTIONS

Match the following.

1. _____ allergen
2. _____ allergy
3. _____ cilia
4. _____ COPD
5. _____ epiglottis
6. _____ larynx
7. _____ pharynx
8. _____ rhinitis
9. _____ trachea

a. result of immune system reaction

b. inflammation of the nasal passages

c. tiny hair-like organelles in the nose and bronchial passageways

d. windpipe

e. substance capable of causing a hypersensitivity reaction

f. condition resulting from something continually blocking oxygen external exchange in the lungs

g. the voicebox

h. small, leaf-shaped cartilage attached to the tongue that prevents substances other than air from entering the trachea

i. part of the throat from the back of the nasal cavity to the larynx

Choose the best answer.

10. The primary function of the respiratory system is to:
    a. transport air to and from the lungs.
    b. supply oxygen to the blood.
    c. exchange oxygen for carbon dioxide.
    d. keep the brain alive.

11. Chronic obstructive pulmonary disease (COPD) is:
    a. an umbrella term for emphysema and chronic bronchitis.
    b. a serious respiratory disease that makes it difficult to breathe.
    c. partially blocked bronchi and bronchioles.
    d. all of the above.

12. The exchange of gases between blood and cells is called:
    a. pulmonary ventilation.
    b. internal respiration.
    c. external respiration.
    d. cellular respiration.

13. Which does not belong to the conducting portion of the respiratory system?
    a. alveoli
    b. bronchioles
    c. nose
    d. pharynx

14. The structure that closes off the larynx is called the:
    a. glottis.
    b. Adam's apple.
    c. epiglottis.
    d. vocal cords.

15. The exchange of gases occurs in the:
    a. trachea.
    b. bronchioles.
    c. alveoli.
    d. bronchus.

16. The volume of air that can be exhaled after normal exhalation is the:
    a. tidal volume.
    b. residual volume.
    c. inspiratory reserve volume.
    d. expiratory reserve volume.

4. The Combat Methamphetamine Epidemic Act of 2005 requires nonprescription products to be sold from behind the pharmacy counter if they contain any of the following products *except*:
   a. dextromethorphan.
   c. pseudoephedrine.
   b. ephedrine.
   d. phenylpropanolamine.

5. Which of the following drugs would be considered the most appropriate for an acute asthma attack?
   a. albuterol
   c. amoxicillin
   b. Singulair®
   d. Flagyl®

ACTIVITY 25-1: Anatomy Worksheet

The Upper Respiratory Tract

Label the following illustration of the upper respiratory tract.

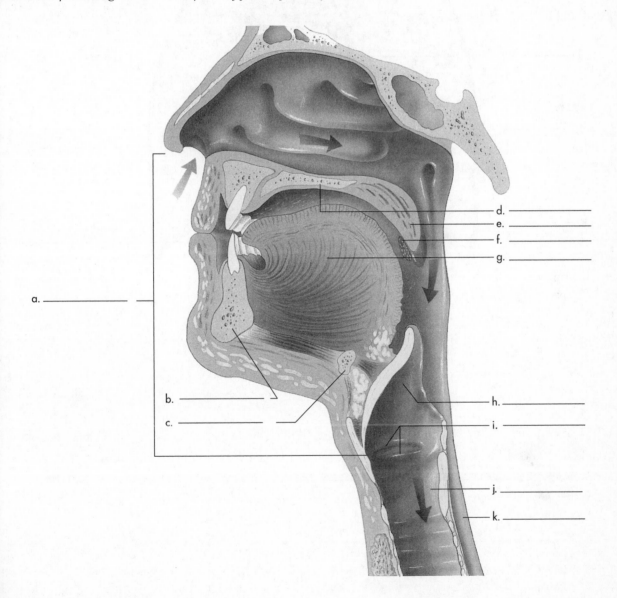

The Lower Respiratory Tract

Label the following illustration of the lower respiratory tract.

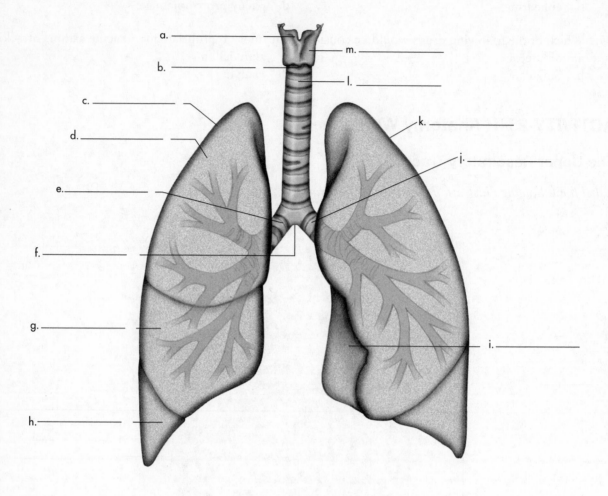

The Lungs

Label the following illustration of the lungs.

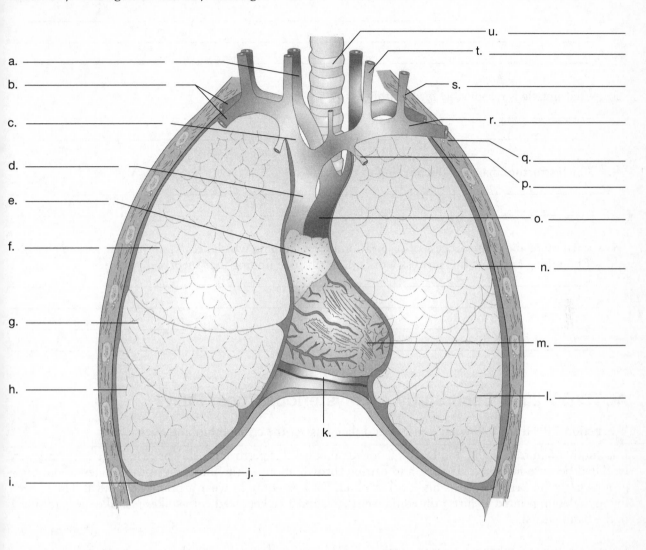

a. _____

b. _____

c. _____

d. _____

e. _____

f. _____

g. _____

h. _____

i. _____

j. _____

k. _____

u. _____

t. _____

s. _____

r. _____

q. _____

p. _____

o. _____

n. _____

m. _____

l. _____

Questions

1. Describe the two main functions of the respiratory system.

   _____

   _____

   _____

   _____

2. What occurs if a part of the body does not receive enough oxygen? What is the medical term for this?

_____

_____

_____

_____

3. What muscle is responsible for breathing?

_____

_____

4. Which structure manages the opening to the trachea?

_____

_____

5. Learn more about the process of respiration by researching which area(s) in the brain are in charge of breathing and how this process works. Describe one finding that surprised you.

_____

_____

_____

_____

ACTIVITY 25-2: Case Study—A Mysterious Chest Pain

Instructions: Read the following scenario and then answer the critical thinking questions.

It is another Saturday night, and Dave's favorite punk band is performing downtown. Dave goes out every weekend because he enjoys dancing and getting thrown about in the mosh pit at the venues where these groups perform. Because this is his favorite band, Dave is going to wear a brand-new outfit he has been dying to debut: printed T-shirt, printed flat sneakers, and a jacket laced with spikes just like the lead singer in the band wears.

Dave is no amateur when it comes to mosh pits. He has been doing this for about two and a half years now and feels like he will be doing it for a lot more years. He even met his girlfriend in the pit six months ago, and she is going to meet him there tonight. Dave arrives just as the band is about to start, so he positions himself near the front. As the band plays, the crowd gets very physical, tossing, jumping, and thrashing. Bodies clash while the music plays. It is a great night for Dave.

The next day Dave experiences some chest pain and some shortness of breath. He shrugs it off, thinking that he may have overexerted himself the night before in all the excitement. As the day progresses, however, his heart begins racing and his chest feels tight. Suddenly the chest pains become more intense, especially while coughing, and Dave takes himself to the emergency room.

At the emergency room, they initially think Dave is having a heart attack, because he is gripping his chest. They listen to his chest and are unable to find breathing sounds in the left lung. An X-ray is ordered so the physicians can see if air is outside the lung. While Dave has his shirt off in the X-ray department, the technician notices a puncture wound in his back. The results of the X-ray are positive for air outside the lung.

1. What is Dave's condition?

_____

_____

2. Based on the scenario, what likely led Dave to acquire this condition?

_____

_____

_____

_____

3. What is the treatment for this condition?

_____

_____

_____

_____

4. How do you think this experience will affect his favorite mosh-pit activity?

_____

_____

_____

_____

ACTIVITY 25-3: Case Study—A New Baby

Instructions: Read the following scenario and then answer the critical thinking questions.

Mr. and Mrs. Kent could not be happier. They have delivered a beautiful baby girl and are ready to raise a child. The nursery is done, the diapers are stacked. Each outfit has been hand-selected, and Mrs. Kent has taken three months off from work to take care of the baby.

A short time after they take the baby home, they notice that the baby's stool is greasy and has a strong, pungent odor. Being new parents, they believe that this is normal. Shortly after this discovery, though, they notice that the baby coughs a lot—they feel it might be excessively. Both Mr. and Mrs. Kent are in excellent health. Mrs. Kent takes the baby to the doctor for a checkup.

The baby presents with incessant coughing, with phlegm production and thick sinuses full of mucus. A stool sample is ordered when Mrs. Kent explains the smelly situation and the baby's diaper is full of diarrhea. The doctor orders an examination of the sputum, blood tests, and a sweat test.

1. What does the doctor suspect might cause these symptoms?

_____

_____

_____

2. Why does the doctor order a sweat test and examination of the sputum?

_____

_____

_____

_____

3. What is the average life span of a person with this disease? From what complication do they usually die?

_____

_____

_____

_____

4. How can this be a hereditary disease, when neither parent has this disease?

_____

_____

_____

_____

5. How do you think this might affect the family's lifestyle choices?

_____

_____

_____

_____

ACTIVITY 25-4: Case Study—Multi-Ingredient Products

Instructions: Read the following scenario and then answer the critical thinking questions.

Everyone in the Hendersen household is sick with a cold. Dad, Mom, 16-year-old Shari, 11-year-old Dan, and 18-month-old Brandy all have severe nasal congestion. Miserable as they are, Mom has made several trips to the local mega-grocery store to purchase one cold remedy after another. She has bought them all, including capsules, gelcaps, disintegrating tablets, and powders that are mixed into liquids.

At first she chose the medication that she remembered seeing advertised in the magazines she read while waiting for her appointments; these seemed familiar and somewhat comforting when they were right in front of her. Later, she started making choices based on the pretty packaging and how many ingredients were in the formulation, figuring the more the better.

Frustrated by all her futile attempts to find a medication that would work, she decides to stop by the pharmacy the next time she visits the mega-grocery store. She asks the pharmacist for a recommendation of the most popular remedy that would help her family. The pharmacist asks if they have any other symptoms besides the nasal congestion and she replies no. He gives her the standard information about plenty of fluids, chicken soup, and saline nose drops. He then tells her that she needs a decongestant; however, there is one family member who will not be able to use it.

1. Based on the information in the scenario, what was Mrs. Kent doing wrong in selecting medications?

_____

_____

_____

_____

2. What is the common cold and how is it contracted?

_____

_____

_____

_____

3. What can be done to avoid spreading a cold to others?

_____

_____

_____

_____

4. Which family member was the pharmacist referring to when he warned that one family member could not use the decongestant? Why?

_____

_____

_____

_____

5. What other medicines might interact with decongestants?

_____

_____

_____

_____

LAB 25-1: Proper Usage and Maintenance of a Nebulizer Machine

Objectives:

Demonstrate the proper use and maintenance of a nebulizer machine.

Demonstrate ability to teach patients how to set up, use, and clean a nebulizer.

Pre-Lab Information:

Gather the materials needed:

- nebulizer machine
- nebulizer kit assembly, including:
  - nebulizer cup unit
  - tubing
  - mouthpiece or mask
  - tee adapter
  - training respiratory treatment or normal saline ampule
  - nebulizer filter
  - warm water
  - mild detergent solution
  - vinegar

Explanation:

If you work as a pharmacy technician in a retail pharmacy setting, you will need to assist patients who require prescribed nebulizer treatments. Many patients do not learn from their physicians how to set up, use, and clean the nebulizer properly; this means that your skilled assistance is critical to them and ensures proper medication compliance.

Activity:
Part One

Procedure: Operating a Nebulizer Machine

1. Open the nebulizer cup unit by turning it counterclockwise. Pour the medication (3 mL training respiratory treatment or normal saline) into the bottom portion of the unit.
2. Close the nebulizer by turning the cup unit clockwise.
3. Connect one end of the tubing to the air outlet located on the nebulizer machine and the other end of the tubing to the nebulizer cup unit.
4. Attach the tee adapter to the top of the nebulizer cup unit.
5. Attach the mouthpiece or mask to one end of the tee adapter, leaving the opposite end open.
6. Connect the nebulizer machine to a power outlet and turn on the machine using the ON/OFF switch. It is normal for the machine to make a loud vibrating sound and to emit a smoking mist from both ends of the tee adapter.
7. The patient should insert the mouthpiece into the mouth, or have a mask secured over the nose and mouth and then breathe normally until the treatment is complete.

8. Upon completion of the treatment, turn the nebulizer machine off and remove the nebulizer kit assembly for proper cleaning.

Part Two

Procedure: Cleaning/Maintenance of a Nebulizer Kit Assembly

1. After each use, the nebulizer kit assembly should be cleaned to avoid possible infection.
2. Clean each component of the nebulizer kit assembly, excluding the tubing, with warm water and a mild detergent solution.
3. Rinse the components with warm water for 30 seconds to remove the detergent.
4. Soak all the parts in a mixture of 3 parts warm water to 1 part vinegar for 30 minutes.
5. Rinse the components with warm water and allow them to air-dry on clean paper towels.
6. The nebulizer filter should be changed every 6 months or as soon as it turns a gray color.

Discussion Questions:

1. Why is it important for pharmacy technicians to be knowledgeable about the operation and maintenance of nebulizer machines?

_____

_____

_____

_____

2. Which patient categories would benefit from using a face mask for administration, as opposed to a mouthpiece?

_____

_____

_____

_____

3. Why is it important that the nebulizer components be cleaned following each treatment?

_____

_____

_____

_____

Student Name: _____

Lab Partner: _____

Grade/Comments: _____

_____

_____

Student Comments: _____

_____

_____

CHAPTER 26

The Cardiovascular, Circulatory, and Lymph Systems

After completing Chapter 26 from the textbook, you should be able to:	Related Activity in the Workbook/Lab Manual
1. List, identify, and diagram the basic anatomical structure and parts of the heart.	Review Questions, PTCB Exam Practice Questions Activity 26-1
2. Explain the function of the heart and the circulation of the blood within the body.	Review Questions, PTCB Exam Practice Questions Activity 26-1
3. List and define common diseases affecting the heart, including the causes, symptoms, and pharmaceutical treatment associated with each disease.	Review Questions, PTCB Exam Practice Questions Activity 26-2, Activity 26-3, Activity 26-4, Activity 26-5
4. Explain how each class of drugs works to mitigate symptoms of heart diseases.	Review Questions, PTCB Exam Practice Questions
5. Describe the mechanism of action of anticoagulants, indications for use, and antidotes for overdose.	Review Questions
6. List a variety of drugs intended to affect the cardiovascular system, their classifications, and the average adult dose.	Review Questions, PTCB Exam Practice Questions
7. List the total cholesterol, LDL, HDL, and triglyceride ranges for an average adult and describe the differences between HDL, LDL, and triglycerides.	Review Questions Activity 26-5
8. Describe the structure and main functions of the lymphatic system, and explain its relationship to the cardiovascular system.	Review Questions, PTCB Exam Practice Questions Activity 26-1

INTRODUCTION

The cardiovascular system, or circulatory system, is responsible for transporting blood to all parts of the body. It includes the heart, arteries, arterioles, veins, venules, and capillaries. The arteries are responsible for carrying oxygen-rich blood to the cells while the veins carry the deoxygenated blood back to the heart and lungs. The lungs and respiratory system work in tandem with the cardiovascular system to sustain life. To accomplish its primary purpose as a pumping mechanism that circulates blood to all parts of the body, the heart relies on a conduction system comprised of nodes and nodal tissues that regulate the various aspects of the heartbeat. In addition, the nervous system plays a vital role in regulating heart rate. The lymphatic system and circulatory system also work closely together as blood and lymph fluid move through the same capillary system. Lymph fluid removes wastes and debris from the body and supports the immune system by filtering out pathogens and draining excess fluid from the body.

The two common diseases affecting the cardiovascular system are congestive heart failure (CHF) and coronary artery disease (CAD). Congestive heart failure occurs when the heart pumps out less blood than it receives, resulting in a weakened and enlarged heart, and in less blood being pumped to feed the other organs. CAD is a condition characterized by insufficient blood flow to the heart. Hypertension, or high blood pressure, and hyperlipidemia, or high blood cholesterol, are two additional conditions that affect the cardiovascular system. Often, both hypertension and hyperlipidemia go undetected, as these conditions do not cause substantial symptoms. As a pharmacy technician, you should also be aware of the most common cardiovascular disorders that require pharmacological treatment, including conditions treated with OTC drugs.

REVIEW QUESTIONS

Match the following.

1. __c__ arterioles
2. __f__ atrioventricular valves
3. __i__ contractility
4. __h__ DOC
5. __j__ DVT
6. _____ dyscrasias
7. __o__ hematuria
8. __d__ hyperlipidemia
9. __m__ interstitial space
10. __k__ leukocyte
11. __a__ venules
12. __q__ plaque
13. __g__ phlebitis
14. __p__ pulmonary edema
15. __e__ proteinuria
16. __n__ semilunar valves
17. __l__ thrombus

a. smallest of veins
b. body tissue spaces
c. smallest of arteries
d. high concentrations of lipids
e. large quantities of protein in the urine
f. tricuspid and mitral valves
g. inflammation of a vein
h. drug of choice
i. ability to contract and the degree of contraction
j. deep venous thrombosis
k. white blood cell
l. blood clot
m. abnormal condition of the body, especially a blood imbalance
n. aortic and pulmonary valves
o. blood in the urine
p. condition in which fluid collects in pulmonary vessels
q. fatty deposits high in cholesterol

Choose the best answer.

18. The human body contains _____ of blood.
    a. 4,300 gallons
    b. 15.6 liters
    c. 5.6 liters
    d. none of the above

19. The heart muscle pumps _____ of blood daily.
    a. 4,300 gallons
    b. 16.6 liters
    c. 5.6 liters
    d. none of the above

ACTIVITY 26-1: Anatomy Worksheet

The Heart

Label the following illustration of the heart.

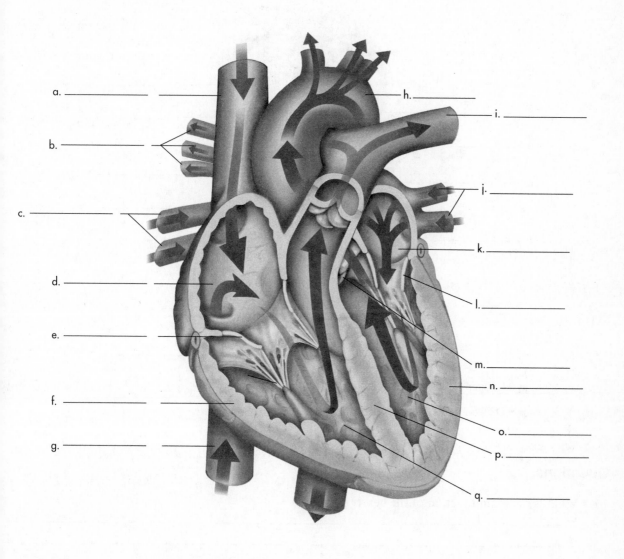

a. _____

b. _____

c. _____

d. _____

e. _____

f. _____

g. _____

h. _____

i. _____

j. _____

k. _____

l. _____

m. _____

n. _____

o. _____

p. _____

q. _____

Pulmonary Circulation

Label the following illustration showing pulmonary circulation.

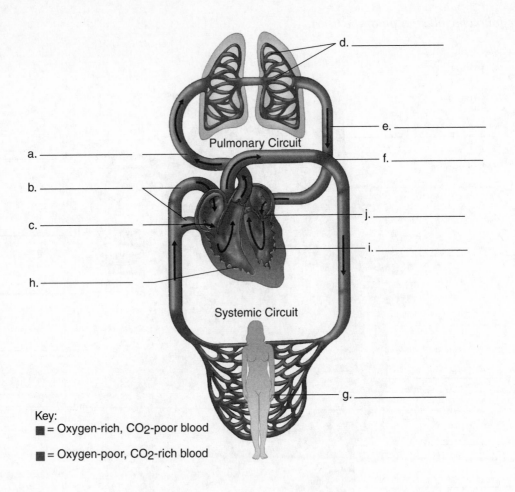

Questions:

1. What is the main function of the heart?

_____

_____

_____

2. What are three functions of blood?

_____

_____

_____

3. Which vessels supply the heart with blood?

_____

_____

_____

4. Describe the process of pulmonary circulation in your own words. Use your textbook or other medical resources to help you.

_____

_____

_____

_____

_____

_____

5. Describe the cardiac cycle in your own words. Use your textbook or other medical resources to help you.

_____

_____

_____

_____

_____

_____

6. How is lymph circulated throughout the body?

_____

_____

_____

_____

ACTIVITY 26-2: Case Study—Leg Pain

Instructions: Read the following scenario and then answer the critical thinking questions.

Eleanor Stark is an active woman who volunteers at the community food bank up to four days a week. Eleanor is a very healthy 62-year-old. Other than docusate sodium for constipation, and an occasional acetaminophen for pain, her only regular medication is estrogen. Eleanor recently returned from a visit to her sister's home, 10 states away, where she traveled by bus. Although it was a long, tiring ride, she thoroughly enjoyed the opportunity to see her sister.

Eleanor is now presenting with pain and tenderness in one leg. She says that it feels hot, and it even looks red-hot and appears to be swelling up more each day. She makes an appointment with her doctor when she can no longer tolerate the pain. It is not long before Eleanor is sent to the hospital and kept there to treat her problem.

1. What problem does Eleanor appear to have?

_____

_____

2. Based on the information given about Eleanor, what could have placed her in a high-risk category for this condition?

_____

_____

3. What is the goal of treatment for this type of condition?

_____

_____

4. When Eleanor becomes an inpatient at the hospital, what will her treatment be?

_____

_____

5. Eleanor is a very active lady and despises being in the hospital for treatment. Is there an alternative to a lengthy hospital stay?

_____

_____

ACTIVITY 26-3: Case Study—A Medical Emergency

Instructions: Read the following scenario and then answer the critical thinking questions.

The ambulance is dispatched to an apartment complex about 45 miles away from the hospital. A neighbor called in, stating that the man next door would not answer the door after she heard a suspicious thump. The ambulance arrives at the Cottonwood Apartment complex at 6:30 a.m. The paramedics pound on the door of apartment 224. They hear a whimper from inside the apartment and the neighbor opens the unlocked door for the emergency personnel. They find a man, about 50 years old, hunched over and clenching his fist against the center of his chest.

The man states that his chest is tight and has been for almost an hour. He does not have pain anywhere else. Medical history questions reveal that the man has high blood pressure and has been prescribed nitroglycerin for chest pain; however, he could not get to it in the bathroom medicine cabinet. He says that the nitroglycerin usually works.

On the way to the hospital, three doses of nitroglycerin 0.4 mg sublingual give him no relief. Oxygen and an IV are started and he is given morphine. Within minutes the pain is subsiding. IV nitroglycerin is started.

1. Why does the clenched fist mean so much to the emergency personnel?

_____

_____

2. How does nitroglycerin work in the body?

_____

_____

3. What safety precaution, in relation to blood pressure, must be considered when using nitroglycerin?

_____

_____

ACTIVITY 26-4: Case Study—A Bad Headache

Instructions: Read the following scenario and then answer the critical thinking questions.

Carmen is a 54-year-old, diabetic, overweight mother of 6 children who range in age from 32 to 7. She has always been a model housewife and mother, preparing all family meals, keeping the house tidy, and helping the children with schoolwork. In addition to taking care of her children, she is also raising two grandchildren, ages 7 and 9. Carmen's medical history includes diabetes, asthma, periodic constipation, heartburn, and mild depression at times.

One evening Carmen develops a mild headache and takes some acetaminophen before retiring to sleep after another long day. By morning, her headache is so bad that her head is throbbing, she is sensitive to light, her ears are ringing, and she sees spots before her eyes. She cannot get out of bed because moving intensifies the headache.

1. What do you suspect is going on with Carmen?

   _____

   _____

2. What tests might be conducted to confirm this diagnosis?

   _____

   _____

3. What lifestyle changes could Carmen make that would make a difference in her health condition?

   _____

   _____

ACTIVITY 26-5: Analyzing Cholesterol Screening Test Results

In Chapter 26 of the textbook, you learned about the role cholesterol plays in causing heart disease, stroke, and other health conditions. Physicians screen their patients to determine their lipid levels: total cholesterol, LDL, HDL, and triglycerides. They then compare these levels against acceptable ranges to determine if a patient may be at risk for developing a heart attack or stroke. They then use this information to decide if the patient requires medication, lifestyle and/or behavioral changes, or a combination of both.

As a pharmacy technician, it is important for you to understand how the cholesterol screening tests work and to be familiar with the different ranges. Your place of employment may also offer free screenings to patients or customers.

Part One

Review the information on cholesterol in Chapter 26 of your textbook. Then, visit the American Heart Association website and locate the information sheet called "What Do My Cholesterol Levels Mean?" (http://www.americanheart.org/presenter.jhtml?identifier=3004817). Now answer the following questions.

1. What does the abbreviation *HDL* mean?

   _____

2. Why is HDL considered "good" cholesterol?

   _____

   _____

3. What is the normal range, for both women and men, for HDL cholesterol?

   _____

   _____

4. What does the abbreviation *LDL* mean?

   _____

5. Why is this considered "bad" cholesterol?

   _____

   _____

6. What is the normal range for LDL cholesterol? What is an optimal range for a person at risk of heart attack or death from heart attack? What is an optimal range for a person with heart disease or diabetes?

   _____

   _____

   _____

7. What are triglycerides, and how are they related to heart disease?

   _____

   _____

8. What is a normal range for triglycerides?

   _____

   _____

Part Two

Now you will review some cholesterol screening test results for three fictitious patients. Review the results, then go to http://www.americanheart.org/presenter.jhtml?identifier=183 to determine the ranges for each patient and answer the related questions.

Patient 1

Mary Smathers, age 53, had her annual physical last week. Here are the results of her cholesterol screening.

Lipid Screen	Result	What is the range for this patient?
Total cholesterol	181	
Triglycerides	56	
HDL cholesterol	74	
LDL cholesterol	96	

1. Based on these ranges, does Mary Smathers appear to be at risk for developing coronary heart disease?

   _____

2. How about her risk of having a heart attack or stroke?

   _____

Patient 2

John Price, age 83, just received the results of his cholesterol screening.

Lipid Screen	Result	What is the range for this patient?
Total cholesterol	242	
Triglycerides	163	
HDL cholesterol	32	
LDL cholesterol	140	

1. Based on these ranges, does John Price appear to be at risk for developing coronary heart disease?

   _____

2. How about his risk of having a heart attack or stroke?

   _____

3. Name five things John can do to improve his lipid result numbers.

   _____

   _____

   _____

   _____

   _____

4. What are some risk factors for coronary heart disease?

_____

_____

_____

_____

Patient 3

Manny Lewis, an overweight smoker in his 50s, also received the results of his cholesterol screening.

Lipid Screen	Result	What is the range for this patient?
Total cholesterol	198	
Triglycerides	153	
HDL cholesterol	37	
LDL cholesterol	119	

1. Based on his levels, what condition is Manny at risk of developing?

_____

_____

2. What specific lifestyle changes should Manny adopt immediately to improve his numbers?

_____

_____

CHAPTER 27
The Immune System

After completing Chapter 27 from the textbook, you should be able to:	Related Activity in the Workbook/Lab Manual
1. Explain how the body's nonspecific and specific defense mechanisms work to keep the body safe from disease-causing microorganisms.	Review Questions Activity 27-1
2. Understand the basic relationships between the immune system and the various body systems.	Review Questions Activity 27-1, Activity 27-4, Lab 27-2
3. List and describe the different types of infectious organisms.	Review Questions, PTCB Exam Practice Questions Activity 27-1, Lab 27-1
4. Compare and contrast HIV-1 and HIV-2 and identify the various subgroups of HIV.	Review Questions, PTCB Exam Practice Questions
5. List the five stages of progression of HIV to AIDS.	Review Questions
6. Explain how the different classes of HIV drugs work.	Review Questions
7. Describe autoimmune disease and identify various types.	Review Questions, PTCB Exam Practice Questions
8. Understand how drug resistance develops and what steps can be taken to stop it.	Review Questions Lab 27-1
9. List and define common anti-infective drug classifications, their mechanisms of action, and their side effects.	Review Questions, PTCB Exam Practice Questions Activity 27-3, Lab 27-1
10. Describe both tuberculosis and malaria and their causes, treatments, and prevention.	Review Questions Activity 27-3
11. Identify the different types and uses of vaccines and how they work in the body.	Review Questions

INTRODUCTION

The immune system protects the body from foreign invaders that would otherwise destroy it, or parts of it, via infection or cancer. The immune system uses numerous kinds of responses to attacks from these foreign invaders, and is amazingly effective most of the time. Its defensive barriers and mechanisms include nonspecific mechanisms, such as the skin, mucus and cilia in the linings of the respiratory and digestive passageways, and the blood clotting process. They also include specific defense mechanisms, such as the white blood cells, thymus gland, lymph nodes, antibodies, and lymphocytes (B-cells and T-cells).

Many different classes of medications affect the immune system. These include drugs for the treatment of HIV/AIDS, tuberculosis, and malaria, as well as for many other conditions and diseases of the immune system. Pharmacotherapeutic treatment of pathogens includes antibacterials, anti-infectives, and antifungals, to name a few. As a pharmacy technician, it is important for you to have a clear understanding of what these drugs are and how they work to protect the body.

In addition to fighting foreign invaders, sometimes the immune system is called upon to help defend against the autoimmune process in cases of autoimmune diseases, like lupus erythematosus or rheumatoid arthritis, in which a person's immune system mistakenly attacks itself. The end result of this defense is often inflammation. These autoimmune diseases are treated both pharmacologically and nonpharmacologically. The pharmacotherapeutic goal of treatment is to reduce inflammation, or to stop or suppress the inflammatory process.

REVIEW QUESTIONS

Match the following.

1. _____ aerobic
2. _____ anaerobic
3. _____ antibodies
4. _____ antigens
5. _____ complement
6. _____ DNA
7. _____ epitopes
8. _____ endocytosis
9. _____ hemopoietic
10. _____ genome
11. _____ lysis
12. _____ macrophage
13. _____ pathogen
14. _____ phagocytes
15. _____ RNA

a. process in which cells take up fluids, particles, and other substances

b. the destruction of cells

c. molecules that trigger an immune response

d. blood-forming

e. nucleic acid that carries genetic information

f. nucleic acid that is needed for the metabolic processes of protein synthesis

g. group of proteins that activate a sequence resulting in the death of a substance

h. white blood cell, found in connective tissue and the bloodstream

i. region on the surface of an antibody that is capable of producing an immune response

j. specialized cells that engulf and ingest other cells

k. a disease-causing organism

l. requires oxygen for life

m. complete hereditary material of an organism

n. does not require oxygen for life

o. proteins that specifically seek and bind to antigens

Choose the best answer.

16. Which of the following is not a defense against infection?
    a. mucus
    b. bone marrow
    c. vertebral column
    d. skin

17. Which of the following is not a deterrent to pathogens?
    a. phagocytes or macrophages
    b. lysozymes
    c. tears
    d. none of the above

18. What causes scabs?
    a. clotting factors
    b. flora
    c. proteins
    d. scabbing gene

19. Which are protozoa that most often consume algae and bacteria?
    a. sporozoans
    b. zooflagellates
    c. cilates
    d. ameboids

20. Which have a specialized opening in the outer edge to capture their prey?
    a. sporozoans
    b. zooflagellates
    c. cilates
    d. ameboids

21. Which are parasites that live inside a host and often cause disease to the host by robbing the host of nutrients?
    a. sporozoans
    b. zooflagellates
    c. cilates
    d. ameboids

22. Which of the following is not a solution to resistance?
    a. Avoid using antibiotics unnecessarily.
    b. Complete each antibacterial regimen; do not have leftover pills.
    c. Use the widest-spectrum antibiotic possible.
    d. Use the common antibiotics first.

True or False?

23. A bacillus, or rod-shaped, bacterium has an approximate measurement of 0.5 to 1 μm in width and from 1 to 4 μm in length.

    T   F

24. Spirillium is comma shaped or resembles part of a wave.

    T   F

25. About 20% of nosocomial bacterial infections (often acquired in hospitals) are resistant to at least one of the most commonly prescribed antibiotics.

    T   F

26. Some organisms are resistant to all FDA-approved antibiotics and can be treated only with experimental and potentially toxic drugs.

    T   F

Match the following.

27. _____ Stage 1
28. _____ hormones
29. _____ Stage 2
30. _____ chemotherapy
31. _____ Stage 3
32. _____ radiation
33. _____ Stage 4
34. _____ antibodies
35. _____ Stage 5
36. _____ surgery

a. opportunistic infections to a CD4 cell count or level below 200 per cubic millimeter of blood

b. usually the first line of treatment for solid tumors

c. last and final stage of wasting to death

d. may be used in conjunction with other treatments

e. signs and symptoms of HIV begin to show

f. uses cytotoxic agents to kill cancer cells

g. infected without presentation of signs or symptoms

h. prevent cancer cells from receiving signals necessary for continued growth and division

i. initial transmission and infection with HIV

j. used to target cancer cells, depriving the cancer cells of necessary signals or causing the direct death of the cells

PHARMACY CALCULATION PROBLEMS

Calculate the following.

1. If cefuroxime 750 mg IV is administered to a patient tid × 3 days, how many grams will the patient receive over the entire course?

2. A patient has a prescription for acyclovir 200 mg capsules. If the scrip reads, "Take one capsule five times daily for 10 days," how many milligrams will the patient take during the entire course of treatment?

3. Statistically, if one out of every four women has the herpes virus, how many women might be infected at a university with 7,500 women enrolled?

4. Your pharmacy marks up all herbal medication 40% above cost. If a bottle of echinacea costs the pharmacy $3.25, what is the retail price?

1. All of the following are types of infectious organisms *except*:
   a. yeasts.
   b. bacteria.
   c. viruses.
   d. lipids.

2. AIDS is the result of infection by which type of infectious organism?
   a. yeast
   b. bacterium
   c. virus
   d. parasite

3. Ciprofloxacin (Cipro®) belongs to what class of antibiotics?
   a. quinolone
   b. sulfa
   c. cephalosporin
   d. aminoglycoside

4. All of the following are considered to be autoimmune diseases *except*:
   a. cystic fibrosis.
   b. Crohn's disease.
   c. lupus.
   d. multiple sclerosis.

5. Which of the following classes of antibiotics is divided into four generations?
   a. penicillins
   b. aminoglycosides
   c. macrolides
   d. cephalosporins

ACTIVITY 27-1: Anatomy Worksheet

A Lymph Node

Label the following illustration of a lymph node.

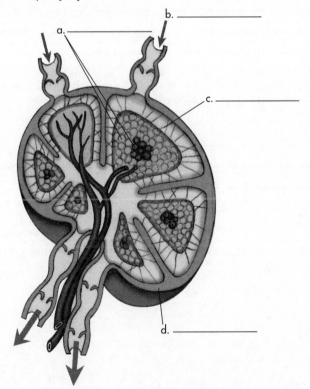

A Virus

Label the following illustration of a virus.

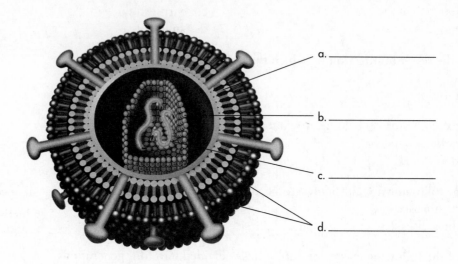

a. _____

b. _____

c. _____

d. _____

Questions:

1. What are nonspecific defense mechanisms? Give five examples and discuss how each one functions.

   _____
   _____
   _____
   _____
   _____

2. How is the cell-mediated response different from the antibody-mediated response? Which type of response plays a role in the effectiveness of vaccinations?

   _____
   _____
   _____
   _____

3. How does the immune system affect or assist the other systems within the body? Match each immune system effect with the correct body system.

Match the following.

1. _____ Provides antibodies found in skin (IgA, IgG, etc.) to assist in immune function of protection.

2. _____ Lymph vessels carry absorbed lipids to the bloodstream.

3. _____ Assists in repair after injuries. Assists in repair of bone. Macrophages (phagocytes) fuse to make bone cells.

4. _____ Tonsils, which are lymphoid tissue, protect against infection at the entrance to the respiratory tract. Lungs remove inhaled and deposited solid material and microorganisms. Plays a supportive role in maintaining and eliminating fluids.

5. _____ Fights blood vessel infections. Returns interstitial tissue fluid to circulation via veins.

6. _____ Fights bladder and kidney infections.

7. _____ Thymus gland secretes thymosin.

8. _____ Produces antibodies to assist in immune system function. Through cytokine- and interleukin-mediated pathways, regulates this system by inducing the release of gonadotropins (luteinizing hormone and follicle-stimulating hormone).

9. _____ Produces *cytokines*, immune hormones that affect the production of other hormones by the hypothalamus.

a. nervous

b. circulatory

c. endocrine

d. renal

e. respiratory

f. musculoskeletal

g. integumentary

h. reproductive

i. digestive

4. Name six kinds of infectious organisms.

_____

_____

_____

_____

_____

_____

ACTIVITY 27-2: Case Study—A Severe Cold

Instructions: Read the following scenario and then answer the critical thinking questions.

Mrs. Tindle has been coming into your retail pharmacy quite frequently in the past four days. She has purchased several OTC multi-ingredient cough/cold remedies. She looks miserable and appears to have a nasty cold. When she returns two days later for more medicine, you comment, "Back so soon?" She states that her son has also been sick and that her husband is beginning to catch the cold also. She tells you that her son was the first one in the family to get sick.

Mrs. Tindle finally takes herself and her 16-year-old son to the doctor's office after 6 days of suffering with multiple symptoms. She presents with sore throat, chills, diarrhea, and vomiting that has worsened. Occasionally she has a fever and takes acetaminophen. Her son presents with symptoms of thick green nasal discharge and a cough that will not quit. He works out a lot and believes that his condition is due to the hard, constant workouts.

Mrs. Tindle explains to the doctor that they have tried "everything" over the counter, including multiple popular cough/cold preparations. They want to know if they can get an antibiotic today.

1. What else would the doctor do to see if this is a bacterial infection that can be treated with an antibiotic?

   _____

   _____

   _____

2. What are the diagnoses for the mother and the son in this scenario? What does the doctor prescribe for each, considering their symptoms?

   _____

   _____

   _____

3. Is there any other treatment option for each person's condition?

   _____

   _____

   _____

4. What is the difference between bacterial and viral infection?

   _____

   _____

   _____

5. Mrs. Tindle returns to your pharmacy upset that she did not receive an antibiotic from the doctor for her cold like her son did for his symptoms. She insists that the pharmacy call and ask her doctor for an antibiotic for her. What do you do?

   _____

   _____

   _____

ACTIVITY 27-3: Case Study—TB

Instructions: Read the following scenario and then answer the critical thinking questions.

A 49-year-old Jamaican male moved to the United States about 10 years ago. His medical history includes a diagnosis of rheumatoid arthritis, for which he is prescribed prednisone 20 mg, methotrexate, and Humira®.

The patient has just returned from Jamaica, where he visited family members, and noticed within days that he was having increasing difficulty breathing, accompanied by a cough. He did not recall being around anyone sick while in Jamaica. The patient becomes very sick with fever and chills and stops taking the Humira®. He visits the doctor, who finds nothing wrong and tells him that the symptoms will disappear in a few days.

A few months later, he visits Jamaica again. Within days of returning, he has a bad cough that produces blood and shortly he ends up in the emergency room. TB is suspected and he is placed into a negative-pressure room. The TB skin test comes up negative, but another type of lung biopsy comes back positive for TB.

1. What are the symptoms of an active TB infection?

_____

_____

_____

2. Given the information provided in the scenario, what could have contributed to the TB infection?

_____

_____

_____

3. Knowing that TB is a communicable disease, what are other public-exposure concerns in this scenario?

_____

_____

_____

4. Could the pharmacy have provided any patient information regarding his other health condition that might have alerted this patient to his high-risk TB category?

_____

_____

_____

5. What is the treatment for this type of condition?

_____

_____

_____

ACTIVITY 27-4: Case Study—Birthday Party Emergency

Instructions: Read the following scenario and then answer the critical thinking questions.

Tommy is an 8-year-old, precocious little boy who is quite a handful for his teachers in school. To his teachers, it seems that Tommy cannot sit still for a minute, and he is always getting into something. Because Tommy is constantly jumping around and unable to focus his attention, the teachers think he might have ADHD. The school convinces Tommy's mother to seek medication for this condition. Tommy also suffers from headaches, asthma, and constant stomach pain that has lasted ever since his mother can remember. At her wit's end, Tommy's mother makes an appointment for him the following week.

Over the weekend, Tommy attends his cousin's birthday party, where all the children are playing and running around. All of a sudden Tommy is on the floor with what appears to be an anaphylactic reaction to something. As people scramble to call an ambulance, Tommy's mother frantically tries to find out from the other children what happened to Tommy. One of the other little boys says that the last thing he saw was Tommy eating a Snickers® candy bar in the kitchen.

1. Drawing from the facts in this scenario, what is the most likely cause of Tommy's anaphylactic reaction?

   _____

   _____

   _____

2. What is an anaphylactic reaction?

   _____

   _____

   _____

3. Tommy has eaten Snickers® bars before, so why did he not have this reaction then?

   _____

   _____

   _____

4. What is the treatment for this condition?

   _____

   _____

   _____

LAB 27-1: Web Research Activity—Understanding the Herpes Virus

Objective:

Learn about the misconceptions about the herpes virus, how it is spread, and ways to reduce transmission of the virus.

Pre-Lab Information:

Go to the website http://www.cdc.gov/std/Herpes/default.htm. Review the main points on this page, including the fact sheet link, to find out what the herpes virus is, how herpes infection is diagnosed, how the virus is spread, and how it is currently being treated. You may be surprised at the statistics provided by the U.S. Centers for Disease Control and Prevention regarding genital herpes.

Explanation:

The herpes simplex virus type 1 and 2 cause the sexually transmitted disease called genital herpes. It affects one in four women and one in five men in the United States—more than 45 million people. Some statistics show that 70% of those who carry the virus do not even know that they have it. This seems to be one of the reasons why this virus is becoming so widespread. Another reason is that most people believe that the virus is spread only during an outbreak. This is untrue, because the virus can be transmitted during sexual activity even if the infected person is not having an outbreak.

Herpes is a painful condition that affects the person physically and psychologically. There is no cure for infection with the herpes simplex viruses, but medical treatments are available. There are a few antivirals that can be used daily to help prevent outbreaks, or intermittently to shorten outbreaks that occur. One medication, valacyclovir, has been shown in clinical studies to actually reduce the risk of transmission. The best prevention is abstinence, but consistent condom use can help reduce the risk.

Activity:

Review the website in the pre-lab section. Study the statistical reports, and review what herpes is, how it is transmitted, and how it can be treated. Use this information to answer the following questions.

1. According to the CDC, how many Americans are infected with the herpes simplex viruses?

   _____

   _____

2. How many women does it affect?

   _____

   _____

3. How is infection with the HSV 1 and 2 virus diagnosed?

   _____

   _____

4. When a person has the first HSV outbreak, how many outbreaks can she or he expect within that first year?

   _____

   _____

5. Can an infected person infect a sexual partner even when no symptoms or lesions are present?

_____

_____

Student Name: _____

Lab Partner: _____

Grade/Comments: _____

_____

_____

Student Comments: _____

_____

_____

LAB 27-2: Web Research Activity—Alternative and Complementary Medicine

Objective:

Familiarize yourself with some alternative remedies for boosting the immune system.

Pre-Lab Information:

- Access the following website: http://nccam.nih.gov/ and search for the following herbs: echinacea, ginseng, astragalus, and goldenseal.

- Access this website for information regarding acupuncture and traditional Chinese medicine (TCM): http://nccam.nih.gov/health/acupuncture/

- http://nccam.nih.gov/health/ayurveda/ will provide information about Ayurvedic medicine from India. These Web pages are sponsored by the National Center for Alternative and Complementary Medicine, which is a legitimate organization for the advancement of alternative and complementary medicine.

Explanation:

China has successfully used herbs and acupuncture for more than 2,000 years to treat many illnesses and diseases. TCM can boost the immune system, relieve pain, and cure other illnesses and diseases. India has used the Ayurvedic system for thousands of years; it consists of herbs, massage, and yoga. Many people in the United States have turned to alternative medicine to complement the mainstream treatments they are receiving from their physicians. There are good aspects and bad aspects to this approach. Currently, the FDA does not evaluate any dietary supplement or herb, so we cannot be sure we are getting the product for which we paid. A lawsuit in 2008 against "Airborne" homeopathic cold supplement made the headlines because the maker claimed that its product would prevent colds. However, its clinical research was not well defined, and the company was sued for $23 million for false advertising. Because the FDA does not regulate dietary supplements in the way that it does medications, some of these types of products cannot be proven to work. Many herbs also have dangerous interactions with prescription and nonprescription medications. However, some independent and clinical research has begun on various herbs and alternative therapies, with varying degrees of success. It may be only a matter of time before science can prove whether some of these treatments are beneficial. If a person makes wise choices, alternative therapies can be usefully and helpfully integrated into modern Western medicine.

Activity:

It is difficult to do Internet research on alternative medicine, because of the abundance of illegitimate websites trying to make money and the lack of scientifically based research on alternative health. Those seeking alternative treatments often get information by word of mouth or by studying on their own. The National Center for Alternative and Complementary Medicine has a fairly well-documented website, which includes many types of alternative therapies, uses for common herbs, and the scientific data that supports (or rejects) the claims for various substances. Research that website for the common immune-system-boosting herbs listed in the pre-lab section. If the herb is not listed directly on that page, type it into the "search" box to find the information you need.

Also, try the other links in the pre-lab section regarding traditional Chinese medicine, acupuncture, and Ayurveda. These are certainly not the only types of alternative or holistic healing. However, building a foundation of knowledge about two of the many cultures that use herbs and alternative techniques acts as a stepping stone in incorporating some of these modalities into our own lives.

Critical Thinking Questions:

1. Do you find any similarities between Ayurvedic medicine and traditional Chinese medicine?

   _____

   _____

   _____

   _____

2. Based on the claims made about the immune-system-boosting herbs, would you try them to improve your health? Explain your answer.

   _____

   _____

   _____

   _____

3. Based on the brief summary of acupuncture, do you feel that people could benefit from this treatment? Why or why not?

   _____

   _____

   _____

   _____

4. If herbal supplements continue to gain popularity in the United States, do you feel that herbal supplements should be monitored or regulated? Explain your answer.

   _____

   _____

   _____

   _____

Student Name: _____

Lab Partner: _____

Grade/Comments: _____

_____

_____

Student Comments: _____

_____

_____

CHAPTER 28
The Renal System

After completing Chapter 28 from the textbook, you should be able to:	Related Activity in the Workbook/Lab Manual
1. List, identify, and diagram the basic parts of the renal system.	Review Questions, PTCB Exam Practice Questions Activity 28-1
2. Explain the functions of the nephron, kidney, and bladder.	Review Questions, PTCB Exam Practice Questions Activity 28-1
3. List and define common diseases and conditions affecting the renal system and explain the mechanisms of action of each class of drugs used to treat each disease.	Review Questions, PTCB Exam Practice Questions Activity 28-2, Activity 28-3, Activity 28-4
4. Explain how homeostasis of fluid and electrolytes affects the body.	Review Questions, PTCB Exam Practice Questions Activity 28-3

INTRODUCTION

The renal system, or urinary system, is a fairly simple system with few components; however, its condition has a grave impact on many parts of the body. Genitourinary tract infections, poor kidney filtration, and water imbalance can indicate or cause diabetes, high blood pressure, or dehydration. The proper functioning of the kidneys is essential to maintain life. The drugs most commonly used to treat diseases of the renal system are anti-infectives and diuretics. The use of strong diuretics that help to remove excess water may also cause a loss of potassium, which may lead to muscle and heart problems. A delicate balance of electrolytes, kidney function, filtration, and waste removal must be maintained at all times during illnesses and while taking medications that affect or treat the urinary tract. As a pharmacy technician, you should be aware of the most common urinary system disorders that require pharmacological treatment, including conditions treated with OTC drugs.

REVIEW QUESTIONS

Match the following.

1. __H__ acidosis
2. __G__ bilirubin
3. __E__ dialysis
4. __A__ Kegel
5. __C__ ketone
6. __J__ palliative
7. __I__ pH
8. __D__ specific gravity
9. __F__ urobilinogen
10. __B__ void

a. pelvic muscle training exercises
b. empty the bladder
c. a by-product of fat metabolism
d. comparison of a substance's density to that of water
e. medical procedure that removes waste from the blood in cases of renal failure
f. produced by the breakdown of bilirubin
g. produced by the breakdown of hemoglobin
h. excessive acid in the body fluids
i. the measure of acidity or alkalinity of a solution
j. reducing the severity of symptoms

Choose the best answer.

11. The specific gravity of water is:
    a. 1.
    b. 2.
    c. 3.
    d. 4.

12. Microscopic kidney cells are known as:
    a. michrons.
    b. nephrons.
    c. nephews.
    d. microns.

13. Which of the following is not a function of the renal system?
    a. filtration of waste from the blood
    b. removal of urine from the body
    c. maintenance of water balance
    d. maintenance of electric balance

14. Phenazopyridine may cause the urine to be colored:
    a. red.
    b. orange.
    c. green/blue-green.
    d. brown/black.

15. Which of the following is not a type of incontinence?
    a. stress
    b. urge
    c. overflow
    d. permanent

True or False?

16. Bilirubin is normally detected in the urine.

    T   F

17. Obesity is not a cause of incontinence.

    T   F

18. Cystitis is an inflammation of the bladder caused in most cases by *E. coli* and staphylococcus.

    T   F

19. Tetracycline is used for UTIs.

    (T)   F

20. Kidney damage can lead to diabetes.

    T   (F)

PHARMACY CALCULATION PROBLEMS

Calculate the following.

1. If a patient needs phenazopyridine 200 mg 1 po tid prn × 4 days, how many tablets should you dispense?

   12 tablets

2. A new prescription has been dropped off for oxybutynin po, 10 mg bid. If the pharmacy only carries 5 mg tablets, how many tablets will be needed for a 30-day supply?

   120 tablets

3. A woman is to receive a trimethoprim/sulfamethoxazole IV for a complicated urinary tract infection. Her dose is 200 mg based on the trimethoprim content. Trimethoprim (TMP)/sulfamethoxazole (SMZ) IV comes as TMP 80 mg/SMZ 400 mg per 5 mL vial. How many mL should be drawn up for the IV?

   $$\frac{80mg}{5 mL} \quad \frac{200 mg}{} \quad 12.5 mL$$

4. A patient took one hydrocodone/APAP tablet po qid × 5 days for pain from kidney stones. How many grams of hydrocodone did the patient receive if each tablet contained 5 mg of hydrocodone and 500 mg of acetaminophen?

   0.1g
   100 mg oxy

5. If 30% of women will have a urinary tract infection in their lifetimes, how many women could this affect if there are 154 million women in the United States?

   46,200,000 woman

1. Which of the following is considered the functional unit of the kidney?
   a. prostate
   b. ureter
   c. bladder
   d. nephron

2. What is the medical term for difficult or painful urination?
   a. dysuria
   b. hematuria
   c. pyuria
   d. anuria

3. The renal system is responsible for all of the following functions *except*:
   a. filtration of waste from the blood.
   b. maintenance of electrolyte balance.
   c. oxygen transport.
   d. maintenance of acid-base balance.

4. All of the following refer to solid mineral deposits that accumulate in the urinary tract *except*:
   a. uroliths.
   b. kidney stones.
   c. UTIs.
   d. calculi.

5. All of the following are used to treat urinary incontinence *except*:
   a. Diovan®.
   b. Ditropan®.
   c. Detrol®.
   d. Urispas®.

ACTIVITY 28-1: Anatomy Worksheet

The Urinary System

Label the following illustration of the urinary system.

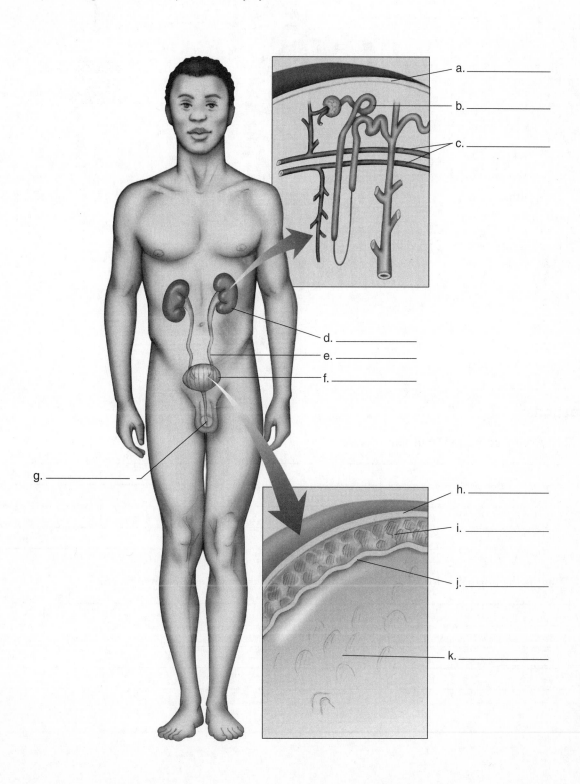

The Nephron

Label the following illustration of the nephron.

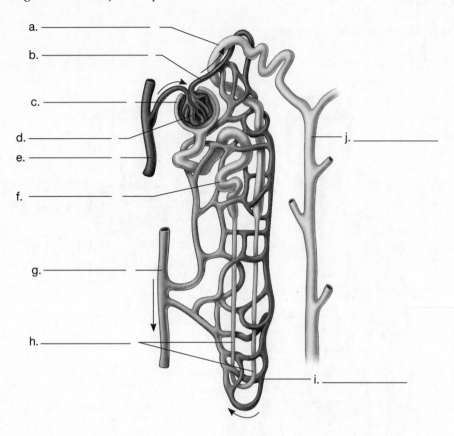

a. _____

b. _____

c. _____

d. _____

e. _____

f. _____

g. _____

h. _____

i. _____

j. _____

Questions:

1. List five functions of the urinary system.

   _____
   _____
   _____
   _____
   _____

2. What is the normal color of urine? Discuss some things that might change its color.

   _____
   _____
   _____
   _____
   _____

3. Use your textbook or other medical reference to learn more about the process of urine formation; then describe it in your own words.

_____

_____

_____

_____

_____

ACTIVITY 28-2: Case Study—UTI

Instructions: Read the following scenario and then answer the critical thinking questions.

Ms. Andelo, a healthy 24-year-old woman, is a periodic customer at the retail pharmacy where you work. She shares the good news that she has been dating a nice young man for about a month and it seems serious. She also lets you know that they have a very physical relationship as well.

Today she is here to pick up some medicine for some symptoms she has been experiencing. Ms. Andelo just came from her doctor's office, where she complained that she is repeatedly experiencing the urge to urinate. However, when she attempts to urinate, it is painful and accompanied by a burning sensation. She is very skittish about the pain and has refrained as much as possible from urinating because of fear. She had hoped it would stop by now. The last time she was able to urinate, she had a spotting of blood but nothing substantial. This has been going on for about four days.

1. What _____ would present if this were a lower urinary tract infection?

_____

_____

_____ Ms. Andelo for a UTI, and for how long?

_____

_____

3. Are any popular alterna_____ able for UTI prevention?

_____

_____

4. Based on the information given in the scenario, what is the probable cause of the UTI?

_____

_____

_____

ACTIVITY 28-3: Case Study—Dialysis

Instructions: Read the following scenario and then answer the critical thinking questions.

Mr. Sanders is a frequent inpatient in the nephrology department where you work as a clinical pharmacy technician. On an outpatient basis, he comes to the hospital for dialysis treatments three times a week. Treatment days can be long ones for Mr. Sanders. By the time he checks in, gets situated, and the dialysis finishes running, several hours pass. He is used to being tired almost all the time, but lately it seems that he is even more tired than usual. For example, even lifting a phone book is sometimes too daunting for him to attempt. Mr. Sanders is also experiencing shortness of breath and an ever-increasing loss of memory. He wonders if this is normal.

Mr. Sanders's other medications include diphenhydramine, warfarin, docusate sodium, calcium, and PhosLo®.

1. Based on the information in this scenario, what condition could Mr. Sanders now have in addition to the chronic renal failure?

   _____

   _____

   _____

2. What treatment is available for this condition?

   _____

   _____

   _____

3. For what reason is Mr. Sanders prescribed the medications diphenhydramine, warfarin, and PhosLo® while he is on dialysis?

   _____

   _____

   _____

ACTIVITY 28-4: Case Study—Incontinence

Instructions: Read the following scenario and then answer the critical thinking questions.

Maryellen Montell is a 42-year-old-woman who recently had a total hysterectomy. Three weeks after this surgery, she is still unable to control urinary leakage, and it occurs at the most inopportune times. She presents with leakage any time she coughs or laughs and sometimes when she climbs stairs.

She comes to the ostomy supply pharmacy where you work, on a very busy day, to pick up some incontinence products, including undergarments. Your co-worker takes in her prescription for the undergarments and begins to process it. She questions Maryellen about sizing. Maryellen replies in a soft voice. Your co-worker tells Maryellen that her insurance will not pay for that size or the brand of "diapers" she needs, and starts to rattle off the list of undergarments your pharmacy does have available. It seems like a lengthy conversation to Maryellen, who just says, "Never mind," and leaves the pharmacy counter in a huff without the prescription. You look at your co-worker, who shakes her head and says, "What was her problem?"

1. According to the description in this scenario, Maryellen exhibits symptoms of which of the four types of incontinence?

_____

_____

_____

2. What happens within the body with this type of incontinence?

_____

_____

_____

3. Is this condition treatable with or without medicine?

_____

_____

_____

4. Given the description of this scenario, why do you think Maryellen left the pharmacy the way she did?

_____

_____

_____

5. If you had taken in the prescription, how would you have handled the transaction differently to help prevent Maryellen from leaving?

_____

_____

_____

CHAPTER 29
The Endocrine System

After completing Chapter 29 from the textbook, you should be able to:	Related Activity in the Workbook/Lab Manual
1. Identify and describe the glands of the endocrine system.	Review Questions, PTCB Exam Practice Questions Activity 29-1
2. Describe the functions of the hypothalamus and pituitary gland, and list other body parts that are affected by these glands.	Review Questions, PTCB Exam Practice Questions Activity 29-1
3. List and define the hormones of the endocrine system and know which gland or organ secretes each hormone.	Review Questions, PTCB Exam Practice Questions Activity 29-1, Activity 29-2, Activity 29-3
4. Describe male and female hormones and some products used for replacement in cases of deficiency of these hormones.	Review Questions, PTCB Exam Practice Questions Activity 29-2, Activity 29-3
5. Identify and describe the major diseases and conditions that affect the endocrine system.	Review Questions, PTCB Exam Practice Questions Activity 29-4, Lab 29-1, Lab 29-2
6. Compare and contrast diabetes mellitus and diabetes insipidus.	Review Questions Activity 29-4, Lab 29-1, Lab 29-2
7. Understand the effects of anabolic steroid use.	Review Questions Activity 29-2

INTRODUCTION

The endocrine system is a collection of glands that produce hormones, substances that help regulate the body's growth, metabolism, and sexual development and function. The hormones, which are released into the bloodstream and transported to tissues and organs throughout the body, influence every cell in some way. The glands of the endocrine system are ductless. The hormones secreted from the endocrine glands are thus released directly into the bloodstream and travel in the body to specific target organs where they exert their effect.

The driving forces of the endocrine system are the hypothalamus, located in the brainstem, and the pituitary gland, which is attached to the base of the hypothalamus. The hypothalamus directs the pituitary gland, which, in turn, controls the thyroid, parathyroid, pancreas, adrenal glands, and the gonads. A complete review of these glands, their secretions, and their effects on body systems illustrates how important the endocrine system is to the proper functioning of the body. For example, every cell in the body depends on thyroid hormones for regulating metabolism.

Some diseases of the endocrine system, such as diabetes, are very familiar to most people; others, such as Graves' disease or Cushing's syndrome, are less common. As a pharmacy technician, you should be aware of the most common endocrine system disorders that require pharmacological treatment, including conditions treated with OTC drugs.

REVIEW QUESTIONS

Match the following.

1. _____ corticosteroid
2. _____ gonads
3. _____ homeostasis
4. _____ hormone
5. _____ isotonic
6. _____ negative feedback
7. _____ polydipsia
8. _____ polyphagia
9. _____ polyuria
10. _____ priapism

a. chemical substance produced by an organ or gland that travels through the bloodstream to regulate the activity of bodily functions

b. process by which the body returns to homeostasis

c. painful, prolonged erection

d. excessive hunger

e. excessive urination

f. a stable and constant environment

g. steroidal hormones produced in the adrenal cortex

h. testes and ovaries

i. characteristic of a solution that has the same salt concentration as that of the blood

j. ingestion of abnormally large amounts of fluid

Fill in the blanks.

11. _____ is the study of the chemical communication system that provides the means to control a large number of physiologic processes.

12. The _____ controls the activity of the pituitary gland.

13. The majority of the thyroid tissue consists of the _____ cells.

14. Thyroid cells combine iodine and the _____ to make T3 and T4.

15. _____ are located on the upper part of each kidney.

Match each drug to its classification.

16. _____ glucocorticoid
17. _____ mineralocorticoid
18. _____ lab-modified estrogen
19. _____ plant-derived estrogen
20. _____ natural hormone

a. testosterone
b. somatostatin
c. estradiol
d. octreotide
e. fludrocortisone

21. _____ secreted hormone
22. _____ androgen
23. _____ brain hormone
24. _____ synthetic form of somatostatin
25. _____ synthetic long-acting somatostatin

f. lanreotide
g. estropipate
h. Premarin®
i. prednisone
j. cortisol

Choose the best answer.

26. Which of the following is not a side effect of anabolic steroids?
    a. edema
    b. chills
    c. jaundice
    d. fever

27. Which of the following is not an irreversible effect of steroids?
    a. body hair
    b. clitoris enlargement
    c. chills
    d. breast shrinkage

28. Which of the following results from insulin resistance combined with relative insulin deficiency?
    a. type 1 diabetes
    b. type 2 diabetes
    c. gestational diabetes
    d. pre-diabetes

29. Which is not a symptom of diabetes?
    a. loss of appetite
    b. frequent urination
    c. increased fatigue
    d. irritability

30. Which type of insulin is the only insulin that can be injected IV?
    a. Humulin N®
    b. R
    c. Lantus®
    d. lente

PHARMACY CALCULATION PROBLEMS

Calculate the following.

1. If the directions for conjugated estrogen cream read, "Apply 0.5 g PV QD," how long will a 60 g tube last?

2. If a diabetic patient gives himself 20 units of insulin tid with meals, how many vials will the patient need for a 30-day supply? The vial contains 10 mL and has a concentration of 100 units/mL.

3. A patient requires a tapering prescription for methylprednisolone 4 mg tablets for a severe allergic reaction. It normally is stocked in a convenience pack, but that form is currently back-ordered. The patient agreed that she could take the tablets in a bottle as long as all the directions are included. The directions read:

Day 1: Take 6 tablets (at once or in divided doses)

Day 2: Take 5 tablets (at once or in divided doses)

Day 3: Take 4 tablets (at once or in divided doses)

Day 4: Take 3 tablets (at once or in divided doses)

Day 5: Take 2 tablets (at once or in divided doses)

Day 6: Take 1 tablet

How many tablets should you dispense?

4. A man takes 0.125 mg of levothyroxine daily for hypothyroidism. How many micrograms would this man take over 30 days?

5. You just received a prescription for desiccated thyroid 180 mg tablets. The computer system only lists the product in grains. How many grains are in one tablet?

PTCB EXAM PRACTICE QUESTIONS

1. Which gland in the endocrine system is responsible for the regulation of calcium in the body?
   a. thymus
   b. thyroid
   c. pituitary
   d. parathyroid

2. Which disease is characterized by the body's failure to produce insulin?
   a. type 1 diabetes
   b. type 2 diabetes
   c. gestational diabetes
   d. pre-diabetes

3. Which insulin is dosed once daily?
   a. NPH
   b. Humalog®
   c. Lantus®
   d. ultralente

4. Graves' disease involves which endocrine gland?
   a. thyroid
   b. parathyroid
   c. pancreas
   d. pituitary

5. Male sex hormones are also referred to as:
   a. estrogens.
   b. progestins.
   c. insulins.
   d. androgens.

ACTIVITY 29-1: Anatomy Worksheet

The Endocrine Glands

Label the following illustration of the endocrine glands.

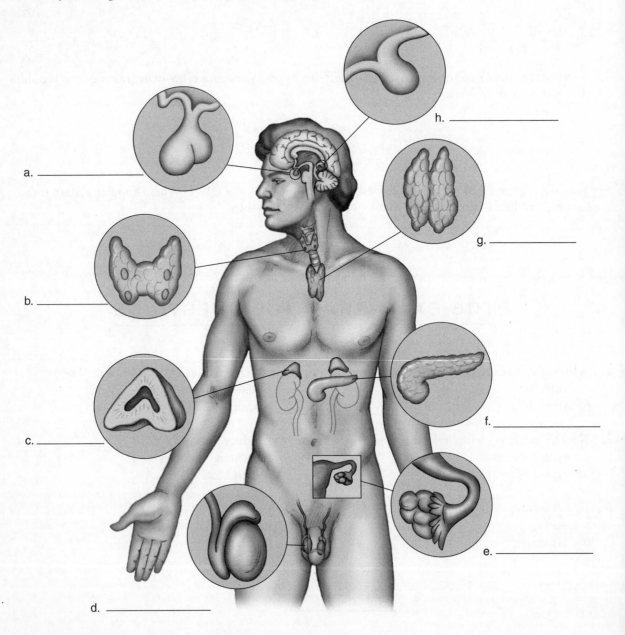

a. _____

b. _____

c. _____

d. _____

e. _____

f. _____

g. _____

h. _____

Now that you have labeled the endocrine glands in the figure, use the following spaces to describe the hormone(s) each gland produces and each hormone's function within the body.

1. _____
   _____
   _____

2. _____
   _____
   _____

3. _____
   _____
   _____

4. _____
   _____
   _____

5. _____
   _____
   _____

6. _____
   _____
   _____

7. _____
   _____
   _____

8. _____
   _____
   _____

ACTIVITY 29-2: Case Study—Anabolic Steroid Use

Instructions: Read the following scenario and then answer the critical thinking questions.

Rob is a 17-year-old male who finally was selected as a defensive tackle for his high school football team. It turns out that Rob is one of the smallest players on the team, but his coach has encouraged him to work out more often and eat certain foods to help him increase his body size and strength. Rob feels the need to be popular with the rest of the high school football team and goes to great lengths to fit in. For example, he works out daily in the well-equipped school gym long after the rest of the team goes home.

Rob is not gaining muscle or strength as fast as he would like, so he resorts to using anabolic steroids to bulk up. Everyone at school is aware of Rob's steroid use, and the athletes typically accept steroid use amongst themselves.

One day, Rob is randomly tested after he assaults another player. During questioning, he is asked to reveal who supplies the steroids that are in his system. Rob brags that he volunteers at a hospital picking up trash, and while in the pharmacy area he walks over to the shelf, out of camera range, and places the capsules in his pocket. He states he has been doing this the entire time and has no other source.

1. What key component(s) in the story reveal that Rob is lying about obtaining the steroids from the pharmacy?

   _____

   _____

   _____

   _____

2. What are some signs of steroid use in a case such as this?

   _____

   _____

   _____

   _____

3. How much pressure (psychologically or otherwise) do you think teenagers like Rob are under to use steroids to meet athletic goals and fit in socially?

   _____

   _____

   _____

   _____

4. What discipline (legal or otherwise) should be applied here, and to whom?

   _____

   _____

   _____

   _____

ACTIVITY 29-3: Case Study—HRT for Men

Instructions: Read the following scenario and then answer the critical thinking questions.

Fifty-year-old Ron thought he was going crazy. Ron has been on hormone therapy for at least nine months now and things were going well for a while. Ron presents to his physician with the following complaint: lately he has been experiencing symptoms that are getting annoying. Although born with a naturally thin body frame and clear, smooth skin, he has developed severe acne and is gaining weight. Ron is certain that these problems are due to the HRT. Also, within the past few weeks Ron has been perspiring more heavily than usual and finds that his perspiration has a foul odor. Ron did not notice that baldness is creeping up also. All these unfavorable symptoms have Ron wondering if HRT is worth the trouble. The physician tells Ron that these symptoms are normal with this type of therapy, and adjusts the dose. As Ron continues HRT therapy, some symptoms persist while others are reduced.

1. Based on the information provided in the scenario, what type of HRT do you think Ron may be on?

    _____

    _____

    _____

    _____

2. What are some other symptoms that Ron might experience, even though they were not mentioned in this scenario?

    _____

    _____

    _____

    _____

3. What psychological effects do you think the patient might be experiencing with body and appearance changes?

    _____

    _____

    _____

    _____

ACTIVITY 29-4: Case Study—Insulin

Instructions: Read the following scenario and then answer the critical thinking questions.

Mrs. Kendall has been coming to your retail pharmacy for years. You always look forward to seeing her. She is a very aware patient who knows exactly what medicine she is taking and for what reason. Your prescription profile shows that Mrs. Kendall only takes about three medications, as she has always been in good health.

Today she presents to your pharmacy a little distraught. It appears that she has been crying, and she is just not herself. She tells you in a sullen voice that the doctor has just prescribed several new medications and that she is there to pick them up. You look at her profile and notice that she has been prescribed diabetes type 1 medications, including a test meter, test strips, other supplies, and insulin.

Even though she appeared to be in picture-perfect health, Mrs. Kendall reveals to you that she has been taking oral diabetes medication for some time, and has ordered her medicine through another pharmacy. She was certain that she could "kick" her diabetes and that she would not need insulin. She makes several negative comments, such as "I don't need any shots" and "This is just so they can get more money out of me!" Obviously Mrs. Kendall is in shock regarding her new diagnosis.

1. What are the considerations regarding proper use of the medications that are being ordered for Mrs. Kendall today at your counter?

   _____

   _____

   _____

   _____

2. Given Mrs. Kendall's fragile state of mind, whose responsibility is it to help her understand the importance of properly treating her disease?

   _____

   _____

   _____

   _____

3. If Mrs. Kendall's disease progresses, what other products might she possibly need from your pharmacy?

   _____

   _____

   _____

   _____

LAB 29-1: Using a Blood Glucose Meter

Objectives:

Demonstrate the procedure for testing blood glucose levels.

Learn what supplies are required to perform blood glucose monitoring.

Pre-Lab Information:

- Review Chapter 29 in your textbook to learn more about diabetes.
- Visit the American Diabetes Association website: www.diabetes.org
- Gather the following materials:
  - blood glucose meter
  - blood glucose meter test strip
  - lancing device
  - lancet
  - control solution (optional)

Explanation:

Approximately 6.6 percent of the U.S. population has diabetes, but about one-third of that group is unaware of their serious medical condition. Diabetes is a disease in which the body does not produce or properly use insulin, a hormone that is needed to convert sugar, starches, and other food into the energy necessary for daily life. The cause of diabetes is not certain, but both genetics and environmental factors (such as obesity and lack of exercise) appear to play roles.

As a pharmacy technician, you need to understand how diabetic patients monitor their blood glucose levels using a blood glucose meter. This knowledge will help you assist customers who have questions about equipment and supplies.

Activity:

In this activity, you will test your own blood glucose levels.

Blood Testing Procedure

1. Wash hands with warm, soapy water.
2. Insert a new lancet into the lancing device.
3. Adjust the lancing device to the appropriate depth to collect a proper sample.
4. Turn on the blood glucose meter and ensure that it is properly coded for the test strips, if necessary. (Follow the specific manufacturer's instructions.)
5. Remove a test strip from the vial and recap the remaining test strips immediately.
6. Insert the test strip into the blood glucose meter.
7. Lance your finger and allow an ample blood drop to form.
8. Place the sample tip/section of the test strip next to the blood drop and hold it there until the blood glucose meter confirms that the blood sample was adequate for testing.
9. Remove the finger from the test strip and wait for the blood glucose meter to display the test results.
10. Discard the used lancet and test strip in a biohazard waste container.

Note: Control solution can be used in place of an actual blood sample for training purposes. For step 7, squeeze a drop of control solution onto the fingertip.

Note: Due to the variety of blood glucose monitors, you should thoroughly read the instructions provided by the manufacturer to ensure that the proper procedures are being followed.

Discussion Questions:

1. What was your blood glucose level? Is your result low, normal, or high?
   _____
   _____

2. How often should type 2 diabetics test their blood sugar?
   _____
   _____

3. Why is it important that used lancets and test strips be thrown away in a biohazard waste container?
   _____
   _____
   _____
   _____

Student Name: _____

Lab Partner: _____

Grade/Comments: _____
_____
_____

Student Comments: _____
_____
_____

LAB 29-2: Simulated Insulin Injection

Objective:

Become familiar with the procedure for giving an insulin injection.

Pre-Lab Information:

Gather the following materials:

- insulin syringe
- vial of normal saline or sterile water
- alcohol swab
- biohazard waste container

Explanation:

Some patients who have type 1 diabetes require daily insulin injections. Giving yourself a daily injection can be emotionally and psychologically difficult, as well as physically demanding.

Activity:

In this exercise, you will experience the process of giving yourself an insulin injection, using saline or sterile water as your "mock" insulin.

Procedure

1. Using a new, unopened vial of normal saline or sterile water, label it as U-100 insulin, 100 units/mL.
2. Calculate the proper dosage in mL needed for 10 units.
3. Select the appropriate size insulin syringe (U-100) to use for injection.
4. Remove the vial cap and swab the rubber diaphragm with an alcohol swab.
5. Pull back the plunger on the syringe to the calculated dosage, for adding air into the syringe.
6. Insert the needle into the vial. Push the plunger in to transfer the air from the syringe to the vial, then invert the vial and pull back on the plunger to draw up the needed volume of solution.
7. Using your thumb and index finger, gently pinch up a section of skin on the side of your abdomen.
8. Insert the needle into the pinched skin. Push the plunger to inject the solution and then remove the syringe.
9. Dispose of the syringe in a biohazard waste container.

Note: Normal saline is the preferred solution for training use, as its pH is close to that of the human body.

Discussion Questions:

1. How did you feel, emotionally, preparing to inject yourself?

   _____

   _____

   _____

   _____

2. How did you feel, physically, as you administered the injection?

_____
_____
_____
_____

3. In what ways will this exercise help you to provide better patient care?

_____
_____
_____
_____

Student Name: _____

Lab Partner: _____

Grade/Comments: _____
_____
_____

Student Comments: _____
_____
_____

CHAPTER 30
The Reproductive System

After completing Chapter 30 from the textbook, you should be able to:	Related Activity in the Workbook/Lab Manual
1. List, identify, and diagram the basic anatomical structures and parts of the male and female reproductive systems.	Review Questions, PTCB Exam Practice Questions Activity 30-1
2. Describe the functions and physiology of the male and female reproductive systems and the hormones that govern them.	Review Questions, PTCB Exam Practice Questions Activity 30-1
3. List and define common diseases affecting the male and female reproductive systems and understand the causes, symptoms, and pharmaceutical treatments associated with each disease or condition.	Review Questions, PTCB Exam Practice Questions Activity 30-2, Activity 30-3, Activity 30-4
4. Describe the indications for use and mechanisms of action of various contraceptives.	Review Questions, PTCB Exam Practice Questions Activity 30-2

INTRODUCTION

The reproductive system is made up of internal reproductive organs, associated ducts, and external genitalia. Its primary function is the reproductive process. Sex hormones are produced in the gonads: in males, in the testes; and in females, in the ovaries.

Although many diseases can affect the reproductive system, a pharmacy technician will most frequently encounter conditions involving contraception, infertility, sexually transmitted diseases (STDs), and benign prostatic hyperplasia (BPH). As a pharmacy technician, it is important for you to be well informed regarding the different types of contraceptives, as well as their side effects and contraindications, and to be familiar with common conditions and disorders of the reproductive system.

REVIEW QUESTIONS

Match the following. Some answers may be used more than once.

1. _____ contraception
2. _____ endometrium
3. _____ hyperplasia
4. _____ oocyte
5. _____ ovaries
6. _____ ovulation
7. _____ ovum
8. _____ STD
9. _____ STI
10. _____ testes

a. reproduction of cells within an organ
b. female reproductive organs that produce eggs
c. process by which an ovarian follicle ruptures and releases an egg
d. sexually transmitted infection
e. male reproductive organs that produce sperm
f. sexually transmitted disease
g. birth control
h. lining of the uterus
i. egg

Choose the best answer.

11. The most abundant and active of the estrogens is:
    a. estrace.
    b. estropipate.
    c. estrodil.
    d. estradiol.

12. Federal law requires that all drugs containing estrogen:
    a. be dispensed with a patient package insert.
    b. also contain progesterone.
    c. be clearly labeled "do not take if pregnant."
    d. have a dispenser.

13. Which of the following will not interact with chemical contraception?
    a. antibiotics
    b. antipyretics
    c. antifungals
    d. antiepileptics

14. Oxytocin causes:
    a. labor contractions.
    b. cramping relief for PMS.
    c. menstruation.
    d. milk production.

15. Endometriosis is a condition characterized by:
    a. fragments of the uterine lining found in other parts of the pelvic cavity.
    b. vaginal odor and discharge.
    c. sterility.
    d. increased fertility.

16. The main function of progesterone is:
    a. to stimulate the development of the uterine lining and the mammary glands.
    b. to maintain the uterine lining if implantation occurs.
    c. to start menstruation.
    d. to give feminine features and characteristics.

True or False?

17. Activities that increase a male's risk for infertility include bicycling.

    T   F

18. Oxidants negatively affect DNA in the sperm.

    T   F

19. Anabolic steroids increase sperm production.

    T   F

20. Many STDs do not cause much harm or severe symptoms.

    T   F

PHARMACY CALCULATION PROBLEMS

Calculate the following.

1. If 0.3% of 2,000,000 women on medroxyprogesterone injection for contraception were to become pregnant, how many women would that affect?

2. If 8% of 5,000,000 women experience PMDD, how many women would that affect?

3. A man has brought in a prescription for prazosin 5 mg capsules. The prescription indicates that he is to take 10 mg bid. How many capsules would you need to dispense for a 90-day supply?

4. For latent syphilis, the recommended treatment is penicillin g benzathine (long-acting), 7.2 million units, divided into 3 weekly intramuscular injections. How many milligrams will the patient receive per dose?

5. A man is receiving 50 mg of testosterone cypionate IM every 2 weeks for hormone replacement. If the clinic stocks testosterone cypionate 100 mg/mL, how many mL of drug will the patient receive over the course of 8 weeks?

PTCB EXAM PRACTICE QUESTIONS

1. Women experiencing premenstrual dysphoric disorder (PMDD) may be treated with all of the following *except*:
   a. antidepressants.
   b. NSAIDs.
   c. testosterone.
   d. oral contraceptives.

2. All of the following classes of drugs may interact with birth control drugs *except*:
   a. antihypertensives.
   b. antifungals.
   c. antiepileptics.
   d. antibiotics.

3. Which of the following medical terms describes the most common cause of male infertility?
   a. oligospermia
   b. azoospermia
   c. dysspermia
   d. aspermia

4. Which of the following drugs is *not* used to treat erectile dysfunction (ED)?
   a. vardenafil
   b. tadalafil
   c. sildenafil
   d. triavil

5. Which of the following is the correct generic name for Flomax®?
   a. terazosin
   b. prazosin
   c. tamsulosin
   d. alfuzosin

ACTIVITY 30-1: Anatomy Worksheet

The Female Reproductive System

Label the following illustration of the female reproductive system.

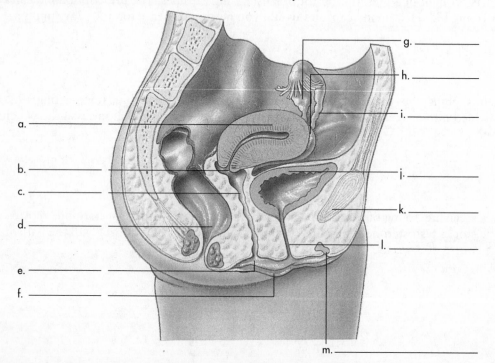

The Male Reproductive System

Label the following illustration of the male reproductive system.

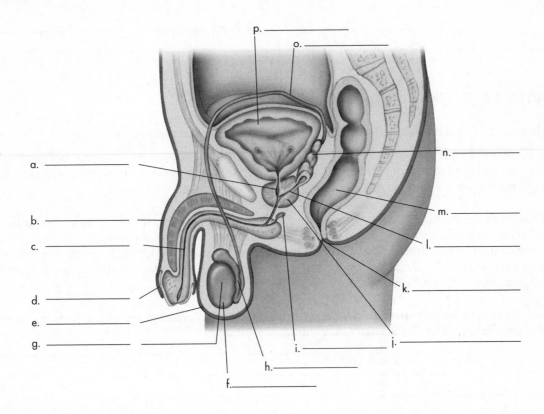

p. _____

o. _____

a. _____

b. _____

c. _____

d. _____

e. _____

g. _____

f. _____

h. _____

i. _____

j. _____

k. _____

l. _____

m. _____

n. _____

Questions:

1. Name the four hormones that are responsible for the female menstrual cycle. Where are these hormones produced within the body?

   _____

   _____

   _____

   _____

2. What is the main hormone that is responsible for male secondary sexual characteristics? Where is it produced within the body?

   _____

   _____

   _____

   _____

3. Name three different forms of contraception, explain how each method works, and give examples of each.

_____

_____

_____

_____

ACTIVITY 30-2: Case Study—Gonorrhea

Instructions: Read the following scenario and then answer the critical thinking questions.

Anna, a 17-year-old high school senior, presents to the community clinic with a vaginal discharge accompanied by pain and burning during urination. Anna just got out of a physically abusive relationship with an 18-year-old male from the same high school after two years of dating.

Anna is scared that something is very wrong with her because of these symptoms, and comes to the clinic to get a checkup in confidence. The doctor who sees her orders lab tests that eventually lead to a diagnosis of gonorrhea. Anna is prescribed some medication for the gonorrhea and is told to notify her sexual partner that he may need to be treated as well. Anna is terrified at the prospect of notifying her abusive ex-boyfriend and does not know what to do.

1. Does Anna have an obligation to tell her ex-boyfriend (and his current partner, if he is involved with someone else)? Can someone else contact him?

_____

_____

_____

2. What are the consequences of this condition for Anna and her past partner if left untreated? How does it affect health?

_____

_____

_____

3. What can Anna do to avoid contracting an STD in the future?

_____

_____

ACTIVITY 30-3: Case Study—Erectile Dysfunction

Instructions: Read the following scenario and then answer the critical thinking questions.

Gary, a 52-year-old hardware store owner, has battled with BPH for months now. He also has other medical conditions, including high blood pressure, which is being treated with oral medications. In his mind, he is much too young for this condition. Originally Gary tried to control his BPH by limiting fluids in the evening, moderating his caffeine consumption, and scheduling void times. He even tried a very popular herbal supplement said to help with BPH. When these were unsuccessful, he was prescribed an alpha blocker. Unfortunately, this did not work either, and he had to have a transurethral resection of the prostate (TURP), a surgical procedure to remove part of the prostate.

After his TURP, Gary experienced erectile dysfunction and his provider prescribed Viagra® to treat the ED. Gary has arrived at your pharmacy today to pick up his first order of Viagra®. Normally when you see Gary at your pharmacy, he is upbeat and always smiling. Today he has his head down. It is difficult to tell if he is sad or not.

1. Do you know any popular herbal supplement that some people claim helps with BPH? What is it (name all you know of)?

    _____

    _____

    _____

2. Based on the information in the scenario, is Gary's ED due to his high blood pressure or the TURP?

    _____

    _____

    _____

3. Can you think of any special customer service needs Gary might have, given his demeanor today?

    _____

    _____

    _____

4. What alpha blockers might have been appropriately prescribed early in the pharmaceutical treatment plan?

    _____

    _____

    _____

ACTIVITY 30-4: Case Study—Oxytocin

Instructions: Read the following scenario and then answer the critical thinking questions.

Thirty-two-year-old Amanda is at least two weeks overdue in delivering her baby. She is in agony and finds it hard to get around. She is certain her water has broken, calls her OB/GYN, and is instructed to head to the hospital.

When Amanda arrives, she is whisked away to begin monitoring her condition. Her blood pressure is slightly elevated, but the contractions are so mild that she really cannot feel them at this point. She is dilated to only three centimeters, although her water has broken.

Hours later, Amanda has advanced to five centimeters and her contractions are stronger; however, she remains at this stage for quite a while. Eventually, her doctor decides to induce labor to move the delivery along. Amanda is given oxytocin before and after the delivery of the baby.

1. What is oxytocin typically used for before the delivery of a baby?

   _____

   _____

   _____

2. What is oxytocin typically used for after the delivery of a baby?

   _____

   _____

   _____

3. In what drug administration form does the pharmacy technician prepare oxytocin for obstetric patients?

   _____

   _____

   _____

4. Oxytocin can also be used to help abort the fetus in cases of incomplete abortion or miscarriage. Do you think it is acceptable to use oxytocin this way? Why or why not?

   _____

   _____

   _____

After completing Chapter 31 from the textbook, you should be able to:	Related Activity in the Workbook/Lab Manual
1. Explain the functions of the nervous system and its division into the central and peripheral nervous systems.	Review Questions, PTCB Exam Practice Questions Activity 31-1
2. Compare and contrast the sympathetic and parasympathetic nervous systems.	Review Questions, PTCB Exam Practice Questions Activity 31-1
3. Describe the function or physiology of neurons and nerve transmission and the various neurotransmitters.	Review Questions Activity 31-1
4. Explain the relationship of the nervous system to the other body systems.	Review Questions Activity 31-1, Activity 31-2, Activity 31-3, Activity 31-4, Lab 31-1
5. Explain the functions of the blood-brain barrier and describe what types of substances will and will not cross it.	Review Questions Activity 31-1
6. List and define common diseases affecting the nervous system and discuss the causes, symptoms, and pharmaceutical treatment associated with each disease.	Review Questions, PTCB Exam Practice Questions Activity 31-2, Activity 31-3, Activity 31-4, Lab 31-1
7. Identify the common drugs used to treat diseases and conditions of the nervous system.	Review Questions, PTCB Exam Practice Questions Activity 31-2, Activity 31-3, Activity 31-4, Lab 31-1

INTRODUCTION

The nervous system is a very complex system that interacts with every other system in the body to ensure homeostasis and regulate the body's responses to internal and external stimuli. The nervous system communicates with all cells in the body through nerve impulses that are conducted from one part of the body to another via the transmission of chemicals called *neurotransmitters*.

The nervous system is divided into two parts, the central nervous system (CNS) and the peripheral nervous system (PNS). The central nervous system includes the brain, the spinal column, and their nerves. The peripheral nervous system is also divided into two parts: the somatic nervous system, which controls voluntary movement of the body through muscles; and the autonomic nervous system, which controls involuntary motor functions and affects such things as heart rate and digestion.

Diseases and conditions affecting the nervous system include anxiety, depression, bipolar disorder, Parkinson's disease, alcohol addiction, and seizures. Pain due to injury or cancer also affects the nervous system. *Neuropharmacology*, or pharmacology related to the nervous system, is one of the most diverse and complicated areas of pharmacology. As a pharmacy technician, you must have a solid understanding of the common diseases affecting the nervous system and the pharmaceutical treatments associated with these diseases.

REVIEW QUESTIONS

Match the following.

1. _____ adjuvant
2. _____ afferent
3. _____ anxiety
4. _____ anxiolytic
5. _____ CNS
6. _____ cerebrospinal fluid
7. _____ EEG
8. _____ efferent
9. _____ gray matter
10. _____ hypotension
11. _____ PNS
12. _____ narcolepsy
13. _____ white matter

a. condition of frequent periods of deep sleep
b. nervous system excluding the brain and spinal cord
c. component of myelinated nerve tissue in the CNS
d. low blood pressure
e. helping or assisting
f. drug used in the treatment of anxiety
g. part of nervous system/brain and spinal cord
h. uncomfortable state of apprehension, worry, and fear
i. nerves sending impulses away from the CNS
j. fluid surrounding brain and spinal cord
k. component of nervous system made up of nonmyelinated nerve tissue
l. nerve sending an impulse toward the CNS
m. graphic record of the electrical activity of the brain

Choose the best answer.

14. Afferent impulses are said to be:
   a. sensory.
   b. integrative.
   c. motor.
   d. perceived.

15. The system by which receptors in the skin send messages to the brain, regulating peripheral blood flow and the sweat glands, is called the:
   a. endocrine system.
   b. lymphatic system.
   c. integumentary system.
   d. renal system.

16. The sympathetic nervous system is governed by the neurotransmitter:
    a. acetylcholine.
    b. synapse.
    c. cytoplasm.
    d. norepinephrine.

17. The _____ is concerned with higher intellect or reasoning, problem solving, parts of speech, movement, and emotion.
    a. occipital lobe
    b. parietal lobe
    c. frontal lobe
    d. temporal lobe

18. Which of the following is not a general property of the blood-brain barrier?
    a. Water-soluble or low-lipid/low-fat-soluble molecules do not penetrate.
    b. Infectious agents cannot open up the BBB.
    c. Large molecules do not easily pass through the BBB.
    d. Highly electrically charged molecules are slowed down.

19. These drugs bind to the GABA-A receptors and increase the actions of GABA.
    a. β-adrenergic blockers
    b. SSRIs
    c. benzodiazepines
    d. MAOIs

Match the following drugs with their categories or treatment uses.

20. _____ clomipramine
21. _____ selegiline
22. _____ perphenazine
23. _____ propranolol
24. _____ carbamazepine
25. _____ venlafaxine
26. _____ methylphenidate
27. _____ paroxetine
28. _____ buspirone
29. _____ alprazolam
30. _____ mirtazapine
31. _____ divalproex
32. _____ caridopa/levodopa
33. _____ methysergide
34. _____ morphine sulfate
35. _____ tacrine

a. non-benzodiazepine
b. atypical antidepressant
c. tetracyclic
d. TCA
e. SSRI
f. β-adrenergic blocker
g. benzodiazepine
h. MAOI
i. anticonvulsant
j. antipsychotic
k. stimulant
l. narcotic used for pain
m. migraine treatment
n. Alzheimer's
o. Parkinson's
p. delays sodium influx

PHARMACY CALCULATION PROBLEMS

Calculate the following.

1. If chlorpromazine 25 mg/100 mL IV is to run over 30 minutes, what is the infusion rate in mL/hr?

2. A patient is to receive 37.5 mg of risperidone long-acting injection. The pharmacy only has 50 mg/2 mL in stock. How many mL are needed for the dose?

3. You need to fill a prescription for duloxetine 30 mg. The directions read "3 caps po QD." The patient only wants a 14-day supply. How many capsules will you need to fill the prescription?

4. If a patient is receiving 0.25 mg of alprazolam tid, how many micrograms is the patient receiving each day?

PTCB EXAM PRACTICE QUESTIONS

1. The drugs Prozac®, Zoloft®, and Paxil® are examples of drugs that selectively inhibit the reuptake of which of the following?
   a. troponin
   b. GABA
   c. serotonin
   d. nortriptyline

2. Which of the following drugs is an indicated treatment for bipolar disorder?
   a. lithium
   b. Librium®
   c. Lasix®
   d. Lyrica®

3. To what class of drugs does Clozaril® belong?
   a. anticonvulsant
   b. antidepressant
   c. antipsychotic
   d. anti-anxiety

4. Which of the following drugs would *not* be used to treat status epilepticus?
   a. Cerebyx®
   b. Ativan®
   c. Celebrex®
   d. Valium®

5. Which of the following drugs would *not* be used to treat Parkinson's disease?
   a. Sinemet®
   b. Aricept®
   c. Parlodel®
   d. Symmetrel®

ACTIVITY 31-1: Anatomy Worksheet

The Nervous System

Label the following illustration of the nervous system.

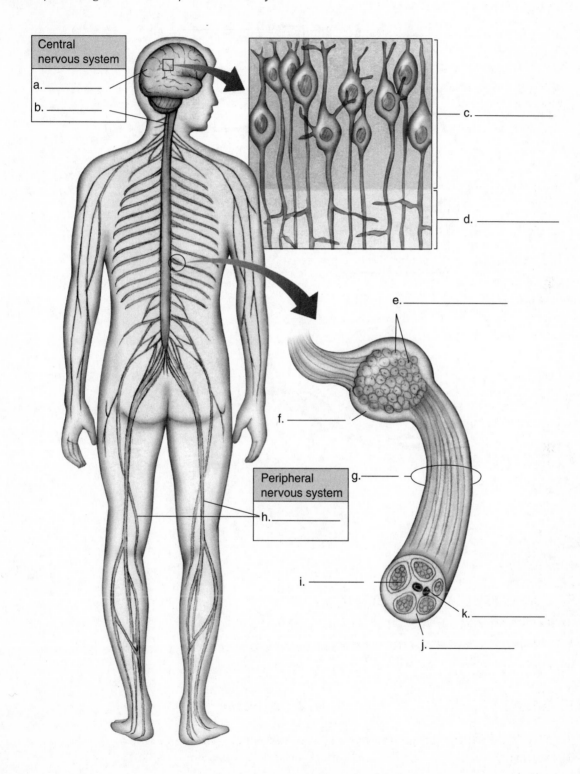

Central
nervous system

a. _____

b. _____

c. _____

d. _____

e. _____

f. _____

g. _____

Peripheral
nervous system

h. _____

i. _____

k. _____

j. _____

The Neuron

Label the following illustration of the neuron.

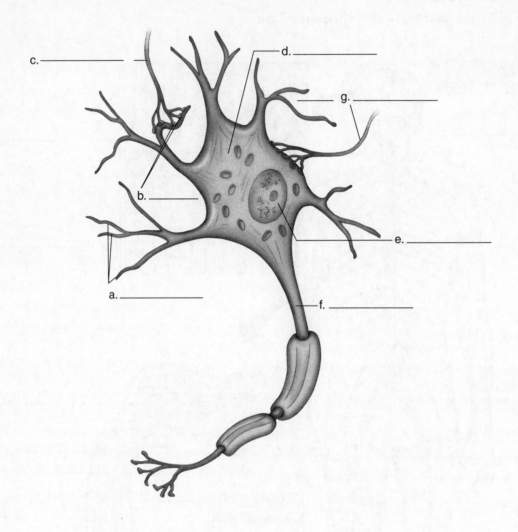

The Brain

Label the following illustration of the brain.

a. _____

b. _____

c. _____

d. _____

e. _____

f. _____

g. _____

h. _____

i. _____

j. _____

k. _____

l. _____

m. _____

n. _____

o. _____

p. _____

q. _____

r. _____

s. _____

t. _____

u. _____

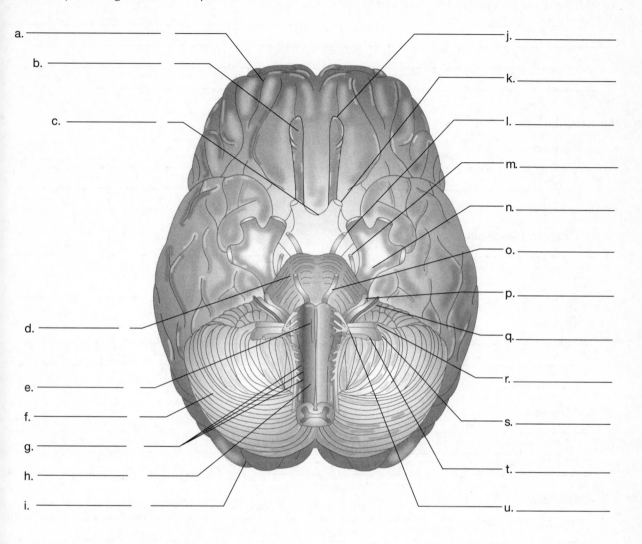

Questions:

1. What are the functions of the nervous system?

   _____

   _____

   _____

   _____

2. Describe how the nervous system affects the following body systems:

   a. Respiratory

   _____

   _____

   _____

   b. Heart/cardiovascular

   _____

   _____

   _____

   c. Skeletal

   _____

   _____

   _____

   d. Muscular

   _____

   _____

   _____

   e. Digestive

   _____

   _____

   _____

   f. Endocrine

   _____

   _____

   _____

   g. Lymphatic/Immune

   _____

   _____

   _____

h. Renal (Urinary)

_____

_____

_____

i. Integumentary

_____

_____

_____

3. Compare and contrast the sympathetic and parasympathetic nervous systems.

_____

_____

_____

_____

4. What are the functions of the neurons? Discuss the process of neurotransmission.

_____

_____

_____

_____

5. What are the functions of the blood-brain barrier? What are some disease states or physical changes that can compromise its integrity?

_____

_____

_____

_____

ACTIVITY 31-2: Case Study—A Change in a Friend

Instructions: Read the following scenario and then answer the critical thinking questions.

Until about eight months ago, you used to play racquetball with Mrs. Vanderbank. At first she missed a game here and there, and then one day she just stated that she hated racquetball and never wanted to play again. This seems to have happened around the same time she stopped taking phone calls from her mother, to whom she had always been close. Reasons she gave included a lack of sleep and energy that was getting worse over time.

Mrs. Vanderbank comes in to pick up her medications one day, and you notice that she has lost an awful lot of weight. You mention that you didn't even know that she was dieting. She replies that she is not, she is just never hungry. Mrs. Vanderbank only weighed 134 lb. a few months ago, and has lost weight since then. She also seems quieter than usual. As a friend, you question her, but she tells you everything is all right.

She is picking up a prescription for fluoxetine. You remember that she was taking sertraline a short time ago but is not now. Another prescription she is picking up is trazodone for sleep. She states that the trazodone is not working, just like the sertraline that did not work.

1. Overall, what disorder do Mrs. Vanderbank's symptoms indicate? Is it major or dysthymic?

_____

_____

_____

2. To what class of drugs do fluoxetine and trazodone belong?

_____

_____

_____

3. As her friend, do you see any conflict of interest in asking Mrs. Vanderbank personal questions while you are at work?

_____

_____

_____

ACTIVITY 31-3: Case Study—The Blue Dog

Instructions: Read the following scenario and then answer the critical thinking questions.

Mr. Ogdahl is a regular at your outpatient pharmacy. At times he exhibits some behaviors that seem rather silly to a lot of folks in other areas where you work. On occasion he seems comfortable enough to have light conversation with you while he waits for his medications.

At times he talks about cartoons that come on in the mornings, specifically the one with the "blue dog." As his visits become more frequent, he seems to talk about the blue dog more and more in a personal sense. He tells you that before he can watch the blue dog each and every morning, he first has to clear off his favorite chair, fold his favorite blanket, scrub his hands until they almost hurt, and pour a cup of orange juice— only orange juice—into a blue cup that matches the blue dog. One time you ask, "Have you ever had apple juice?" and he seems to become upset and rigid, reinforcing that only orange juice will do.

The medicine he has refilled every month like clockwork is oxazepam. One day he tells you that he was prescribed this medicine after cognitive behavior therapy failed.

1. To what class of drugs does oxazepam belong?

_____

_____

_____

2. Based on the short description in the scenario, what seems to be Mr. Ogdahl's condition?

_____

_____

_____

3. In what mental disorder category does this condition fall?

_____

_____

_____

4. How can you explain to other people that Mr. Ogdahl's thoughts are not silly?

_____

_____

_____

ACTIVITY 31-4: Case Study—Pain Relief for Cancer

Instructions: Read the following scenario and then answer the critical thinking questions.

Mrs. Eddleton is a 37-year-old housewife with cancer who asks to speak to a pharmacist for a recommendation. She explains that some days her pain from cancer is debilitating. The pain used to subside after she took her tablet and not return until just before the next dose was due; now, though, the pain is constant. Mrs. Eddleton reads extensively about her condition, hoping to discover a pain medication that will work.

She has regular follow-up visits at the pain management clinic, where they have been prescribing oral morphine three times a day for pain over the last year. She has tried several other pain medications before the morphine. Lately even the morphine has not brought relief. She asks the pharmacist if there is an option where she would not have to take the medicine three times a day and might control the pain a little better. She has read that an opioid patch is available to help with pain like hers.

1. To what patch could Mrs. Eddleton be referring?

_____

_____

_____

2. How is the patch used by the patient, and for what type of pain?

_____

_____

_____

3. Do you know of anything Mrs. Eddleton could do, outside of or in conjunction with taking medication, to ease the pain?

_____

_____

_____

4. Do you think it is acceptable for patients to be proactive in their own medication therapy in ways such as research?

_____

_____

_____

LAB 31-1: Web Research Activity—Alternative Therapies for Sleep and Mood Disorders

Objective:

Search the Internet to discover nonpharmaceutical treatments for disorders such as anxiety, insomnia, and depression.

Pre-Lab Information:

Search the Internet for information regarding the following herbs: chamomile, ginseng, hops, kava kava, skullcap, St. John's wort, and valerian. http://www.herbaltransitions.com/MateriaMedica.html and http://www.sagemountain.com/the-formulary.html contain information regarding these herbs using the common names given.

Pay particular attention to the uses of and precautions regarding these herbs. In addition, access http://www.nlm.nih.gov/medlineplus/druginfo/natural/patient-melatonin.html for reliable information regarding the uses of melatonin.

Explanation:

Many people are turning to holistic medicine or alternative therapies to treat their mood disorders and insomnia. Many do not like the side effects of prescription medications used for these disorders. Some medications for insomnia and anxiety are controlled substances, become less effective over time, and have addictive potential. This has caused a resurgence in the use of herbal medications and other alternative therapies for these disorders. Although the data on the efficacy of some of these treatments is unclear, some alternative medications and treatments show great promise. With any medication, whether herbal, prescription, or OTC, it is always wise to determine if the substance can interact with any other medications a patient is currently taking. If a person is taking a prescription antidepressant, it is not recommended that he or she add an herbal remedy to the regimen if the herb has "natural" antidepressant properties. This can increase the risk of serotonin syndrome, which can be a major medical concern. Some herbs have adverse effects of their own. They are not completely free from side effects merely because they are "natural."

People are also turning to alternative therapies and modalities such as massage therapy, yoga, meditation, and feng shui to help them cope with their mood disorders. Massage therapy and yoga can relax tight muscles, calm the nerves, increase concentration, and confer a host of other benefits. Meditation can help with relaxation, insomnia, and anxiety. Feng shui is a traditional Chinese practice that is supposed to positively influence *qi* (or *chi*), the energy that is within us and all around us. Feng shui employs the methods of traditional Chinese medicine, yin and yang, color, direction, and a host of other things to lift mood, relieve anxiety, and even improve finances. Most often, feng shui use can be recognized by beautiful, but unusual, interior/exterior arrangements, use of color, art, textures, and plants. Feng shui is becoming more popular in the United States, with books, television specials, and even community college courses offered on the subject. Alternative modalities are preferred by those who do not wish to take any kind of medication or herbal remedy, as they have no side effects when used properly.

Activity:

Review the websites recommended in the pre-lab section. The herbs/natural supplements named in that section are commonly used in the United States for various conditions affecting the nervous system. Locate these supplements on the websites to determine which conditions they treat, and if any side effects can occur. Many of these herbs are used to treat a variety of conditions that overlap, such as anxiety and insomnia. You can read about some nonmedical treatments in the preceding explanation section as well.

Questions:

1. What are some alternative treatments for insomnia? Are there any side effects to these treatments? Explain.

_____

_____

_____

_____

2. What are some alternative treatments for anxiety? Are there any side effects to these treatments? Explain.

_____

_____

_____

_____

3. What are some alternative treatments for depression? Are there any side effects to these treatments? Explain.

_____

_____

_____

_____

Student Name: _____

Lab Partner: _____

Grade/Comments: _____

_____

_____

Student Comments: _____

_____

_____

CHAPTER 32
Pediatric and Neonatal Patients

After completing Chapter 32 from the textbook, you should be able to:	Related Activity in the Workbook/Lab Manual
1. Discuss the differences between neonatal and pediatric patients.	Review Questions, PTCB Exam Practice Questions Activity 32-2
2. Explain how the processes of pharmacokinetics in pediatric patients affect drug dosing.	Review Questions, PTCB Exam Practice Questions Activity 32-4, Lab 32-1, Lab 32-2
3. Discuss pediatric drug administration and dosage adjustment considerations.	Review Questions, PTCB Exam Practice Questions Activity 32-4, Lab 32-1, Lab 32-2
4. List two common childhood illnesses and diseases in pediatric patients.	Review Questions, PTCB Exam Practice Questions Activity 32-1, Activity 32-2, Activity 32-3, Activity 32-4

INTRODUCTION

There are many differences between pediatric patients and adults. Pediatric patients are not just small adults, and you must consider a number of factors other than the obvious one of body weight when administering medication. *Neonates* are newborn babies from birth to 1 month of age, whereas *infants* are between the ages of 1 month to 2 years. Finally, a *child* is considered to be between 2 years and 12 years of age.

There are very significant physiologic differences among pediatric patients, and the pharmacokinetic processes known as absorption, distribution, metabolism, and excretion occur quite differently in children compared to adults because a child's organ systems are not yet fully developed. Providing medication therapy to pediatric patients can present a challenge if these differences are not considered. As a pharmacy technician, you need to understand some of the pharmacological differences among neonatal, infant, and pediatric patients; special medication administration considerations; and some of the common disorders that these special patients encounter.

REVIEW QUESTIONS

Match the following.

1. _____ absorption

2. _____ asthma

3. _____ distribution

4. _____ infants

5. _____ intramuscular

6. _____ excretion

7. _____ lipid-soluble

8. _____ metabolism

9. _____ neonate

10. _____ pH

11. _____ pharmacokinetics

12. _____ water-soluble

a. drugs that pass readily into cell membranes composed of mostly fatty substances, such as the brain

b. chemical alteration of drugs or foreign compounds in the body

c. scale that measures the alkalinity or acidity of a substance

d. study of the processes of absorption, distribution, metabolism, and excretion of drugs

e. from birth to 1 month of age

f. drug is absorbed into the bloodstream, then distributed out to the various organs and tissues

g. entrance of a drug into the bloodstream

h. respiratory disease characterized by wheezing and shortness of breath

i. elimination of a drug from the body, usually through urine, feces, or the respiratory system

j. between the ages of 1 month and 2 years

k. drugs composed mostly of water and can be excreted by the kidneys.

l. within a muscle

True or False?

13. The skin of a neonate is thinner than that of an adult.

  T　　　F

14. The neonate's digestive system is less acidic than an adult's.

  T　　　F

15. A dose that is appropriate for an infant may not be appropriate for a neonate.

  T　　　F

16. The liver and kidneys have the smallest blood supply and receive a lower concentration of a drug than other organs.

  T　　　F

17. Children usually have a lower percentage of body water and a higher percentage of body fat than adults.

  T　　　F

18. Pediatric patients are at risk of drug accumulation and possible toxicity.

  T　　　F

19. Children (ages 2 to 12 years) metabolize certain drugs more rapidly than adults.

  T　　　F

20. Steroids can stunt pediatric growth and tetracycline can stain permanent teeth and affect bone development.

    T   F

21. Clark's Rule uses a child's weight to determine a correct dose.

    T   F

22. Before the age of 3 years, a child will probably have at least one ear infection.

    T   F

PHARMACY CALCULATION PROBLEMS

Calculate the following.

1. Using Young's Rule, calculate a dose of acetaminophen for a 10-year-old child who weighs 65 lb., when the usual adult dose is 500 mg.

2. Using Clark's Rule, calculate a dose of ibuprofen for a 9-year-old boy who weighs 60 lb. The usual adult dose is 800 mg.

3. A child is prescribed antibiotic otic drops for a double ear infection. The product comes in a 10 mL bottle. The directions state "2 gtts AU qid × 10D." How many bottles will be required for the entire course?

4. A woman's state health plan for her child covers three out of the four prescriptions needed, with a $2.00 co-pay for each prescription. The fourth prescription is nonformulary and has a usual and customary price of $24.99. How much will the customer pay for all four prescriptions?

5. A prescription for sulfamethoxazole/trimethoprim suspension has been presented to the pharmacy. The pediatric patient is to take one teaspoonful by mouth twice daily for seven days. How many milliliters will be needed to last seven days?

PTCB EXAM PRACTICE QUESTIONS

1. Newborn children from birth to one month of age are referred to as:
   a. neonates.
   b. infants.
   c. adolescents.
   d. babies.

2. Drug distribution, metabolism, and excretion are quite different in which of the following populations, compared to adults, because their organ systems are not fully developed?
   a. children and adolescents
   b. elders
   c. infants and adolescents
   d. neonates and infants

3. What is one of the most common chronic childhood conditions, affecting nearly 6 million children under the age of 18 each year in the United States?
   a. strep throat
   b. conjunctivitis
   c. appendicitis
   d. asthma

4. What is a serious condition that can occur if strep infections are not treated properly?
   a. chickenpox
   b. measles
   c. rheumatic fever
   d. whooping cough

5. Which of the following is *not* a recommended pediatric dosage form of Tylenol®?
   a. suppository
   b. injection
   c. elixir
   d. drops

ACTIVITY 32-1: Case Study—Tummy Troubles

Instructions: Read the following scenario and then answer the critical thinking questions.

Ashley is the cutest little 4-year-old girl you could ever meet. She's a just a ball of light—always bouncing around, happily picking flowers for her grandma and trying to catch all the kittens in the neighborhood. You know Ashley through her mom, who visits the pharmacy where you work to have her prescriptions filled from time to time. Ashley has even brought you flowers!

Ashley is a dancer in the school play and has been rehearsing her part for weeks. She is very excited to have such a big part and cannot wait to show her family what a good dancer she will be on stage!

Ashley is quite finicky when it comes to food. Like most children her age, she has her favorites (chicken and peanut butter), but will do anything she can to avoid eating the things she does not like. More concerning to her mom, though, is the fact that she can hardly get Ashley to drink anything. Other kids usually like juice or some other liquid, but Ashley will barely drink even water.

One day during the school rehearsal, Ashley complains to the teacher that she has a really bad bellyache and asks for her mom. The teacher sends her to the infirmary, where the school nurse has her lie down. Later, when Ashley has a bowel movement, it hurts so much that she cries out. Mom comes running and notices hard, pellet-like stools in the toilet. Mom comes to the pharmacy and requests a recommendation from the pharmacist for Ashley's problem. In spite of the pharmacist's recommendation, Ashley continues to have cramping abdominal pain with frequent and painful bowel movements.

1. Ashley is experiencing what condition, sometimes found in children as well as adults?

_____

_____

2. What do you think the pharmacist might have recommended when the mother went to the pharmacy? Is Senokot® a good choice?

_____

_____

_____

_____

3. Typically, how long does the treatment for Ashley's condition last?

_____

_____

_____

_____

4. How is treatment stopped?

_____

_____

_____

_____

5. What might be done in an acute instance of Ashley's condition?

_____

_____

_____

_____

ACTIVITY 32-2: Case Study—A Visit to the ER

Instructions: Read the following scenario and then answer the critical thinking questions.

Mr. and Mrs. Swanson are 30-something, healthy parents. Both work and manage to spend quality time with their 8-month-old baby boy. Even though they both work, the weekends are dedicated to various activities. They take walks, go to the beach, and even have picnics together where the baby lies out on a blanket in the grassy neighborhood park.

One day the Swansons find themselves taking their baby boy into the emergency room, after he appears to have had a really bad cold for far too long. It seems like the baby caught the same cold that Mrs. Swanson's sister had at the same time. The sister baby-sits while the Swansons are at work during the day.

Their baby boy has had a stuffy nose and cough for more than a week now. Today they notice that he is wheezing laboriously and his skin is slightly bluish in color. A quick temperature check confirms that he has a fever. Baby is cranky, fussy, and cries constantly when he is not coughing. Upon arrival at the hospital, the doctor takes a sample of fluid from the baby's nose and orders an X-ray of the chest. A sound check reveals crackling sounds from the lungs. A short time later the baby is admitted into an isolation room.

1. From the description in this scenario, what most likely is the baby's diagnosis and complication?

_____

_____

_____

2. Why is the baby's skin discolored?

_____

_____

_____

3. How is the baby treated for his condition(s)?

_____

_____

_____

_____

4. How can the family prevent future outbreaks of this condition?

_____

_____

_____

_____

5. Name some differences between neonatal and pediatric patients.

_____

_____

_____

_____

ACTIVITY 32-3: Case Study—A Bad Cough

Instructions: Read the following scenario and then answer the critical thinking questions.

Tanya Bankert is a young, smart, and proud single mother. In spite of what others have told her, she has done a fantastic job raising her 14-month-old male infant. No doubt some days are harder than others, but Tanya knows that she and the baby are going to make it.

Tanya is leery of giving children medicine for every little sniffle, and takes a "wait and see" attitude when things come up. When her child sneezes, she does not run out to the doctor for antibiotics.

Tanya's infant develops a cold, which is not that uncommon, and she treats it gently for a few days. When the infant boy develops a cough, Tanya decides to wait and see if it will go away on its own. Tanya does little things like using a cool-mist humidifier in her son's room and giving him plenty of fluids, but she has read the public warnings against using cold medicines for children and does not seek out any of these treatments.

Within another day or two, the coughing sound changes. It begins to take on the characteristics of a peculiar "barking" sound that sounds like a seal begging for food. Then, the infant seems to have great difficulty breathing and is scared. She immediately takes him into the emergency room. The doctors take the infant's medical history, get a description of his symptoms, and listen to his lungs. The doctors hear prolonged inspiration or expiration and decreased breath sounds. Tanya is anxious to know what this is.

1. Based on the information in this scenario, the infant has what temporary condition?

_____

_____

_____

_____

2. How long does this coughing typically last?

_____

_____

_____

_____

3. What childhood vaccines are available to help prevent the most dangerous forms of this condition?

_____

_____

_____

_____

4. The doctor examines the infant and finds a red, swollen, inflamed airway with bacteria present. What does this mean, and what is the treatment plan in this situation?

_____

_____

_____

_____

ACTIVITY 32-4: Case Study—Accidental Heparin Overdose in Infants

In 2006, three premature infants died at a hospital in Indianapolis due to an accidental heparin overdose. A pharmacy technician stocked an automated dispensing unit with adult-strength heparin (10,000 units per dose) instead of the 10 unit heparin-lock flush. A nurse who removed the adult-strength heparin from the machine assumed that it was the 10 unit dose, and then administered the heparin to three infants, who later died. In 2008, actor Randy Quaid's twin babies received a 2,000-fold overdose of heparin in a California hospital, again because a pharmacy technician stocked adult-strength heparin in a pediatric unit. In this instance, the twins survived.

Many errors were committed by both the pharmacy and the nursing staff in these tragic cases. Unfortunately, these are not isolated instances: both hospitals had had overdoses of heparin occur in the past. One main concern is the packaging of the heparin. The labeling of the two products is so similar that it is easy to mistake one for the other. The wrong heparin should never have gotten out of the pharmacy if a series of double-checks had been in place, or if bar-coding technology had been in use. The nursing staff should have double-checked the dosage on the packaging before administering the heparin, but it is often assumed—and justifiably so—that the pharmacy stocked the correct product. At the time of this writing, the Quaids are currently suing the drug company for negligence. Labeling is being changed to differentiate between products, and hospitals are putting a system of checks into place from pharmacy to medical unit. Why does it always take terrible events like these to stimulate corrective action?

Critical Thinking Questions:

1. Who do you feel should take responsibility for these accidental overdoses?

   _____
   _____
   _____
   _____

2. Do you think that a pharmacy technician should be liable for negligence?

   _____
   _____
   _____
   _____

3. What would you like to see done to prevent mistakes like this from happening at your workplace?

   _____
   _____
   _____
   _____

LAB 32-1: Pediatric Cough/Cold Medications and the FDA

Objective:

Research the FDA drug advisory for the use of cough and cold medications in children.

Pre-Lab Information:

- Review Chapter 32 in your textbook.
- Explore the following FDA website: http://www.fda.gov/cder/drug/advisory/cough_cold_2008.htm

Explanation:

Parents and other caregivers often have questions about cough and cold medications. As a pharmacy technician, it is important for you to understand the FDA's drug advisory for use of these drugs in children.

Activity:

Review the FDA's online drug advisory (http://www.fda.gov/cder/drug/advisory/cough_cold_2008.htm) and answer the following questions.

1. To what age group does this drug advisory apply?

   _____

   _____

   _____

   _____

2. The FDA recommends *not* using cough and cold medications in the age group identified in question #1. What eight recommendations does the FDA make for the use of cough and cold medications in children older than those to whom the advisory applies?

   _____

   _____

   _____

   _____

Student Name: _____

Lab Partner: _____

Grade/Comments: _____

_____

_____

Student Comments: _____

_____

_____

LAB 32-2: Pediatric Dosing

Objective:

Practice using Clark's Rule and Young's Rule to determine doses for pediatric patients.

Pre-Lab Information:

- Review Clark's Rule and Young's Rule in Chapter 32 of your textbook.
- Review Chapter 14, "Dosage Calculations," in your textbook.

Explanation:

As a pharmacy technician, you may be asked to calculate or check pediatric doses using Clark's Rule and/or Young's Rule.

Activity:

Use Clark's Rule and/or Young's Rule to answer the following questions.

1. A 2-year-old weighing 40 lb. needs phenytoin. The adult dose is 250 mg tid. Using Clark's Rule, how much phenytoin will this child need for each dose?

   _____

   _____

   _____

   _____

2. An infant needs furosemide. She weighs 20 lb. and the adult dose is 40 mg bid. Using Clark's Rule, how much furosemide will this child need for each dose?

   _____

   _____

   _____

   _____

3. A 6-year-old needs theophylline. The adult dose is 100 mg tid. Using Young's Rule, what is the correct dose for this child?

   _____

   _____

   _____

   _____

4. A 10-year-old needs phenobarbital. The adult dose is 60 mg bid. Using Young's Rule, what is the correct dose for this child?

   _____

   _____

   _____

   _____

Student Name: _____

Lab Partner: _____

Grade/Comments: _____

_____

_____

Student Comments: _____

_____

_____

CHAPTER 33
Geriatric Patients

After completing Chapter 33 from the textbook, you should be able to:	Related Activity in the Workbook/Lab Manual
1. Discuss the physiological changes that occur in geriatric patients.	Review Questions, PTCB Exam Practice Questions Activity 33-2, Activity 33-3
2. List several factors that affect pharmacokinetic processes in geriatric patients.	Review Questions, PTCB Exam Practice Questions Activity 33-1, Activity 33-2, Activity 33-5, Activity 33-6
3. Discuss polypharmacy and noncompliance in geriatric medication therapy.	Review Questions, PTCB Exam Practice Questions Activity 33-1, Activity 33-5, Activity 33-6
4. Discuss Medicare Part D and its effects on medication dispensing to the geriatric population.	Review Questions
5. Explain ways in which geriatric medication dispensing will change in the future, and how extended life expectancy will change pharmacy practice.	Review Questions Activity 33-5, Activity 33-6

INTRODUCTION

The number of geriatric patients is increasing, and will affect pharmacy practice in very significant ways. There are nearly 40 million Americans who are 65 years of age or older. Currently, geriatric prescriptions account for the greatest percentage of medication orders filled. Some experts have reported that 50 percent of all OTC products sold today, and 30 percent of prescription medications, are consumed by the elderly. Other factors, such as physiological changes, polypharmacy, multiple diseases, and noncompliance (a patient's refusal or inability to follow a prescribed drug regimen), also affect geriatric medication therapy. As a pharmacy technician, you need to understand the unique factors involved in caring for geriatric patients.

REVIEW QUESTIONS

Match the following.

1. _____ absorption

2. _____ adverse effects

3. _____ bioavailability

4. _____ distribution

5. _____ excretion

6. _____ geriatric

7. _____ half-life

8. _____ metabolism

9. _____ noncompliance

10. _____ OTC drugs

11. _____ polypharmacy

12. _____ side effects

13. _____ toxicity

a. drug poisoning that can be life-threatening or extremely harmful

b. chemical change of drugs or foreign compounds in the body

c. when a patient does not follow a prescribed drug regimen

d. amount of a drug that is available for absorption

e. amount of time it takes the body to break down and excrete one-half of the drug

f. population over the age of 65

g. elimination of a drug from the body

h. undesirable and potentially harmful drug effects

i. entrance of a drug into the bloodstream

j. drug effect other than the intended one; usually undesirable but not harmful

k. administration of more medications than clinically indicated

l. abbreviation for over-the-counter; drugs that can be purchased without a prescription

m. entrance of a drug from the blood to organs and tissues

Choose the best answer.

14. The number of _____ patients is increasing and will affect pharmacy practice significantly in several ways.
    a. adolescent
    b. mental
    c. cancer
    d. geriatric

15. Because the kidneys, liver, and brain are the organs that require the most blood flow to function properly, the _____ and _____ processes slow as people age.
    a. metabolism, excretion
    b. metabolism, absorption
    c. excretion, absorption
    d. kidneys, liver

16. Which of the following is a common reason for noncompliance by the elderly?
    a. dosing schedule is confusing
    b. difficulty understanding or remembering what the drug is
    c. inability to afford the drug
    d. all of the above
    e. none of the above

True or False?

17. Organ size generally increases in the elderly, as do blood flow and cardiac output.

    T   F

18. The patient must sign up for Medicare within 3 months of becoming eligible (3 months before reaching age 65 or 3 months thereafter).

    T   F

19. By the year 2050, the elderly population will increase to approximately 72 million.

    T   F

20. The elderly are projected to consume as much as 85 percent of all OTC medications by the year 2010.

    T   F

PHARMACY CALCULATION PROBLEMS

Calculate the following.

1. A normal adult requires 0.1 mcg/kg/min of remifentanil for continuous IV infusion. However, in geriatric patients the dosage should be reduced by half. How many micrograms will a 192 lb. geriatric patient receive over 10 minutes?

2. If an elderly patient with reduced renal function is to receive a 50% reduction in the usual dose of digoxin 0.25 mg, how many micrograms of digoxin should this patient receive?

3. Zaleplon 10 mg is usually given qhs. If a geriatric patient is prescribed half of this dose, how many milligrams will the patient receive over a 14-day period?

PTCB EXAM PRACTICE QUESTIONS

1. Adults experience a decrease in many physiological functions between the ages of:
    a. 18 to 30 years.
    b. 20 to 40 years.
    c. 30 to 50 years.
    d. 50 to 70 years.

2. Which of the following are physiological changes that occur with aging?
    a. increased renal blood flow
    b. increased hepatic blood flow
    c. increased cardiac output
    d. increased body fat

3. Which of the following drugs can cause elderly patients to become dizzy, unsteady on their feet, and possibly fall if the dosage is not adjusted appropriately?
    a. benzodiazepines
    b. diuretics
    c. acetaminophen
    d. ibuprofen

4. Which of the following drugs requires a lower dose in geriatric patients due to reduced renal blood flow?
   a. aminoglycoside antibiotics
   b. thiazide diuretics
   c. penicillin
   d. aspirin

5. Which of the following is a reason for the greater incidence of adverse drug reactions in elderly individuals?
   a. increased cardiac output
   b. decreased intestinal motility
   c. increased kidney function
   d. decreased drug metabolism in the liver

ACTIVITY 33-1: Case Study—Organization

Instructions: Read the following scenario and then answer the critical thinking questions.

Mrs. Muffet is everyone's favorite customer in the grocery chain retail pharmacy where you work. She is an endearing, 78-year-old, white-haired woman whom everyone calls "grandma." After buying her eggs and milk, she will stop by and say hello even if she is not there to pick up any prescriptions. Mrs. Muffet is a widow with no living relatives. As the years go by, Mrs. Muffet, like a lot of people her age, forgets things all the time. She often comments that she would forget she had a cat if it did not meow.

Mrs. Muffet takes a total of nine tablets, some three times a day. Today she comes to the pharmacy to have three more prescriptions filled that her doctor just prescribed. One of the medications she is picking up is prednisone, on a 21-day tapering dose schedule. The medication regimen specifies various tablet amounts at various dosing times, but the instructions are very difficult to follow. This is in addition to all the other medications she takes, including heart, blood pressure, cholesterol lowering, furosemide, potassium, stool softener, thyroid, PPI, aspirin, and a few inhalers.

Recently your pharmacy became concerned when Mrs. Muffet told everyone that sometimes she forgets if she has taken her medications. When she cannot remember, she just takes the "next bunch" in case she did not get them. You feel that there are some things you can do to help Mrs. Muffet get better organized.

1. What are some special concerns in the elderly population that are exhibited in Mrs. Muffet's case?

   _____
   _____
   _____
   _____

2. How can the pharmacy help with the tapering-dose instructions for Mrs. Muffet's prednisone?

   _____
   _____
   _____
   _____

3. What else can be done to help Mrs. Muffet get organized with her medications?

   _____
   _____
   _____
   _____

4. Can you think of any other resources that might be able to help someone like Mrs. Muffet with her daily needs?

_____

_____

_____

_____

ACTIVITY 33-2: Case Study—Three Age-Related Issues

Instructions: Read the following scenario and then answer the critical thinking questions.

Mrs. Crendall and her husband have been regular customers at the retail pharmacy where you work for more than 15 years. They started coming to the pharmacy when they were in their early 60s, and say they have received the best care and customer service there and that is what keeps them coming back. Jokingly, Mrs. Crendall comments that they will be bringing in more and more business as they get older and are customers for life!

Over the years, most of the normal things that occur with aging bodies have happened to the Crendalls. They move a little slower, hunch over a little more than usual, cannot remember every little detail of the day, and sometimes need a little help in the bathroom to move Mother Nature along. Also, both Mr. and Mrs. Crendall are feeling the effects of aging on their eyes. Their vision is failing at different rates, but they nonetheless both have difficulty seeing various things that are small and detailed.

They come to your pharmacy today, together as always, and bring up a problem. Knowing that great customer service is always provided, they are certain that the pharmacy can help with solutions. There are three issues to address. One is that even though their insurance mandates it, they can no longer physically cut tablets in half. They do not have the strength in their hands any longer and even when they manage to break a tablet, it is usually a powder when they are done. The second issue is that they can no longer read the prescription labels. Between them, they have so many that they do not even know what the drugs are for any more. The third issue is that every time they pick up their medications, it seems that some have changed. What was once a green tablet last month is a pink one this month. They are very confused by the constant changes.

1. What are some options available to assist with the Crendalls' tablet-cutting problem?

_____

_____

_____

_____

2. Vision is a major problem for some elderly patients. What options can you think of to help with their vision problems in this scenario?

_____

_____

_____

_____

3. Do many pharmacies recognize the special needs of the elderly patient, and create ways to assist this population with such issues as the ones described in the scenario?

_____

_____

_____

_____

4. How can you help with the confusion over the changing appearance of medications at each fill?

_____

_____

_____

_____

ACTIVITY 33-3: Case Study—Limited Mobility

Instructions: Read the following scenario and then answer the critical thinking questions.

Jack is a 68-year-old who gets around quite well with his wheelchair. He resisted getting the chair as long as he could, but severe knee, hip, and leg problems made it almost impossible for him to walk. Almost everyone who sees him thinks he is helpless and feels sorry for him. However, Jack does not feel that way. He is very independent, running his own errands via mass transportation, and he even teaches a swimming class for wheelchair-using seniors at the YMCA.

Jack requires a lot of ostomy supplies and orders through the ostomy and medical supply area of a pharmacy where you work. From time to time he needs to be refitted for such things as catheters, wafers, leg bags, and "diapers." Over the years Jack has gained some weight as he has slowed down. Jack is stubborn and refuses to get one of those "old-people electric scooters for lazy people."

With just his trusty wheelchair, Jack has managed to pick up his supplies from the pharmacy and take the bus back to his home with no problems. With his weight gain and further aging, though, Jack has had difficulty manipulating the oversized packages and boxes, and finds that he is becoming weaker, too. Although Jack really enjoys coming by the pharmacy to say hello, he finds he can no longer manage this task no matter what he does.

1. What solutions can you offer Jack to get him his ostomy supplies?

_____

_____

_____

_____

2. Do you think Jack is a good candidate for an electric scooter? If so, what could you do to help Jack understand that it would make life easier?

_____

_____

_____

_____

3. How can you help Jack not feel so helpless when he comes to the pharmacy?

_____

_____

_____

_____

4. What emotional impact do you think the circumstances in this scenario might have on Jack, or any elderly patient?

_____

_____

_____

_____

ACTIVITY 33-4: Case Study—Walk-In Clinic

Instructions: Read the following scenario and then answer the critical thinking questions.

A 63-year-old woman weighing 108 pounds has a circulation disorder and low blood pressure. She is taking medication that controls her blood pressure, and she has been walking around the block every day to get a little exercise. She was having some difficulty falling asleep at night, so she went to a walk-in clinic to ask the doctor about it. The doctor wrote her a prescription for zolpidem 10 mg, and said that she should take one tablet every night at bedtime to help her fall asleep. Over the next few days, she began to have blurred vision, urinary retention, dizziness, and confusion. She also felt very drowsy during the day, had difficulty concentrating, and began having coordination problems.

1. What do you think caused her new symptoms?

_____

_____

_____

_____

2. How could these symptoms have been prevented?

_____

_____

_____

_____

ACTIVITY 33-5: Geriatric Dosing Exercise

Many types of medications require a reduction in the standard adult dose when used for the geriatric population. As a pharmacy technician, you need to familiarize yourself with some of the common classifications that affect the elderly and which doses must be reduced. You should also become knowledgeable about the physical changes that occur as we age.

As our bodies age, we experience many changes. Decreased metabolism and excretion, slowed digestion, and increased fat stores are among the many physiological changes that occur. These are some of many factors that affect how certain drugs are processed. Drugs often stay in an elder's system for a longer period of time, build up to toxic levels in the body, and produce unwanted adverse effects. Kidney function declines over time, and the kidneys play a major role in excretion. Clinical pharmacists and physicians can predict how well or poorly certain medications are excreted by a patient by measuring the amount of creatine produced and filtered. Two laboratory values that are often measured are serum creatine and creatine clearance. These are obtained through a urine sample. The serum creatine level is used to predict the creatine clearance, which indicates the level of kidney function. These two values are very useful tools, but if a patient has very low body fat and has muscle atrophy, these values will not be accurate. The serum creatine and creatine clearance values are usually used in conjunction with another formula, which takes into account the patient's age, weight, and gender. This formula is called the *Cockroft-Gault Equation*.

Physicians and pharmacists need to use caution when using certain drug classes for the elderly. At normal adult doses, these drugs build up in the system and can cause many adverse affects. Some medications can affect the central nervous system, motor functions, cardiovascular system, and gastrointestinal system. Effects can be mild to severe. The dose of almost any type of medication that causes sedation should be reduced. These types include anesthetics, antihistamines, benzodiazepines, non-benzodiazepine hypnotics, narcotics, antipsychotics, and certain antidepressants. If given at normal adult doses, most sedatives (e.g., alprazolam) or sleep medications (e.g., zolpidem), can build up over time, causing excessive drowsiness, dizziness, and confusion. These side effects can also set the individual up for a bad fall, resulting in a hospital stay to repair a fractured hip. Usually, a simple reduction in dose is adequate to maintain appropriate levels in the geriatric body.

Activity:

The following questions state a normal adult dose for a medication. Using the information given, you will calculate the appropriate reduced dosage for a geriatric patient.

1. The normal adult dose of propofol IV required to maintain anesthesia is 12 mg/kg/hr. If a geriatric patient weighs 80 kg, find the infusion rate in mg/hr if you have to reduce the dosage by 50%.

2. If a normal adult dose of diphenhydramine is 50 mg, what is the geriatric dose if it is to be reduced by 50%?

3. A geriatric patient is prescribed trazodone tid. The maximum daily dosage allowed for geriatrics is 75 mg. How many milligrams should be given for each dose?

4. A physician determines that her elderly patient requires a 25% reduction in the normal daily dose of sertraline 100 mg. How many milligrams will be given per dose?

ACTIVITY 33-6: Web Research Activity—Medication Noncompliance by the Elderly

Noncompliance by the elderly patient is an important issue that you should be familiar with as a pharmacy technician. Older patients often take several medications each day and frequently have a difficult time managing the large number of drugs they are sometimes prescribed.

Activity:

Visit the AdultMeducation Web site (http://www.adultmeducation.com/index.html) and answer the following questions about medication noncompliance by older adults.

1. According to the Web site, what are the five dimensions of medication adherence?

_____

_____

_____

_____

2. What are the five broad components of the social and economic factors that influence noncompliance by the elderly?

_____

_____

_____

_____

3. What are two barriers in the healthcare system that influence noncompliance by the elderly?

_____

_____

_____

_____

4. What are four condition-related barriers to medication compliance by the elderly patient?

_____

_____

_____

_____

5. What are five therapy-related barriers to medication compliance by the elderly patient?

_____

_____

_____

_____

6. What are two broad patient-related barriers to medication compliance by the elderly patient?

_____

_____

_____

CHAPTER 34
Biopharmaceuticals

After completing Chapter 34 from the textbook, you should be able to:	Related Activity in the Workbook/Lab Manual
1. Name at least two drugs developed by using recombinant DNA technology, and outline their uses.	Review Questions, PTCB Exam Practice Questions Activity 34-1, Activity 34-2, Activity 34-3, Activity 34-4, Lab 34-1
2. Discuss the four steps in the genetic engineering process.	Review Questions Activity 34-4, Lab 34-1
3. Explain briefly how a company gets approval for a biopharmaceutical drug from the FDA.	Review Questions Activity 34-4, Lab 34-1
4. Discuss why biopharmaceuticals, genetic engineering, and stem cell research are important in the future of pharmacy and the practice of medicine.	Review Questions Activity 34-1, Activity 34-2, Activity 34-3, Activity 34-4, Lab 34-1

INTRODUCTION

Biopharmacology is the branch of pharmacology that studies the use of biologically engineered drugs. *Biopharmaceuticals* are substances created using biotechnology. They can be proteins like antibodies, and even consist of DNA and RNA. Research is being conducted to find new therapeutic medications, or biopharmaceuticals, to treat such life-threatening diseases as AIDS, various cancers, and Parkinson's disease.

Large majorities of biopharmaceuticals are derived from existing life forms, such as plants and animals, although they are produced by means other than direct extraction from a biological source. Genetic engineering is another way to create new drugs; stem cell research also offers opportunities to discover new therapeutic treatments, and is making significant strides in the development of new medications used today. As a pharmacy technician, you should be familiar with some of the concepts of biopharmacology, their impact on the pharmaceutical industry, and their role in the future of pharmacology.

REVIEW QUESTIONS

Match the following.

1. _____ allergenic
2. _____ biologics
3. _____ biopharmaceuticals
4. _____ biopharmacology
5. _____ biotechnology
6. _____ Gaucher's disease
7. _____ GMO
8. _____ MS
9. _____ neutropenia
10. _____ rheumatoid arthritis
11. _____ transformation
12. _____ vector

a. autoimmune disease that causes chronic inflammation of the joints

b. organism that does not itself cause disease, but spreads disease by distributing pathogens from one host to another

c. alteration of an organism itself or the cell in the genetic engineering process

d. disease in which there are an abnormal number of the white blood cells that are responsible for fighting infections

e. substances created using biotechnology

f. substance that can cause an allergic reaction

g. use of biological substances or microorganisms to perform specific functions, such as the production of drugs, hormones, or food products

h. branch of pharmacology that studies the use of biologically engineered drugs

i. organism whose genetic material has been altered using the genetic engineering techniques known as recombinant DNA technology

j. disease in which fatty materials collect in the liver, spleen, kidneys, lungs, and brain and causes the person to be susceptible to infections

k. chronic, inflammatory disease of the white-matter areas of the brain and spinal cord in the central nervous system

l. medicinal products such as vaccines, blood products, allergenics, and proteins

True or False?

13. Biopharmaceutical drugs are used for therapeutic or diagnostic purposes and are defined as pharmaceuticals derived from life forms.

    T   F

14. It takes approximately 15 years for a drug to move from the experimental stage to the pharmacy.

    T   F

15. During the first, preclinical phase, the company files an Investigational New Drug Application with the FDA.

    T   F

Match the following.

16. _____ abatacept
17. _____ Humira®
18. _____ anemia from cancer therapy
19. _____ etanercept
20. _____ Remicade®
21. _____ breast cancer
22. _____ Gaucher's disease
23. _____ genital warts
24. _____ Pulmozyme®

a. adalimumab
b. Crohn's disease
c. trastuzumab
d. Epogen®
e. rheumatoid arthritis
f. Enbrel®
g. cystic fibrosis
h. Cerezyme®
i. Alferon N®

PHARMACY CALCULATION PROBLEMS

Calculate the following.

1. A patient who has RA has been prescribed infliximab 2.5 mg/kg for her first dose. Calculate the number of milligrams the patient will receive if she weighs 140 lb.

2. Etanercept is usually dosed at 50 mg SC twice a week for 3 months for severe plaque psoriasis. How many grams will a psoriasis patient receive over 3 months?

3. Find the dose of abatacept needed if a patient weighs 195 lb. According to the manufacturer's recommendation, a patient weighing less than 60 kg should receive a 500 mg dose. If a patient weighs between 60 and 100 kg, the patient should receive a 750 mg dose. If the patient weighs more than 100 kg, the patient should receive a 1,000 mg dose.

4. A patient is to receive rituximab 700 mg IV in 250 mL 0.9% sodium chloride. If the IV is to be infused at 100 mg/hr, how long will it take for the IV to be completely infused?

PTCB EXAM PRACTICE QUESTIONS

1. Which of the following medications was among the first to use recombinant DNA technology?
   a. Lovenox®
   b. Pancrease®
   c. Humulin®
   d. Plavix®

2. Which of the following biotechnology drugs is used to treat breast cancer?
   a. Orencia®
   b. Herceptin®
   c. Humira®
   d. Remicade®

3. When a biopharmaceutical company has completed the preclinical phase, what does it file with the FDA?
   a. DEA
   b. ANDA
   c. BDEA
   d. INDA

4. Which of the following biotechnology drugs is used to treat Crohn's disease?
   a. Enbrel®
   b. Orencia®
   c. Remicade®
   d. Humira®

ACTIVITY 34-1: Case Study—Darbepoetin ALFA

Instructions: Read the following scenario and then answer the critical thinking questions.

Mrs. Critten has had a great life. She has been married for 42 years, has four wonderful children and a miniature poodle that she loves dearly. Sometime in the past decade, during one of her annual checkups, Mrs. Critten was found to have cancer. It was a slow-growing, chronic type, but one that would, over time, cause her to easily catch infections as it progressed.

Eventually Mrs. Critten's cancer progressed to the point where chemotherapy was considered for treatment. She weighed the pros and cons and decided to begin treatment. Treatment would not cure her condition, but it could help extend her life while maintaining a good quality of life.

Mrs. Critten experienced a few side effects common to chemotherapy patients, such as nausea and vomiting, hair loss, and anemia. She was prescribed medication for the nausea and vomiting that typically lasted a few days after each treatment, wore wigs for the increasing hair loss, and was prescribed a synthetic form of erythropoietin called darbepoetin alfa (an erythropoiesis-stimulating agent (ESA)). This medication increases the number of red blood cells and is typically used for the treatment of anemia in cancer patients undergoing chemotherapy.

1. What drug form of this medicine is available?

_____

_____

_____

_____

446 **CHAPTER 34** *Biopharmaceuticals*

© 2009 Pearson Education, Inc.

2. What are the black-box warnings for this medication?

_____

_____

_____

_____

3. How long will Mrs. Critten's treatments with darbepoetin for anemia last?

_____

_____

_____

_____

4. How long does it take to feel the benefits of darbepoetin?

_____

_____

_____

_____

5. Can this medication be mixed into an IV solution?

_____

_____

_____

_____

ACTIVITY 34-2: Case Study—Avonex®

Instructions: Read the following scenario and then answer the critical thinking questions.

Monte Evans is a 27-year-old African-American male who loves volunteering at the boys' and girls' community center. He has worked with adolescent children for many years, both for counseling and as a Big Brother. He thrives on planning different events for the many different children he helps. Monte feels that he can make a difference to impressionable young people. Anyone you ask will tell you that Monte spends most of his time and energy planning activities for this specific age group.

For a while now, Monte has been having intermittent problems such as muscle weakness, lack of coordination, loss of the sense of touch, and pain in his muscles. Sometimes he has only one of these symptoms, sometimes more, and sometimes none. He is baffled until he visits his doctor and is diagnosed with multiple sclerosis. The doctor begins immediate treatment with Avonex® (interferon beta-1a). Mr. Evans brings his prescription to your pharmacy to have it filled.

1. What is multiple sclerosis?

_____

_____

_____

_____

2. What is Avonex®?

_____

_____

_____

_____

3. How is Avonex® mixed for use?

_____

_____

_____

_____

4. Mr. Evans calls your pharmacy to order a refill of his Avonex®, but he needs it mailed to him. What special considerations are there regarding delivery?

_____

_____

_____

_____

ACTIVITY 34-3: Case Study—Etanercept

Instructions: Read the following scenario and then answer the critical thinking questions.

Mrs. Agarstier is an aging star of the stage. In her earlier years she starred in many Off-Broadway shows—or, as she puts it, "*way* off Broadway." Although she was never truly famous, it was not because she did not try hard. Mrs. Agarstier loved to act and dance. She would rehearse for hours, day after day, polishing an already perfect routine. She would bend, stretch, and pirouette with ease and grace. When she needed to, she could act out an entire six-person scene by herself. She often reminisces about these times and wishes they were not so far away.

Mrs. Agarstier has rheumatoid arthritis. For years she struggled with the pain, mainly in her hands. Lately her hands look deformed; they are no longer the pretty, graceful hands of a stage star.

During the course of her disease, treatment therapies have included analgesics, NSAIDs, cortisones, and DMARDs. Each has had its benefits and each has had its disadvantages. Now that her hands are deformed and painful, the doctor would like to start Mrs. Agarstier on etanercept.

1. What is rheumatoid arthritis?

_____

_____

_____

_____

2. What is etanercept?

_____

_____

_____

_____

3. What two formulations are available for etanercept?

_____

_____

_____

_____

4. Along with infliximab and adalimumab, etanercept is in a class of drugs known as what?

_____

_____

_____

_____

ACTIVITY 34-4: Web Research Activity—FDA and Biopharmaceuticals

Research into and development of biologics have grown exponentially in the past decade. Currently, many biologics are being used to treat arthritis, diabetes, and immune-system disorders. The many advances being made in this field are accompanied by increasing debate over ethics, religion, and governmental regulations. This area of medicine will continue to develop and grow in the 21st century, so pharmacy technicians need to be familiar with these types of products.

Activity:

Review Chapter 34 in your textbook. Then go to http://www.fda.gov/cder/biologics/qa.htm and examine the "Frequently Asked Questions" section. Access http://www.fda.gov/cber/index.html for a variety of topics related to biopharmaceuticals, including cellular and gene therapy.

After reviewing the chapter in the textbook and the websites, answer the following questions regarding biopharmaceuticals and the FDA.

1. How does a biological product differ from a medication?

_____

_____

_____

_____

2. Which division of the FDA regulates biopharmaceutical products?

_____

_____

_____

_____

3. What types of products are considered biological in nature?

_____

_____

_____

_____

4. What are some of the requirements for licensing a new biological product?

_____

_____

_____

_____

LAB 34-1: Biopharmaceuticals, Genetic Engineering, and Stem Cell Research

Objective:

Review the biopharmaceutical industry and concepts of genetic engineering and stem cell research.

Pre-Lab Information:

- Review Chapter 34, "Biopharmaceuticals," in your textbook.
- Visit the following websites:
  - http://www.fda.gov/consumer/updates/genetherapy101507.html
  - http://stemcells.nih.gov/info/basics/basics1.asp
  - http://www.follistim.com/Consumer/FollistimAQCartridge/RecombinantDNAtechnology/index.asp

Explanation:

Genetic engineering, stem cell research, and the biopharmaceutical industry have been responsible for very exciting developments in the treatment of several human diseases. It is important for pharmacy technicians to have an understanding of how these treatments differ from other therapies. This exercise is designed to give you the opportunity to explore this promising area of medicine.

Activity:

Using the following websites, research and answer the following questions.

Human Gene Therapy

Visit http://www.fda.gov/consumer/updates/genetherapy101507.html

1. What is a human gene therapy product?

   _____
   _____
   _____
   _____

2. How do these products work?

   _____
   _____
   _____
   _____

3. What is the potential impact of these products for consumers?

   _____
   _____
   _____
   _____

4. What is the FDA's role in regulating these products?

_____

_____

_____

_____

5. Have any gene therapy products been approved yet?

_____

_____

_____

Stem Cells

Visit http://stemcells.nih.gov/info/basics/basics1.asp.

1. What is another term used to describe cell-based therapies?

_____

_____

2. What are the two kinds of human or animal stem cells that scientists use in research?

_____

_____

_____

_____

3. What disease is highlighted in the website as having a very promising future treatment based on stem cells?

_____

_____

_____

_____

Recombinant DNA

Visit http://www.follistim.com/Consumer/FollistimAQCartridge/RecombinantDNAtechnology/index.asp

1. What is Follistim® used to treat?

_____

_____

_____

_____

2. Recombinant technology begins with the isolation of what?

_____

_____

_____

_____

3. What is a vector?

_____

_____

_____

_____

4. What happens to the vector before it is introduced into host cells to express the protein?

_____

_____

_____

_____

Student Name: _____

Lab Partner: _____

Grade/Comments: _____

_____

_____

Student Comments: _____

_____

_____